Veterinary Parasitology

Veterinary Parasitology

Editors :

Dr. R. Katoch, M.V.Sc, Ph.D
Professor & Head

Dr. R. Godara, M.V.Sc
Assistant Professor

Dr. Anish Yadav, M.V.Sc, Ph.D
Associate Professor

Division of Veterinary Parasitology
Faculty of Veterinary Sciences and Animal Husbandry
Sher-e-Kashmir University of Agricultural Sciences and
Technology of Jammu, R.S. Pura-181 102, Jammu

SSPH

SATISH SERIAL PUBLISHING HOUSE
403, Express Tower, Commercial Complex, Azadpur, Delhi-33 (India)
Phone : 011-27672852, Fax : 91-11-27672046
E-mail : info@satishserial.com, hkjain1975@yahoo.com
Website : www.satishserial.com

Published by :

SATISH SERIAL PUBLISHING HOUSE

403, Express Tower, Commercial Complex, Azadpur, Delhi-110033 (INDIA)
Phone : 011-27672852 Fax : 91-11-27672046
E-mail : info@satishserial.com, hkjain1975@yahoo.com

ISBN 978-93-81226-89-6

Typeset at: Harminder Kharb *for* Laxmi Art Creation # 9971212252
Printed at: Salasar Imaging Systems, Delhi-110035

Preface

In India, the subject of Veterinary Parasitology has undergone a vast change and has grown with numerous advancements during last three decades. The different parasitic diseases like fasciolosis, GI nematodosis, myiasis and trypanosomosis cause heavy economic losses to livestock industry of India. The molecules used for chemotherapeutic control has also shown resistance in changed scenario of intensive Livestock production industry and has emerged as new threat. The data regarding new disease like cryptosporidiosis is emerging fast in Veterinary and Medical Sciences. The changing food habits of Indian will make them more prone to zoonotic diseases of parasitic origin as data pertaining to meat-borne diseases is lacking which requires more of research work in years to come. Inspite of large number of references for presence of parasite of zoonotic importance in stray dogs and cats, the data of disease in human is lacking. The student of Veterinary Parasitology are dependent of foreign books which lack important information regarding epidemiology and control measures to be adopted in India's context.

In the present book attempt has been made to combine viewpoints of different workers in particular field gathered from the literatures published in last three decades by scientist in India and abroad and necessary conclusion have been derived after reviewing the work of particular parasitic disease in Indian context.

The chapters of present book will help post-graduate students and researchers in discipline of Veterinary Parasitology. The book will also be used by policy makers to adopt recent diagnostic methods and control measures for important parasitic diseases of livestock industry. The book will also be of use to medicos as particular reference to zoonotic forms and role of animals in transmission of these diseases to man.

Editors

Preface

Contents

Chapter 1

Acaricide Resistance : An Insight on Development Status and Management

N.K. Singh and Jyoti
Department of Veterinary Parasitology, College of Veterinary Science, GADVASU, Ludhiana-141 004, India

Ticks and tick-borne diseases (TTBDs) are a major problem to livestock health in the world and its severity depends on region, species involved, agents, host population, socioeconomic and technological advances in control measures (Solis, 1991). Losses attributable to ticks are caused either directly through tick worry, blood loss, damage to hides and udders and the injection of toxins, or indirectly through mortality or debility caused by the diseases transmitted by or associated with the ticks. Ticks rank first as arthropod vectors of protozoa, rickettsiae, bacteria and viruses, causing diseases in nonhuman vertebrates and rank second only to mosquitoes as vectors of pathogens to humans (Zhou *et al.*, 2009). The problem of TTBDs has been ranked high in terms of their impact on the livelihood of resources of poor farming communities in developing countries including India. The global economic loss due to tick infestation has been estimated as US$14,000 to 18,000 million annually and the cost of management of TTBDs in livestock of India is as high as US$ 498.7 million per annum (Minjauw and McLeod, 2003). The most common combined effect of TTBDs in Indian dairy system is reduction in milk yield i.e. loss of 14% of the lactation (McLeod and Kristjanson, 1999) and quality of hides for leather industry (Biswas, 2003).

Control of tick infestation has been difficult because ticks have few natural enemies. The use of chemical acaricides is at present the major and most widely used tick control strategy in the world. However, use of acaricides had limited efficacy in reducing tick infestations and is often accompanied by serious drawbacks, including the selection of acaricide resistant ticks, environmental contamination and contamination of milk and meat products with drug residues. Resistance is emerging as the one of the biggest problems, because the availability of new antiparasitic drugs is becoming scarcer (Fragoso *et al.,* 1999).

Definition of resistance

Resistance is defined as the capacity acquired by individuals of a parasite population that allows them to survive doses of chemicals which are generally lethal to a normal population (Nari and Hansen, 1999). Cross-resistance (CR) is the mechanism used by resistant insect species to survive the chemically related insecticide exposure, using a generic detoxification pattern (Metcalf, 1989). Multiple resistance (MR) is the use of various mechanisms to the action of several classes of chemically unrelated insecticides (Metcalf, 1989). For example, Parkhurst strain of *Rhipicephalus microplus,* (resistant to synthetic pyrethroid), Ultimo strain of *R. microplus* (resistant to synthetic pyrethroid, organophosphates and amitraz).

The main problem faced by entomologists is the resistance to chemicals, due to the presence of CR and MR between insect pests, progressive decrease in effective insecticides and high cost of developing new insecticides. There is an exponential growth pattern between the discovery of new insecticides and the development of strains resistant to these new products, for DDT (dichloro diphenyl dichloroethane) resistance appeared 6.3 years after entering the market, for lindane after 5 years, for organophosphate (OP) after 4 years, for carbamates after 2.5 years and for synthetic pyrethroids (SP) resistance appeared after only 2 years (Metcalf, 1989).

Resistance is not universal, and is most widespread and diverse in the one-host cattle tick (e.g. *R. microplus*). In other one host cattle ticks (e.g. *R. decoloratus),* resistance can be a severe problem, but these ticks are less widespread and less important than *R. microplus*. Resistance to acaricides has been much slower to develop in the two- and three-host ticks (e.g. *Rhipicephalus, Amblyomma, Hyalomma* and *Ixodes*), where longer generation times, less acaricidal exposure of the immature tick stages and the presence of alternative hosts might have helped to reduce selection pressure.

The resistance of ticks to acaricides is an inherited phenomenon and occurs due to continuous selection pressure. It results from the exposure of populations of ticks to chemical acaricides and subsequent survival and further propagation of ticks that are less affected by the acaricide. The higher reproductive rates of ticks that have heritable resistance factors, and the resulting increase in the proportion of these ticks in the population which carry genes for these factors is called selection. Also, insecticide resistance is a dynamic, multidimensional phenomenon dependent on biochemical, physiological, genetic and ecological factors. All of these vary with species population and geographical location.

Development of resistance

The development of resistance is an evolutionary process that occurs by genetic selection. Several insect species have survived naturally to adverse conditions, through a process of gradual adaptation to maintain order in ecosystems (Rosario and Hernandez, 2001). When an insecticide is used extensively, resulting in a strong selection pressure to eliminate susceptible individuals, the insecticide becomes the most important selection agent. In contrast to the slow evolution of resistance to toxic substances produced by plants in nature, the development of resistance to synthetic insecticides has been extremely fast, probably because the insects can utilize compounds developed in defence against allelo-chemicals or plant pathogens (Rosario and Hernandez, 2001). The speed with which resistance develops in a population depends mainly on the initial frequency of resistance genes, selection intensity, the degree of dominance of the gene and the relative ability of the genotype (Stone, 1972). In general, the frequency of resistance genes is very low in populations that have been under selection pressure. The rate of natural or spontaneous mutation to other genes is low (1/100,000 to 1/1,000,000) (Fragoso and Soberanes, 2001). The development of resistance is divided into following three phases.

Establishment phase : It arises when the resistant allele appears in a population; usually this process takes place by natural mutations and independently to selection pressure.

Development phase : Is the phase of increasing number of resistant individuals and occurs by the preferential survival rate of resistant ones after the use of chemicals. This process can follow two selection modes.

a) *Rapid :* Occurs when the gene that confers resistance is dominant or partially dominant and allows selection of heterozygotes.

b) *Slow :* When the alleles are recessive or are ineffective in isolation.

Emergency phase : Occurs by a high rate of selection pressure in a short phase and the resistant allele is common enough in the population to demonstrate a reduction in the effectiveness of the acaricide.

Evolution of resistance to acaricides

The involvements of the factors directly influencing the development of resistance evolution are classified as:

Genetic : Include the frequency of resistant (R) alleles, number of R alleles, dominance, insight, expression and interactions of R alleles (Goeters and Tabashnik, 2000). The rate of change in allele frequency at any given locus in a closed population is a function of allele frequency, dominance, and the relative fitness of the various genotypes. Dominance is a decisive factor on the genes that confer resistance. The degree of dominance of the gene influences the increase of resistant individuals in a population under selection pressure. When the resistant allele was recessive, the resistant population increases after nine generations (F9), whereas when the R allele was dominant the increase of resistant individuals occurs in the four generation (F4).

Biological : Include biotic aspects of the pest and number of generations, number of offspring per generation, monogamy, polygamy, and shelter survival chance (Bourguet *et al.*, 2000). It should be noted that most of the factors mentioned can not be controlled by man and the importance of certain previously quantified is only feasible when the resistance is already a problem on the farm and not before its evolution. The presence of survival shelters slows the increase in the frequency of resistant allele because some susceptible individuals occur outside the treatment, which helps perpetuate the susceptible alleles in a larger population (Goeters and Tabashnik, 2000). The impact of immigration has a major impact both on the frequency of resistant allele and in population growth. The delay in the evolution of resistance usually results from the constant influx of susceptible individuals to help cancel the evolution that has been made by the selection of insecticides.

Operational chemical : Includes the chemical nature of the pesticide, the initial use of pesticides, residue persistence, formulation, application type, application threshold, and threshold selection, selection of state of life and alternate selection (Georghiou and Taylor, 1977). These factors can be enlisted as following:

- Treatment frequency–the more often the ticks are exposed to the chemical, the more likely they will develop resistance to it. Treatment of European cattle in eastern Australia every three weeks has resulted in rapid development of acaricide resistance.
- Under-dosing risks tick survival, enhancing tolerance/resistance to the chemical.
- Persistent use of one chemical group for tick control.

The nature of the acaricide also influences the development of resistance and characteristic of an 'ideal' acaricide are as follows:

- Has a high level of toxicity towards all stages of the life cycle of cattle ticks.
- Can be easily administered by a number of methods, such as pour-on, plunge dip, spray dip or injection.
- Is cost-effective.
- Is rapidly metabolized and excreted to reduce the level of chemical residue in the animal, which requires long withholding periods and export slaughter intervals.

Mechanisms of resistance

The control of cattle ticks presently relies heavily on "no ticks/no tick-borne diseases" theory of disease control and encourages the heavy use of chemicals to control the tick vectors and this has lead to the development of resistance in ticks to these chemicals (Roulston *et al.*, 1981). As resistance to chemicals developed for a class of acaricides, a new class was introduced to alleviate the problems. Meanwhile introduction of new insecticides in the market became almost negligible largely because of the high costs associated with research, development, registration and the prognosis of a limited effective lifespan of the new insecticide (Feyereisen, 1995). Acaricide resistance to several classes of acaricides has been rapidly increasing as a result of excessive selection pressure by long term and intensive use of acaricides (Foil *et al.,* 2004). Resistance to acaricides in *R. microplus* has occurred in every region of the world where chemical control has been used to control ticks on cattle (FAO, 2004).

The livestock producers often experience multi-species resistance in ticks exposed to acaricides (Morales *et al.,* 1999) which involved both multiple tick species (e.g. *Amblyomma variegatum* and *R. microplus*) and multiple taxa (e.g. *R. microplus* and *Haematobia irritans*). The impact of insecticides/acaricides resistance is 2-fold: (1) the insecticide/ acaricides 'treadmill' leads to the introduction of a huge arsenal of highly toxic chemicals in the environment, and (2) an immediate increase in the dosage of the insecticide/ acaricides, thus compounding the problems of resistance and environmental contamination (Feyereisen, 1995).

The plasticity of the genome of insects has facilitated the development of resistance to insecticides and allows the development of future insecticide resistance (Rosario and Hernandez, 2001). During the past several years there has been a large number of studies aimed at understanding the biochemical and genetic processes of insects and arthropods developed to counteract the intoxication produced by the insecticide. Diverse resistance mechanisms have been identified in several strains of cattle tick *R. microplus* around the world and multi mechanism appears to be the common phenomenon in acaricides resistant tick population. According to the type of response to pesticide resistance has been grouped into four categories:

Resistance behaviour : It is when the insect adjust their behaviour to avoid contact with the insecticide.

Penetration resistance : It is a modification of the insect exoskeleton to inhibit or retard the penetration of the chemical, and generally has to do with the concentration of lipids that facilitate or retard the penetration of pesticides through this structure.

Metabolic resistance : It is the detoxification of the insecticide by enzymatic processes by the modification of metabolic pathways of the insect. The most important metabolic resistance involves multifunctional oxidases, glutathione S-transferase and esterase (Miller, 1998). This type of resistance involving DDT and SP, which can be assessed by means of inhibitors or synergies that may act to restore some or most effective pesticide. Liu and Scott (1998) mention that in metabolic resistance mechanisms, the most common include SP detoxification by over expression of cytochrome P450 enzymes. P450 enzymes (mixed function oxidase, cytochrome P450 monooxygenases) are a complex family of enzymes and play an important role in the adaptation of insects to toxic compounds and are involved in the metabolism of all commonly used insecticides (He *et al.*, 2002).

Target site insensitivity : Is modifying the site of action of insecticide to decrease the sensitivity of the chemical. When this is the cause of resistance, regular resistance levels are very high (1000x) as compared to the detoxification (50x). In order to increase knowledge about the causes of action site insensitivity as a mechanism of resistance molecular biology techniques are used. In most cases, it is likely that the genes that confer resistance are already present at very low levels in the tick population before the introduction of a new acaricide. The rate at which a resistant allele becomes established in the population and the time it takes for the break down of the control process of ticks is dependent upon many factors. These include the frequency of the original mutation in the population before treatment, the mode of inheritance of the resistant allele (dominant, co-dominant or recessive), the frequency of acaricide treatment, the concentration gradient of the acaricide and the proportion of the total tick population that is not exposed to the acaricide (*refugia*).

The main sites of action for SP are voltage-gated sodium channels in the nervous system (Liu *et al.*, 2000). The gene encoding the sodium channel in insects was identified in *Drosophila* spp. (Loughney *et al.*, 1989). The amino acid sequences of the alpha subunits encoded by the gene analyzed together are very similar. Each gene consists of four repeated homologous domains (I-IV) with six transmembrane segments (S 1-6) in each domain. Recent studies showed that point mutations in the gene sequence for the sodium channel are responsible for insecticide resistance (kdr) and super kdr type (which has an additional mutation that confers higher level of resistance) in insects (Miller *et al.*, 1999). In *R. microplus,* the pattern of kdr resistance was determined through mutations in the sodium channel and has identified point mutations in domain II in SP-resistant strains. Furthermore, Guerrero *et al.* (2001) detected the presence of an amino acid substitution Phe-Ile in the domain III S6 segment of the sodium channel resulting in a change in the structure of the channel with the projection altered stereochemistry of the binding site of the channel which gives the tick resistance property by target site modification.

Genetic and biochemical studies have contributed immensely to our understanding of resistance. The classically recognized mechanisms of resistance such as behavioral resistance, reduced penetration or absorption, sequestration and detoxification all contribute to decrease the dose of the acaricide, whereas decreased target site sensitivity or a modification of target site number will contribute to render a dose of acaricide ineffective.

Diagnosis of acaricide resistance

Resistance is usually first recognized as a failure of treatment to eliminate tick burdens from cattle. Although failure of treatment is often the result of incorrect preparation or application of acaricide, the persistence of ticks after frequent, correctly applied treatments indicates that acaricide resistance is likely.

In selecting a suitable laboratory test for acaricide resistance, the following requirements must be satisfied. The test should be sensitive enough to identify resistance early in its emergence. It should also cover the full range of chemical groups that are in use, including the most recently developed active ingredients. The diagnostic test should be simple and inexpensive. It should provide a rapid and reliable result, and be suitable for standardization among laboratories in many countries. The tests for the diagnosis of acaricide resistance fall under bioassays, biochemical and molecular tests.

Bioassays : The most widely used *in vitro* tests are bioassays applied to larvae and engorged female ticks.

Larval Packet Test (LPT) : Was developed in a series of tests with tick *R. microplus* for many years at CSIRO, Australia and was adopted by the FAO as the main diagnostic test for resistance in ticks and further promoted in the form of the FAO Acaricide Resistance Testing Kit. In LPT, live larvae are exposed to filter paper impregnated with acaricides for different time periods, depending on the acaricide. LPT can be used to detect resistance to organophosphates, pyrethroids and amidines.

Larval Immersion Test (LIT) : This larval bioassay (Shaw, 1966) has not been widely used for the diagnosis of resistance and has not been promoted by FAO. Usually a diagnosis is made in about six weeks, the same time required for larval packet test. Comparative studies conducted conclude that the results of immersion test are in good agreement with the results of larval packet test.

Adult Immersion Test (AIT) : This test was described and developed by Drummond *et al.* (1973), to determine the efficacy of new acaricides against several species of ticks. A questionnaire circulated by the FAO Working Group on Parasite Resistance (WGPR) revealed that the method most widely used in laboratories involved with the diagnosis of resistance was the AIT (FAO, 2004). The AIT is a bioassay applied to engorged, female ticks and the main disadvantage is that they require large numbers of engorged females and several weeks are required to get results. Two variants of AIT are being used viz. the classical AIT (with different concentrations of product) and a standardized AIT that uses discriminating doses (AITDD).

Biochemical testing : The correct use of biochemical methods for resistance detection at a mechanistic level can provide a powerful tool for analyzing field and laboratory populations with the aim of improving resistance detection and management. However, these biochemical assays are not complete substitutes for the standard susceptibility tests which are used to measure resistance.

Biochemical testing is basically the use of synergists that inhibit enzymes responsible for metabolic detoxification and, therefore, its effect can be reconstructed, partially or totally, the effectiveness of acaricide to tick strain showed a pattern of behaviour of resistance by metabolic detoxification. Examples of inhibitors include: 1) 1,1-bis-(p-chlorophenyl) ethanol (chlorfenethol) an inhibitor to DDT, 2) O-ethyl O-4-nitrophenyl phenylphosphonate (EPE-oxon), an inhibitor of carboxylesterase for malathion, 3) S,S,S,-tributyl phosphorotriothionate (DEF), an inhibitor of esterases to organophosphorus, and 4) piperonyl butoxide, a microsomal oxidase inhibitor, for carbamates and synthetic pyrethroids (Oppernorth, 1984).

Two variants of the test of the estimation of enzyme levels are in use viz. filter paper and microtitre plate method. The filter paper or nitrocellulose membrane assays are quantified visually or using a densitometer, but provide a permanent record which can be rechecked in future. The microtitre plate tests allow the same tick to be used for all assays and are quantified visually or with a spectrophotometer and hence is more commonly used.

Molecular tests : This test is to determine resistance by detecting the alteration in sequence of the genes encoding the site of action of acaricides in ticks. Gene specific assay such as the sodium channel PCR assay and PCR- RFLP is unequivocal in determining the acaricides resistance. The sodium channel assay of San Felipe and Corrales population from Mexico of *R. microplus* clearly showed that the target site resistance is present in the most of the individuals, which will render pyrethroid acaricides ineffective, as they rely on sodium channel function disruption for their toxicity (Foil *et al.*, 2004). Several pyrethroid resistant population of *R. microplus* has been surveyed for mutated sodium channel gene and only the single amino acid changing mutation which the PCR is designed to detect, has been found (He *et al.*, 1999; Jamroz *et al.*, 2000). The main advantage of these tests is that they provide results within hours, and a disadvantage is that it can identify genotype or resistance mechanisms associated with mutations. Thus, a tick population with a mechanism of resistance conferred by mutation or based on enzyme mechanisms/metabolic resistance can be genotyped as susceptible, if this does not have the specific mutation detected by PCR.

Distribution of acaricide resistance

Worldwide scenario

The prevalence of resistance to acaricides varied between regions, depending mainly on the local ecology of ticks and application of acaricide. Resistance to arsenical, organochlorines and cyclodiene acaricides was reported in tick populations during the year 1930 to 1960 in different areas of the world (Wharton, 1976). Later during 1960-1970s, the development and widespread use of organophosphorus (OP) acaricides resulted in the development of resistance to many of the chemicals (Weilgama, 1980). Likewise the development and use of synthetic pyrethroids during the time period ranging from 1970 to 1980 and onwards was followed inevitably by development of resistance to some of these compounds in different regions of the world (Brun, 1992; WHO, 1992; Benavides *et al.*, 2000; Jonsson *et al.*, 2000).

Resistance of *R. microplus* to diazinon was reported from Columbia, Mexico and Huila (Benavides, 1995; Oritz *et al.*, 1995; Romero *et al.*, 1997). Arantes *et al.* (1996) reported resistance to trichlorophon from Brazil and similar findings were made by Benavidis (1995) from Columbia. Ortiz *et al.* (1995) reported resistance to dioxanthion and chloropyriphos in Mexico. Coronado (1995) and Romero *et al.* (1997) reported resistance to chlorfenviphos from Venezuela and Columbiana, respectively. Resistance to coumaphos has also been reported (Rosario *et al.*, 1997).

Rodriguez-Vivas *et al.* (2006) reported the resistance to organophosphates and pyrethroids in *R. microplus* ticks in Yucatan state of Mexico against discriminating doses of deltamethrin, cypermethrin, flumethrin, chlorfenvinphos and coumaphos. Resistance to the formamidine acaricide, amitraz has also been observed in Mexico in recent years (Soberanes *et al.*, 2002; Rodriguez-Vivas *et al.*, 2006). Many of the Mexican isolates of *R. microplus* have now become resistant to multiple acaricides (Li *et al.*, 2004). The resistance of ticks to acaricides has also been described from tropical zones in Africa, South America, Australia and France (WHO, 1992; Benavides *et al.*, 2000; Jonsson *et al.*, 2000). Development of resistance in *R. microplus* to synthetic pyrethroids has also been reported in several American countries (Fragoso *et al.*, 1995; Ortiz, *et al.*, 1995) including resistance to cypermethrin in the east Argentinean tick infested region.

Hagen *et al.* (1999) analyzed tick samples from different countries in Central America and found varied prevalence of resistance against synthetic pyrethroids. In Costa Rica and Brazil, Alvarez *et al.* (1999) and Furlong (1999) found prevalence resistant to synthetic pyrethroids in ticks.

Indian scenario

Resistance in ticks against different acaricides had been reported by several workers from various parts of the country. Among the various acaricides used in India for the control of ticks in livestock, γ–BHC was first against which resistance was reported in *R. microplus* (Chaudhary and Naithani, 1964; Khan and Srivastava, 1977), followed by dieldrin (Sangwan *et al.*, 1993), sevin (Basu and Haldar, 1997) and lindane (Kumar, 1999). As per the report published by FAO (2004), the tick population in India has developed resistance against all the available acaricides.

Synthetic pyrethroids particularly deltamethrin and cypermethrin have been used extensively for tick control in most parts of country for the past decade leading to tick populations resistant against both the acaricides. Ticks (*R. microplus*) collected from dairy farms at Ludhiana, Punjab, when subjected to AIT with a discriminating dose (AITDD) revealed a very high degree of resistance against deltamethrin (96.67%) and cypermethrin (93.33%) (Singh *et al.*, 2010). The results of AIT revealed that 94.92, 91.53, 88.14, 96.61 and 88.14% of *R. microplus* adult female ticks from Ludhiana, Punjab were resistant at 0.0025,

0.005, 0.0075, 0.01 and 0.0125 percent concentration of deltamethrin, respectively. Further, the reproductive index varied from 0.52-0.57 in treated ticks, and the hatching percentage of eggs laid by the treated ticks was almost similar to those of the control ticks (Singh *et al.*, 2012).

Recently, Vatsya and Yadav (2011) conducted a study to monitor the status of deltamethrin resistance in field populations of *R. microplus* from different geographical locations of Uttarakhand state in northern India. The highest 50% lethal concentration (LC50) was recorded for the Kashipur population of ticks [0.0175%; resistance factor (RF) = 34.26] followed by Nagla (0.00273%; RF 5.35), Dehradun (0.00266%; RF 5.21), Pantnagar (0.002402%; RF 4.71), Almora (0.00164%; RF 3.21), and New Tehri (0.00104%; RF 2.04) when compared with the reference susceptible Pithoragarh strain (LC50 0.00051%; RF 1.0). Also, the *in vitro* evaluation revealed three tick populations to have deltamethrin-resistant phenotypes (RF>5); two populations to be tolerant (RF 3–5) and one population to have susceptible phenotypes (RF<3). Synergism studies revealed the likely involvement of monoxygenases and esterases in the imparting resistance in Nagla and Dehradun isolates.

The resistance status of *R. microplus* to "Diazinon" was evaluated in 20 locations situated at various agro-climatic regions of India using AIT. The minimum effective concentration of Diazinon in laboratory reared acaricide susceptible IVRI-I strain of *R. microplus* and was determined as 635.2 ppm. The discriminating dose (DD) was worked out as 1270.4 ppm and was tested on female ticks collected from organized and unorganized farms located at different agro-climatic regions of India. On the basis of the data generated on three variables viz. mortality, egg masses and reproductive index, the resistance level was categorized as I, II, III and IV. The average resistance factor (RF) of 6.1 (level II) was recorded in the ticks collected from the northern sub-temperate trans-gangetic plains while high average RF values of 26.65 (level III) was recorded in the ticks collected from tropical middle-gangetic plains (Kumar *et al.*, 2011).

Sharma *et al.* (2012) conducted a cross sectional study to assess the resistance against synthetic pyrethroids in *R. microplus* collected from 27 areas located in 6 agro-climatic regions of India using adult immersion test and larval packet test. The minimum effective concentration of deltamethrin in laboratory reared acaricide susceptible

IVRI-I strain of *R.* (*B.*) microplus was determined as 29.6 ppm in AIT and 35.5 ppm in LPT, whereas it was determined 349.1 and 350.7 ppm, respectively in AIT and LPT for cypermethrin. Out of 27 areas of tick collection, 18 (66.6%) areas showed resistance against deltamethrin and cypermethrin. Among 18 areas, resistance to deltamethrin at level I was detected in 8 areas (resistance factor = 2.0-4.9), at level II in 9 areas (RF = 5.2- 11.8), at level III in one area (RF = 34.9) and at level IV in one area (RF = 95.7). The resistance to cypermethrin was detected in 16 areas and the level of resistance was detected at level I in 10 areas (RF = 2.06-4.64) and at level II in 6 areas (RF = 5.13- 9.88). They observed that the middle gangetic and trans-gangetic regions had higher density of resistant ticks where intensive cross-bred cattle population is reared and the synthetic pyrethroids are commonly used.

Impact of resistance on the production costs of acaricides

One of the most important technological achievements of the twentieth century is the development of increasingly effective drugs in controlling a wide range of parasitic species. For the pharmaceutical industry involved in constant development of chemicals there is an increasing concern regarding the frequent development of resistance and consequently, the presence of residues in products of animal origin (Nari and Hansen, 1999). Normally, the presence of residues is a response to increased frequency of application and/or dosage of drugs, which can affect international trade (Kunz and Kemp, 1994). Multiple cross-resistance adversely affect the life of the new insecticides and the effectiveness of new products even before positioning in the market.

In 1997, worldwide sales of endoparasiticides (36%), endectocides (25%) and ectoparasiticides (39%) were US $ 3,100 million (Mackenzie, 1998). A moderate loss of efficiency (usually not displayed at field level) represents heavy losses in terms of cost-efficiency of pest control. Metcalf (1989) mentioned that for development of a new pesticide it is required to test many potential products. In 1956, about 1,800 compounds were evaluated, while in 1984, it tested 22,000. Nari and Hansen (1999) report that the cost of developing a new pesticide is 100-230 million US dollars in a process that can take more than 10 years since the discovery of a candidate to its availability in the market.

Resistance management

Acaricide resistance has usually been managed after emergence, by the use of new products. New, very effective, long-acting available acaricides, as well as new labour-saving techniques for acaricide application (pour-on, injection, boluses and tags) help in dealing with the problem of resistance. This is encouraging, but increasing problems with chemical residues are imposing much more stringent requirements for registration and are affecting the use of both old and new acaricides.

In the past, substantial research has been directed at understanding resistance mechanisms and developing alternative methods to combat resistance (other than the obvious method of changing to a new group of chemicals) (Nolan and Schnitzerling, 1986). However, the main objective of resistance management lies in trying to reduce the number of applications throughout the year by using resistant zebu breeds or 'indigenous' cattle. In some situations, there is no justification for using acaricides to control ticks (Sutherst *et al.*, 1979). Where acaricides are required, particularly on European breeds or 'improved' cattle, careful (i.e. strategic) timing of treatments can reduce the number of treatments and these should be undertaken before production losses occur. Treatments should be continued and should end only when tick numbers decline to low levels, to prevent large numbers of ticks being exposed to sub-optimal acaricide concentrations. Promoting correct acaricide application has proved far from easy, and promoting resistance-delaying strategies is even more challenging. Also, in view of the difficulty of performing long-term field trials or extrapolating laboratory experiments to the field (Nolan *et al.*, 1989), the problem of resistance management has been addressed mainly by simulation modelling (Sutherst and Comins, 1979).

Some basic management and biosecurity principles can be used to reduce the chances of development of acaricide resistance such as:

- Always use the recommended strength in dips as printed on the chemical label by the manufacturer.
- If using a plunge dip, always re-dip your stirrer cattle.
- Never under-dose animals during treatment with pour-on or injectable applications. Treat the mob at the rate of the heaviest animal, reducing the chance of under-dosing.

- Import only tick-free livestock on to your farm. If this is unavoidable, treat livestock on arrival and only turn out tick-free cattle on to the paddock.
- If you suspect poor tick kill, notify your nearest concerned authority for investigation and testing.

Extensive experience in the field has led to suggestions that the use of strictly managed, uninterrupted, short-interval treatments at recommended concentrations is a reliable means of avoiding or delaying resistance. However, it has also been proposed that intermittent use of high concentration acaricides to kill ticks with resistant alleles may provide a basic means of delaying resistance (Sutherst *et al.*, 1979). Clearly, different interpretations exist regarding optimum acaricide treatment strategies. In practice, uninterrupted, short-interval treatment regimes often break down for various reasons and, in any case, the costs of such treatment are becoming prohibitive for many farmers.

The use of rotation or alternation of different groups of pesticides which have no cross-resistance has been proposed although rotation does not always show theoretical advantage. Alternating acaricides reduces the selection pressure from any one chemical, but this assumes that no resistance already exists and that the frequency of resistant individuals to each chemical used will decline during the application of the alternate acaricides. This decline would occur only if there is a fitness cost associated with resistance, or if refugia of untreated pests allow immigration of susceptible individuals to dilute resistance alleles (Roush and Daly, 1990). For tick control, prolonging the active life of a particular acaricide (or acaricide group) which was favoured for its long protection period, high efficacy, low cost or lack of residue problems could be a great advantage. Under current practice, such acaricides are used heavily, and resistance usually develops within a few years, rendering the product worthless.

The use of mixtures of acaricides for delaying resistance in ticks shows promise in modelling studies. Success of mixtures is based on the expectation that one individual is unlikely to carry resistant alleles for two acaricides with different modes of action. For insects, which have been more intensively studied, the potential of a mixture of two insecticides to delay resistance required a number of conditions to be fulfilled (Curtis *et al.*, 1993). There must be no pre-existing resistance to either insecticide in the mixture, and each insecticide should be applied at optimal and not halved, concentrations. The different insecticides must be compatible in mixtures and of equal persistence; otherwise a sub-lethal concentration of residual deposit of one component would select resistant heterozygotes. Finally, some susceptible insects must escape treatment and dilute the population of resistant survivors for maximum benefit to be gained from mixtures (Roush, 1993). For ticks, information is needed on the proportion of the population to be left untreated. The additional costs, toxicity of mixtures to the host and residue problems would also have to be reconsidered. Use of mixtures to delay acaricide resistance requires more research. Problems with instability, formulation difficulties and costs have mitigated against the use of additives (including mixtures) and synergists (Nolan and Schnitzerling, 1986). Further, quarantine of an area where resistance has been detected, followed by eradication of the resistant strains, is an ideal solution.

Increased concentration is another tactic which has been used successfully in controlling DDT-, OP- and SP-resistant strains of *R. microplus* (Nolan *et al.*, 1989). This also helped to prolong the life of OP acaricides, but new strains eventually emerged which could not be controlled by increased concentrations. This strategy is not always successful in controlling strains. Doubling amitraz concentration, for example, gave little improvement in control of the amidine-resistant Ulam strain of *R. microplus*. Potential host toxicity and chemical residue problems now need to be reconsidered before an increased concentration could be used for resistance management.

The use of botanical/herbal acaricides is also a promising alternative particularly in Indian scenario. The ethno-veterinary and medical knowledge offers a range of herbs to be evaluated for their insecticidal and acaricidal property. Certain plants and herbs are known to possess insecticidal, growth inhibiting, anti-moulting and repellent activities. The evaluation of botanical acaricides in crude extract form and subsequent isolation and characterization of the key active components, have a great scope for commercialization. India possesses 45,000 plant species of which 15,000–20,000 have proven medicinal value and have lands not suitable for agriculture activities. The tested/yet to be tested locally available plant extracts prepared from the perennial plants can easily be grown in these unutilized lands. Once the active principle of the effective components is known the same can be commercially produced and marketed. Besides the cost effectiveness, the environment friendly products will have low mammalian toxicity, less residual effect in animal products and have the potential to reduce or replace the chemical acaricide use. Besides, since botanical acaricides consist of number of active molecules against ticks, the chances of selection of resistance tick population is expected to be slower than commonly used acaricides where single point mutation is rendering an insecticide ineffective (Ghosh *et al.*, 2006)

The principle of integrated control of ticks and tick-borne diseases-through the use of vaccines, tick-resistant cattle, promoting enzootic stability, and the optimal timing of acaricide treatments to reduce costs and increase sustainability of control-will inevitably signal a move away from frequent, uninterrupted acaricide treatments. In the face of these changes, greater knowledge is required of the potential for increased resistance problems and of techniques for delaying resistance to conserve existing acaricides. This need has become more acute with the realization that few, if any, of the existing acaricides (old or new) will be completely free of residue problems.

Conclusions

Although the control of ticks relies heavily on the use of chemicals, the selection of resistant tick strains to the available compounds is a serious threat to the sustainability of this approach. It is, thus, recommended to revise the existing methods and consider other tick control strategies that could best address the problem of acaricide resistance which is almost inevitable. The necessity to develop a sustainable and integrated scheme, in which the isolated methods may be individually inadequate but together with others may exert a vigorous synergy, is justified. This method consists of the use of tick-resistant cattle breeds, pasture management, habitat modification and immunization in combination with rational use of acaricides. Although difficult to materialize in developing countries like India, the prospect of this approach is considerable, as it is the most sustainable method and keeps enzootic stability undisturbed. Further, resistance management almost inevitably continues to involve the implementation of strategies after resistance has occurred and therefore has to operate in a crisis situation. The paradox is, of course, that once resistance has emerged, most of the best options for managing it are no longer effective. Since, the options for controlling resistant ticks are limited there is clearly a need for governments, advisory agencies, and the pharmaceutical and farming industries to cooperate to either prevent or at least facilitate the earliest possible detection of resistance. Hence, surveys on acaricide resistance need to be carried out in major livestock production areas in the country in order to gather a comprehensive database on the magnitude of the problem at a national scale.

References

Alvarez, V., Bonilla, R. and Chacon, R. (1999). Status of resistance in *B. microplus* (Canestrini, 1887) to organophosphates and pyrethroids in Costa Rica. *Rev. Cien. Vet.*, 22: 41-60.

Arantes, G.J., Marques, A.O. and Honer, M.R. (1996). The cattle tick *B. microplus*, in the municipality of Uberlandia. MG: analysis of its resistance to commercial acaricides. *Rev. Bras. Parasitol. Vet.*, 4: 89-93.

Basu, A. and Haldar, D.P. (1997). A note on the effect of continuous use of Sevin 50 WP on some cattle ticks. *J. Vet. Parasitol.*, 11: 183-184.

Benavides, O.E. (1995). *Boophilus microplus* tick resistance to acaricides in Colombia: A summary of the present situation. In: 3rd international seminary on Animal Parasitology. Acapulco, Guerrero, Mexico, Oct. 11–13.

Benavides, O.E., Rodriguez, S.C. and Romario, A. (2000). Isolation and partial characterization of the Mexican strain of *B. microplus* (Canestrini) multi resistant to different acaricides. *Ann. N.Y. Acad. Sci.*, 916: 668-671.

Biswas, S. (2003). Role of veterinarian in the care and management during harvest of skin in livestock species. Proceedings of National Seminar Leather Industry in Today's perspective. Kolkata, India.

Bourguet, D., Genissel, A. and Baymond, M. (2000). Insecticide resistance and dominance levels. *J. Econ. Entomol.*, 93: 1588-1595.

Brun, L.O. (1992). Resistance to deltamethrin in *B. microplus* (Canestrini) (Acari: Ixodidae) in New Caledonia. *J. Aust. Entomol. Soc.*, 31: 301–302.

Chaudhary, R.P. and Naithani, R.C. (1964). Resistance to BHC in the cattle tick *Boophilus microplus* in India. *Bull. Entomol. Res.*, 55: 405-410.

Coronado, A. (1995). Current status of the tropical cattle tick *B. microplus* in Venezuela. In: 3rd International Seminary on Animal Parasitology Acapulco, Guerrero, Mexico, Oct. 11-13, pp. 22-28.

Curtis, C.F., Hill, N. and Kasim, S.H. (1993). Are there effective resistance management strategies for vectors of human disease? *Biol. J. Linnean Soc.*, 48: 3-18.

Drummond, R.O., Ernst, S.E., Trevino, J.L., Gladney, W.J. and Graham, O.H. (1973). *Boophilus annulatus* and *B. microplus*: laboratory test of insecticides. *J. Econ. Entomol.*, 66: 130–133.

FAO (2004). Guidelines resistance management and integrated parasite control in ruminants. Module 1: Ticks: acaricide resistance: diagnosis, management and prevention, pp. 1–53.

Feyereisen, R. (1995). Molecular biology of insecticide resistance. *Toxicol. Lett.*, 82: 83-90.

Foil, L.D., Coleman, P., Eisler, M., Fragoso-Sanchez, H., Garcia-Vazquez, Z., Guerrero, F.D., Jonsson, N.N., Langstaff, I.G., Li, A.Y. and Machila, N. (2004). Factors that influence the prevalence of acaricide resistance and tick-borne diseases. *Vet. Parasitol.*, 125: 163–181.

Fragoso, S.H., Ortiz, E.M., de Labra, V., Ortiz, N.N., Rodriguez, M., Redondo, M., de La Fuente, J. and Hernandez, P.V. (1999). Evaluation of the vaccine against the tick Bm86 (Gavac) for the control of *B. microplus*. Proceedings of IV International Seminar of Animal Parasitology. Puerto Vallarta, Jalisco, Mexico, pp. 47-50.

Fragoso, S.H., Ortiz, E.M., Soberanes, C.N., Santamaria, V.M. and Ortiz, N.A. (1995). Epidemiologia de la resistancia a ixodicides en garrapatas *Boophilus microplus* en la Republica Mexicana. In: 3rd International Seminary on Animal Parasitology Acapulco, Guerrero, Mexico, Oct. 11-13, pp. 45-57.

Fragoso, S.H. and Soberanes, C.N. (2001). Control of SP resistance in the light of current knowledge. Proceedings of XXV Congress Buiatrics. Veracruz, Veracruz, Mexico. Mexican Association of Doctors specializing in cattle, AC, pp. 40-48.

Furlong, J. (1999). Diagnosis of the susceptibility of the cattle tick *B. microplus* to acaricides in the state of Minas Gerais, Brazil. Proceedings of IV International Seminar of Animal Parasitology. Puerto Vallarta, Jalisco, Mexico, pp. 41-46.

Georghiou, G.P. and Taylor, C.E. (1977). Operational Influences in the evolution of insecticides resistance. *J. Econ. Entomol.*, 70: 653-638.

Ghosh, S., Azhahianambi, P. and de la Fuente, J. (2006). Control of ticks of ruminants, with special emphasis on livestock farming systems in India: present and future possibilities for integrated control-a review. *Exp. Appl. Acarol.*, 40:49–66.

Goeters, F.R. and Tabashnik, B.E. (2000). Roles of selection intensity, major genes and minor genes in evolution of insecticide resistance. *J. Econ. Entomol.*, 93: 1580-1587.

Guerrero, F.D., Davey, R.B. and Miller, R.J. (2001). Use of an allele-specific polymerase chain reaction assay to genotype pyrethroid resistant strains of *B. microplus* (Acari: Ixodidae). *J. Med. Entomol.*, 38: 44–50.

Hagen, S., Kopp, J. and Liebisch, A. (1999). Study of acaricide resistance in cattle tick *B. microplus* in Central America. Proceedings of IV Inter-national Seminar of Animal Parasitology. Puerto Vallarta, Jalisco, Mexico, pp. 33.

He, H., Chen, A.C., Davey, R.B., Ivie, G.W. and George, J.E. (2002). Characterization and molecular cloning of glutathione S-transferase gene from the tick, *Boophilus microplus* (Acari: Ixodidae). *Insect Biochem. Mol. Biol.*, 29: 737-743.

He, H., Chen, A.C., Davey, R.B., Ivie, G.W. and George, J.E. (1999). Identification of a point mutation in the para-type sodium channel gene from a pyrethroid-resistant cattle tick. *Biochem. Biophys. Res. Com.*, 261: 558–561.

Jamroz, R.C., Guerrero, F.D., Pruett, J.H., Oehler, D.D. and Miller, R.J. (2000). Molecular and biochemical survey of acaricide resistance mechanisms in larvae from Mexican strains of the southern cattle tick, *B. microplus*. *J. Insect Physiol.*, 46: 685-695.

Jonsson, N.N., Mayer, D.G. and Green, P.E. (2000). Possible risk factors on Queensland dairy farms for acaricide resistance in cattle tick (*B. microplus*). *Vet. Parasitol.*, 88: 79–92.

Khan, M.H. and Srivastava, S.C. (1977). *In vitro* tests with some ixodicides against cattle tick, *B. microplus*. *Indian J. Anim. Hlth.*, 16:137-140.

Kumar, S. (1999). Studies on acaricides resistance in common ixodid ticks of Punjab. M.V.Sc thesis submitted to Punjab Agricultural University, Ludhiana.

Kumar, S., Paul, S., Sharma, A.K., Kumar, R., Tewari, S.S., Chaudhuri, P., Ray, D.D., Rawat, A.K. and Ghosh, S. (2011). Diazinon resistant status in *Rhipicephalus (Boophilus) microplus* collected from different agro-climatic regions of India. *Vet. Parasitol.*, 181: 274-281.

Kunz, S.E. and Kemp, D.H. (1994). Insecticides and acaricides: Resistance and Environmental Impact. *Sci. Tech. Rev. OIE.*, 13: 1249-1286.

Li, A.Y., Davey, R.B., Miller, R.J. and George, J.E. (2004). Detection and Characterization of amitraz resistance in the southern cattle tick, *B. microplus* (Acari: Ixodidae). *J. Med. Entomol.*, 41: 193-200.

Liu, N. and Scott, J.G. (1998). Causes increaser transcription of cytochrome P450 CYP6D1-mediated insecticide resistance in house fly. *Insect Biochem. Mol.*, 28: 531-535.

Liu, Z., Valles, M.S. and Dong, K. (2000). Novel point mutations in the germ cockroach for sodium channel gene associated with knockdown resistance (kdr) to pyrethroid insecticides. *Insect Biochem. Mol.*, 30: 991-997.

Loughney, K., Krebs, R. and Ganetzky, B. (1989). Molecular analysis of the para locus, a sodium channel gene in *Drosophila*. *Cell*, 58: 1143-1148.

McLeod, R. and Kristjanson, P. (1999). Tick cost: economic impact of ticks and TBD to livestock in Africa, Asia and Australia. International Livestock Research Institute, Nairobi, Kenya.

Metcalf, R.L. (1989). Insect resistance to insecticides. *Pestic. Sci.*, 26: 333-358.

Miller, T.A. (1998). Mechanism of resistance to pyrethroid insecticides. *Parasitol. Today*, 4: 8-12.

Miller, R.J., Davey, R.B. and George, J.E. (1999). Characterization of pyrethroid resistance and susceptibility to coumaphos in Mexican *B. microplus* (Acari: Ixodidae). *J. Med. Entomol.*, 36: 533-538.

Minjauw, B. and McLeod, A. (2003). Tick-borne diseases and poverty. The impact of ticks and tick-borne diseases on the livelihood of small scale and marginal livestock owners in India and eastern and southern Africa. Research report, DFID Animal Health Programme, Centre for Tropical Veterinary Medicine, University of Edinburgh, UK, pp. 59–60.

Morales, S.G., Fragoso, S.H. and Garcia, V.Z. (1999). Control de la resistencia en garrapatas y moscas deimportancia veterinaria y enfermedades que transmiten. Proceedings of IV International Seminar of Animal Parasitology, Puerto Vallarta, Jalisco, Mexico, pp. 264.

Nari, A. and Hansen, H.J. (1999). Resistance of ecto and endoparasites: current and future solutions. 67th general meeting, International Organization of Epizootics. Paris, France.

Nolan, J. and Schnitzerling H.J. (1986). Drug resistance in arthropod parasites. In: Chemotherapy of parasitic diseases (W.C. Campbell & R.S. Rew, eds). Plenum Press, New York, pp. 603-620.

Nolan, J., Wilson, J.T., Green, P.E. and Bird, P. (1989). Synthetic pyrethroid resistance in field samples in the cattle tick (*B. microplus*). *Aust. Vet. J.*, 66: 179–182.

Oppenorth, J.F. (1984). Biochemistry of insecticide resistance. *Pestic. Biochem. Phys.*, 22: 187-193.

Ortiz, E.M., Santamaria, V.M., Ortiz, N.A., Soberanes, C.N., Osorio, M.J., Franco, B.R., Martinez, I.F., Quezada, D.R. and Fragozo, S.H. (1995). Caracterizaci6n de la resistencia de *B. microplus* en Mexico. In: 3rd International seminary on animal parasitology Acapulco, Guerrero, Mexico, Oct. 11-13 pp. 58–70.

Rodriguez-vivas, R.I., Alonso-Diaz, M.A., Rodriguez, A.F., Fragoso, S.H., Santamaria, V.M. and Rosario, C.R. (2006). Prevalence and potential risk factors for organophosphate and pyrethroid resistance in *B. microplus* ticks on cattle ranches from the state of Yucatan, Mexico. *Vet. Parasitol.*, 136: 335-340.

Romero, N.A., Benavides, O.E., Herrera, G.C. and Parra, T.M.H. (1997). Resistance of the tick *B. microplus* to organophosphate and synthetic pyrethroid acaricides in the department of Huila. *Rev. Colomb. Entomol.*, 23: 9-17.

Rosario, C.R. and Hernandez, O.R. (2001). Chemical evolution of resistance to acaricides. Proceedings of Training Workshop, diagnosis of resistance to acaricides in *B. microplus* ticks. Jiutepec, Morelos, Mexico, pp. 23-30.

Rosario, C.R., Miranda, M.E., Garcia, V.Z. and Ortiz, E.M. (1997). Detection of esterase activity in susceptible and organophosphate resistant strains of the cattle tick *B. microplus* (Acari: Ixodidae). *Bull. Entomol. Res.*, 87:197–202.

Roulston, W.J., Wharton, R.H., Nolan, J., Kerr, J.D., Wilson, J.T., Thompson, P.G. and Schotz, M. (1981). A survey for resistance in cattle ticks to acaricides. *Aust. Vet. J.*, 57: 362–371.

Roush, R.T. (1993). Occurrence, genetics and management of insecticide resistance. *Parasitol. Today*, 9: 174-179.

Roush, R.T. and Daly, J.C. (1990). The role of population genetics in resistance research and management, in Pesticide Resistance in Arthropods (R.T. Roush & B.E. Tabashnik, eds). Chapman Hall, New York and London, pp. 97-152.

Sangwan, A.K., Chhabra, M.B. and Singh, S. (1993). Acaricide resistance status of common livestock ticks in Haryana. *Indian Vet. J.*, 70: 20-24.

Sharma, A.K., Kumar, R., Kumar, S., Nagar, G., Singh, N.K., Rawat, S.S., Dhakad, M.L., Rawat, A.K.S., Ray, D.D. and Ghosh, S. (2012). Deltamethrin and cypermethrin resistance status of *Rhaipicephalus (Boophilus) microplus* collected from six agro-climatic regions of India. *Vet. Parasitol.*, 188: 337-345.

Shaw, R.D. (1966). Culture of an organophosphorus resistant strain of *B. microplus* and an assessment of STI resistance spectrum. *Bull. Entomol. Res.*, 56: 389-405.

Singh, N.K., Haque, M., Jyoti and Rath, S.S. (2012). Deltamethrin resistance in *Rhipicephalus microplus* in Ludhiana. *Indian Vet. J.*, 89: 23-25.

Singh, N.K., Jyoti, Haque, M., and Rath, S.S. (2010). Studies on acaricide resistance in *Rhipicephalus (Boophilus) microplus* against synthetic pyrethroids by adult immersion test with a discriminating dose. *J. Vet. Parasitol.*, 24: 207-208.

Soberanes, M.J., Santamaria, V.M., Fragoso, S.H., and Gracia. Z.V. (2002). First case reported of amitraz resistance in the cattle tick *B. microplus* in Mexico. *Tec. Pecu. Mex.*, 40: 81-92.

Solis, S.S. (1991). *Boophilus* ticks ecology: Perspectives of a panorama. Proceedings of II International Seminar on Animal Parasitology and Tick-borne diseases, Morelos, Mexico, pp. 19-30.

Stone, B.F. (1972). The genetics of resistance by ticks to acaricides. *Aust. Vet. J.*, 48: 345-350.

Sutherst, R.W. and Comins, H.N. (1979). The management of acaricide resistance in the cattle tick, *B. microplus* (Acari: Ixodidae), in Australia. *Bull. Entomol. Res.*, 69: 519–537.

Sutherst, R.W., Norton, G.A., Barlow, N.D., Conway, G.R., Birley, M. and Comins, H.N. (1979). An analysis of management strategies for cattle tick *(B. microplus)* control in Australia. *J. Appl. Ecol.*, 16: 359-382.

Vatsya, S. and Yadav, C.L. (2011). Evaluation of acaricide resistance mechanisms in field populations of *Rhipicephalus (Boophilus) microplus* collected from India. *Int. J. Acarol.*, 37: 405-410.

Weilgama, D.J. (1980). Susceptibility of *Boophilus annulatus* in Sri Lanka to certain acaricides. *Ceylon Vet. J.* 28: 36-42.

Wharton, R.H. (1976). Tick borne livestock diseases and their vectors. Acaricide resistance and alternative method of tick control. *World Anim. Rev.*, 20: 8-15.

WHO (1992). Vector resistance to pesticides. Fifteenth report of the WHO expert committee on vector biology and control. Tech. Rep. Ser. No.818, Geneva, pp. 58.

Zhou, J., Liao, M., Ueda, M., Gong, H., Xuan, X. and Fujisaki, K. (2009). Characterization of an intracellular cystatin homolog from the tick *Haemaphysalis longicornis*. *Vet. Parasitol.*, 160: 180–83.

❑❑❑

Chapter 2

Ancylostomosis : An Overview

R. Katoch, R. Godara, Anish Yadav and Shilpa Sood*
Division of Veterinary Parasitology, *Division of Veterinary Pathology
Faculty of Veterinary Sciences and Animal Husbandry
Sher-e-Kashmir University of Agricultural Sciences and Technology-Jammu,
R.S. Pura-181 102

Introduction

India is world's 12th largest economy and also the fourth largest in terms of purchasing power parity adjusted exchange rates. The economic reforms of 1991 have led to the growth of more than 7% in late 2000s. The country became second faster growing economy in the world in 2008 and the service sector contributes more than half of India's GDP. The rise in industrial and service sectors swelled the population of urban India, inturn also lead to development of slums. There is also increase in urban garbage. There is no proper disposal methodology of garbage presently exist in India. It becomes important source of survival for urban stray dogs.

The dog ownership can be seen as an economic indicator. The 7-10% economic growth per annum in India has led to changing lifestyle patterns in the form of rise of nuclear families and double income house hold. This has also encouraged the growth of dog ownership in urban India. India has one of the world's lowest rate of dog ownership i.e. 4 dogs/1000 people. That's quickly changing, though, with the total number of pups swelling by 58% between 2007 and 2012 according to market research firm Euro Monitor International. The total dog population in India is estimated to be around 30 million with 1:35 dog to human ratio (Varshney and Sharma, 2003). Out of which more than 30% falls under stray category. As per 18th Livestock Census, Department of Animal Husbandry, Dairying and Fisheries, Ministry of Agriculture, the annual growth rate of rural dog population is 2.9%, urban dog population is 6.67%, and the overall growth of dog population in India is 3.37%.

In urban India, they are seen in large numbers in streets,at market places, near abattoirs, butcher shops, food outlets and near garbage bins. In rural India,the stray dogs and vultures are the main scavengers for livestock carcasses as there is no standard method for disposal of livestock carcasses exist in rural India. The dead livestock in rural India is thrown in designated area confined to outskirts of villages wherein it is mainly scavenged by stray dogs, fox and vultures. These urban and rural stray dogs are never dewormed and carry heavy infection of helminthic parasites (Agnihotri *et al.*, 2008; Kachhawaha and Tanwar, 2007; Deka *et al.*, 2008). Beside the majority of urban dog owners lack public health awareness and allow their dogs to defecate in public places like playgrounds, parks, roadside and kitchen gardens. They do not follow any standard method of faecal disposal neither they are go for regular faecal examination and deworming schedule. These owned dogs are dewormed once a year by veterinarian when they visit clinics for vaccination. Thus, the owned dogs also carry heavy infection of helminths (Sharma *et al.*, 2006).

The people do not see the positive aspects of urban stray dogs. They reduce chain snatching and other robbery on the streets. Because of them, the organic garbage in the dustbins does not rot. No doubt a zero garbage India will reduce the urban stray/feral dog number dramatically. An observational report from Wellington Cantonment, Coonoor, Tamil Nadu by Health Superintendant in 2010 states that since they started door to door collection of garbage in the civilian area of the cantonment, the dog population in that used to be very big has drastically declined.

Canine parasitic zoonoses poses a low prioritized public health problem in developing countries such as India, where conditions are conducive for transmission and epidemiology of canine parasitic zoonoses among tea growing communities in North-east India demonstrated the endemicity of the problem (Traub *et al.*,2002). In animal husbandry sector, the funds are provided for enhancing production and animal health segment is ignored. It is given priority when those diseases have impact on poverty alleviation or posse's significant zoonotic threat to human population. Actually diseases which cause high mortality i.e. bacterial and viral origin are given more importance as control measures for them are also feasible and are cost effective, whereas diseases of parasitic origin are neglected. Animal birth control by different agencies to control stray dog population, will indirectly help to control zoonotic diseases of parasitic origin.

Intestinal helminths are one of the main entero-pathogens of dogs, especially in newly whelped or neonate (Blagburn *et al.*, 1996). Some of these helminths are responsible for important zoonotic diseases (Aiello and Mays, 1998). The fecal deposits of owned and stray dogs contaminate public places and rural field with eggs and helminthic larvae of different species of zoonotic parasites (Andresiuk *et al.*, 2007) and play an important role in transmission of these diseases although particular implication of each population is not clearly established (Eguia-Aguilar *et al.*, 2005). The transmission of these zoonotic helminths could be through direct contact or through indirect contact via infected food and water (Lappin, 2002). The distribution and intensity of helminthic infections are influenced by climate, geographical location, host-related factors and economic status of population and it is necessary to analyse the situation in every city (Oliveira-Sequeira *et al.*, 2002; Pierangeli *et al.*, 2003). Temperature, humidity, type of soil, rainfall and certain chemical, and biological conditions favour the development, survival and transmission of infective stages to man. Thus, it is of utmost importance to analyze seasonal prevalence of helminths of pet and stray dogs in a region (Lorenzini *et al.*, 2007). In different countries of world, the prevalence of helminthic eggs in dog faeces has been carried out (Coggins, 1998; Oge and Oge, 2001) members.

Among all infections, hookworms are worldwide in distribution and have high frequency. They principally infect the small intestine of dogs. All hookworms have large buccal cavity directed obliquely dorsally giving "hooked" appearance. The female worms lay typical strongylid eggs which appear in the feces during morula stage of development. The subfamily Ancylostominae and Bunostominae are parasitise carnivores and herbivores, respectively, whereas omnivores are infected by both the subfamilies. *Ancylostoma* has sharp teeth and *Uncinaria* has cutting plates in buccal cavities. The ventral margin of stoma of *Ancylostoma* is armed by one pair teeth in *A. braziliense* and 3 pairs of teeth in *A. caninum*. *Ancylostoma braziliense* is smaller in size as compared to *A. caninum*. (*A. braziliense* male 7.7 to 8.5 mm, female 9-10.5 mm, *A. caninum* male 9-12 mm, female 15-20 mm).

Ancylostoma caninum matures only in dogs and *A. tubaeforme* matures only in cats. *Ancylostoma braziliense* matures both in dogs and cats. *Uncinaria stenocephala* matures in dogs, cats and foxes. *Ancylostoma caninum* is a parasite of dog which has recently been confirmed to develop in the human gut (but without maturing sexually), thus providing novel insights in host-parasite interaction (Prociv and Croese, 1996). *Ancylostoma* eggs and larvae are destroyed by freezing whereas those of *Uncinaria* are very resistant to cold. *Ancylostoma caninum* larvae do not develop to the infective stage at temperature below 15^{0}C. The effect of temperature on the development of eggs has been studied by McCoy (1930). Thus, in India they can develop all through the year except for few winter months in Northwestern region of the country.

The larvae of nematodes commonly respond to chemicals, temperature, torch light and electric potential. They mainly seem to use chemotactic mechanism to find their host for food in the soil. The typical infective larvae are enclosed within two cuticles and their behavior does not vary as they do not feed, defecate, oviposit, mate or undergo morphogenesis. Literature reveals scanty information on infective larvae which penetrate the host's skin and identify their host. Although some skin penetrating infective larvae tend to climb to the top of prominent particles of soil or on grass, but the mechanism controlling this have not yet been analyzed, some workers have reported photo-tactic response or thermal stimuli as the cause in case of infective larvae of hookworms. *Ancylostoma caninum* infective larvae don't respond to light, air, current, sound and vibration.

The stimuli inducing penetration of the host's skin are not well studied. Lipid content in skin does not affect percent entry of infective larvae of *A. tubaeforme*;however, its decrease in skin reduces the entry of infective larvae of *N. americanus*. Heat may also be considered a penetration stimulus as it stimulates thermo-tactic movements in hookworms. Tegan *et al.* (2004) reported pore forming haemolysin from larvae and adult stages of *A.caninum*.

In *A. caninum* eggs are shed in the faeces about 2 weeks after ingestion of larvae and about a month after penetration of skin by larvae. However, not all larvae mature. Some invade skeletal muscle cells (Little, 1978) or gut wall and enter an arrested stage of development. The arrested larvae later become reactivated in response to obscure cues and migrate either to small intestine, where they mature, or to the mammary gland, where they are shed in the milk and infect pups. The arrested larvae are regularly reactivated during the last two weeks of pregnancy. *Ancylostoma caninum* is much more pathogenic for dogs than *A. braziliense* or *U. stenocephala* as it causes higher blood loss per worm (Miller, 1966; Georgi *et al.*, 1969). However, the severity of clinical signs is highly dependent on the age and nutritional status of the host and its worm burden. In pups and immunosuppressed hosts, even light to moderate infections with *A.caninum* can result in significant anaemia, hypoproteinaemia and bloody diarrhoea, and may be fatal (Bowman,2009). A bitch exposed to only one substantial oral percutaneous infection will shed *A. caninum* larvae in her milk for next three lactations, although number of larvae reduces in subsequent lactations (Miller, 1970).

Epidemiology

In India, scanty reports are available from all parts of the country. From eastern part,Chakarvarty *et al.* (1971) examined 1191 faecal samples of dogs in Guwahati and recorded hookworm ova in 777 dogs. Similarly, Baruah and Gogoi (1989) reported 31.52% positivity of dog faecal samples for hookworm ova in Guwahati. Deka *et al.* (1995) based on fecal examination reported *Ancylostoma* to be one of the predominant helminthes parasite in dog's in Lakhimpur region of Assam. Singh and Das (2004) have recorded *Ancylostoma* eggs in 10 samples of soil collected from residential complex and rural areas of Tezpur, Assam. Similarly, Yadav and Tandon (1989) reported *Ancylostoma* eggs in significant number in soil samples collected from children's park, house yards and places in piggeries. Kumar and Sahai (1972) observed 72.7% dogs positive for *A.caninum* in Patna, Bihar. Dasgupta *et al.* (1973) reported 40.02% positivity of hookworm ova in 219 dogs examined in Calcutta. On contrary, Mitra *et al.* (1990) recorded only 26.6% positivity for hookworms. Bhutia *et al.* (1995) on the basis of faecal examination reported 22% incidence of hookworms in dogs in Sikkim. Traub *et al.* (2002) revealed that *A. caninum* is most common infection in dogs in tea growing community area of Assam. Recently, Sharma *et al.* (2006) have reported 22% positivity of hookworm ova in dogs in Patna region.

From northern fertile plains and Northwestern Himalayas few reports are on record. Singh *et al.* (1977) reported 35.5% and 44% infection of hookworm in dogs in Haryana and Delhi, respectively.The highest prevalence 72-90% was observed in rainy season and the lowest in winter season. Pal *et al.* (1979) reported 14.5% incidence of hookworms in dogs in Delhi. Chhabra and Mahajan (1978) reported 42.4% dog's positive for hookworms in Chandigarh. Bhatia *et al.* (1988) on the basis of gastrointestinal tract examination reported 96% tracts of dogs harboring *A. caninum* worms in Mathura. In Ludhiana region, Sandhu *et al.* (1997) and Sushma *et al.* (2001) have reported 33.1% and 31.5% positivity of hookworm ova in dog faecal samples, respectively. Recently, Singh *et al.* (2012) based on fecal examination reported 22.14% incidence of *Ancylostoma* in dogs in small animal clinics of the university, Ludhiana, Punjab, examined in small animal clinics of the University. Katoch *et al.* (2006) recorded hookworm ova in 19.05% dogs examined in Palampur.

Katoch *et al.* (2007) also recorded hookworm ova in 20.7% dog's faecal samples from Jammu region. Recently, Aijaz (2010) has reported 21.1% positivity of hookworm's ova in dog faecal samples from Jammu region.Vatsya *et al.* (2010) reported *Ancylostoma* eggs in 13.68% dogs in tarai region in Uttarakhand.

In southern peninsula, Hedge and Jagannath (1974) examined 712 digestive tracts of dog in Bangalore and recorded *A. caninum* as the most common nematode. Gokak (1990) reported 31% positivity of hookworm ova in fecal samples of dog examined in veterinary hospital Belgaum, Karnataka. The highest infection (50%) was recorded in 1-12 month old age group of dogs in playgrounds, animal sheds, veterinary hospitals and college campus with eggs of *Ancylostoma,* followed by 1-5years age group (42%) and above 5years age group (8%). Breedwise highest infection was recorded in Alsatian (37%) and the lowest in crossbreds. Murleedharan *et al.* (1994) have reported *Ancylostoma* to be most predominant infection in dogs in Karnataka. D'Souza *et al.* (2002) reported 10.6% contamination of soil samples. Mamatha *et al.* (2005) have also reported high frequency of *A. caninum* (65.71) in stray dogs in and around Bangalore.

Srijayant *et al.* (1987) examined 2915 dogs in Madras veterinary college hospital and observed 578 dogs positive for *Ancylostoma.* The prevalence was highest in dogs under two and over eight years of age. The infection was more in purebreds as compared to crossbreds. Balasubramaniam *et al.* (2001) reported 86.8% infection of *Ancylostoma* in dogs in Nammakal, Tamilnadu. Recently, Sarvana (2011) have retrieved *A.caninum* with endoscope from one year old Spitz.

Life Cycle of Hookworms

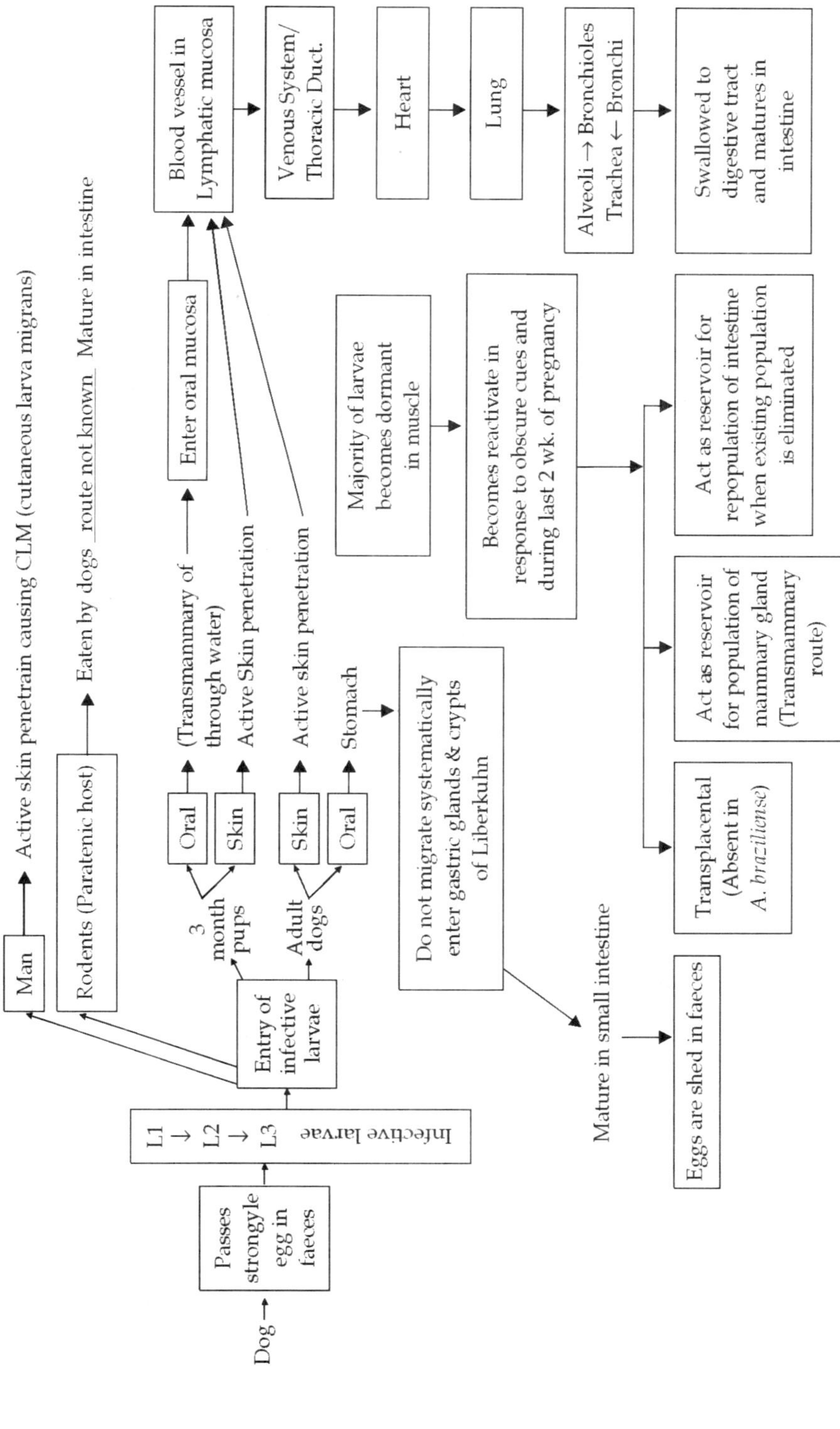

Mohan (1984) observed 39.13% incidence of ancylostomosis in dogs examined from in and around Guntur, Andhra Pradesh and have recorded *A.caninum* and *A.braziliense* species. Rao (2002) have observed 12.98% dogs positive for *A.caninum* in and around Kakinada of Andhra Pradesh. Female dogs had higher frequency (16.28%) as compared to male dogs (8.68%). Breed wise Pomeranian showed highest prevalence rate (17.44%). The prevalence rate was higher in dogs less than one year of age (79%) as compared to 1-5 years (12.8%) and more than 5years age group (8.2%).

Jacob and Pillai (1991) have reported high frequency of *A.caninum* in dogs in Thrissur, Kerala as they observed 45 positive out of 55 dogs examined. Recently, Das *et al.* (2009) have also reported high incidence of hookworm from stray and pet dogs in Puducherry based on faecal examination. The EPG of hookworm eggs ranged in 1200 to 5200 in stray dogs.

From western part of the country Jani *et al.* (1995) reported 26.9% dogs positive for hookworm ova in Gujarat. Contrary to it,Jani (2004) reported 65.91% positivity of *A. caninum* in dogs in Gujarat. Kachhawaha and Tanwar (2007) recorded hookworm ova in 92.9% percent dogs in town located in western desert, Jodhpur. They recorded mean EPG of 1363.85±26.18 with a range of 900 to 1800. Recently, Godara *et al.* (2010) have reported 13.3% dog's positive for hookworm eggs in Jaipur.

Central Indian also revealed high frequency (64.81%) of *A.caninum* with EPG in range of 700-2400 in dogs in Jabalpur. The mixed infection of *A. caninum, Toxocara* and *Dipylidium caninum* with mean egg per gram of *Ancylostoma*was 951.43±88.66 (Nath *et al.*, 2011). In contrary, Qadir *et al.* (2011) reported that 10.25% dogs were positive for hookworm infections from Jabalpur. Asati *et al.* (1999) recorded an average frequency of 20.76% of hookworm eggs infeces of dogs from Indore, Dewas and Mhow cities of Madhya Pradesh. Khante *et al.* (2009) reported 20% and 25.1% incidence of *A.caninum* in adults and pups, respectively, in non-descript dogs in Nagpur, Maharashtra.

Godara *et al.* (2010) have mentioned that the ability to limit the number of hookworms maturing in small intestine is influenced by age, premunition and acquired immunity. Thus, as they growolder they become more resistant to hookworms whether or not they experience infection. They have further stated that ability to compensate for blood loss due to hookworms is influenced by the hemophilic capacity, state of nutrition and the presence or absence of other stresses.

The season is concerned; the majority workers have reported high prevalence during monsoon (Mitra *et al.*,1990; Chakaravarty *et al.*, 1971), although its presence has been noted all through the year (Aijaz *et al.*, 2010).

Clinical forms, control and immunoprophylaxis

Bowmen (2009) have reported four clinical forms of canine hookworm disease. Per acute hookworm disease in neonates occurs due to transmammary infection wherein 50 to 100 adult worms prove fatal. Diagnosis is difficult, clinical signs are important i.e. soft to liquid feces which is dark in colour due to blood. Anthelmintic along with supportive therapy is desired. For control treat bitches with fenbendazole @ 50 mg/kg, but from 40th day of gestation to 14th day of lactation (Burke and Roberson, 1983). Acute hookworm disease occurs due to sudden exposure of susceptible older pups to large number of infective larvae (oral or skin penetration). Large numbers of strongyle eggs are observed in faecal sample and clinical signs appear later on, and such cases respond dramatically to anthelmintic therapy. Hookworm disease is seen in older dogs show anaemia and emaciation. High protein diet along with iron injection, vitamins and anthelmintic may show effective results. In severe cases, blood transfusion is also desired. Hazarika and Roychoudhary (1985) recorded decline in total serum protein from 6.82g/dl to 3.52g/dl within 30 days after oral administration of infective larvae of *A. caninum* in parasite free local bred dogs. Migasena *et al.* (1972) have reported that *A. caninum* infection do affect absorption of amino-acids, carbohydrates and fat from small intestine. The entry of infective larvae through skin in dogs results in acanthosis and hyper keratinization. Serpentine migratory tracts are observed in interdigital spaces. Footpads become soft and spongy and separation of pad may occur leading to claw deformity and thickening of the distal phalanges (Kalofen, 1987). Literature reveals high frequency of hookworms in stray and pet animals but data regarding cutaneous larva migrans in humans is lacking.

Literature reveals use of irradiated infective larvae, excretory and secretary antigens from infective stages and use of recombinant protein with varying degree of protection. Steves *et al.* (1973) vaccinated ten weeks old pups twice by subcutaneous inoculation of x-irradiated *A.caninum* larvae and challenged by hookworm infective larvae showed 88 to 95% reduction of hookworm burden as compared to unvaccinated group. Miller (1978) discussed difficulties of producing sterile vaccine derived from faecal origin. The sterile vaccine was found to have longer shelf life at 10-15°C with special packaging and storage facilities of six months than crude vaccine. The vaccine was compatible with canine distemper vaccine and the common dog anthelmintics. The successful field trials saw the commercial launching of vaccine in 1973, but in 1975 its sale was discontinued owing to poor uptake of the product by veterinarians who were used to controlling the disease by anthelmintic therapy. The effect of molecular variation in antigen from geographically separated parasite populations should be considered during vaccine development (Shan Qiang *et al.*, 2000). Boag *et al.* (2003) induced protective immunity to hookworm infection following vaccination with irradiation attenuated third stage larvae with significant reduction in both worm and fecal egg counts following a challenge infection. Vaccination with irradiated infective larvae and challenge with infective larvae stimulated a dominant antibody response to antigen less than 20kDa in excretory/secretary extract from adult parasites. The vaccination with irradiated *A.caninum* third stage larvae induces a Th2 protective response in dogs and excretory and secretary molecules released during this development stage are likely target of this response (Fujiwara *et al.*, 2006).

Zhan *et al.* (2004) reported anti-*Ancylostoma caninum* surface associated antigen-1 protein partially inhibited (46.7%) invasion of hookworm larvae into dog skin. Bethony *et al.* (2005) vaccinated dogs with most abundant infective larvae secreted antigen and challenged with infective larvae of *A.caninum* exhibited significant reduction in faecal egg counts and intestinal hookworm burden. Zhan *et al.* (2005) observed that vaccination of dog with glutathione S-transferase from adult *A.caninum* resulted in 39.4% reduction in the mean worm burden and 32.3% in egg counts following infective larval challenge. Zhan *et al.* (2008) reported that an immunodominant hookworm antigen encoding a tissue inhibitor of metalloproteinase have a possible role in the parasite-host relationship of canine hookworm infection. Recently, Zhan *et al.* (2008) reported an enzymatically inactivated haemoglobinase from *N.americanus* induces neutralizing antibodies against multiple hookworm species and protect dogs against heterologous hookworm infection. Loukas *et al.* (2005) vaccinated dogs with recombinant cysteine protease from the blood-feeding stage of the canine hookworm *A.caninum* which induced high titre of antigen-specific antibody response and adult hookworm recovered from vaccinated dogs were smaller than control group. Marked decrease in fecal egg count and female hookworm was also recorded in vaccinated group.

Conclusions

The thrust areas recommended for future research in Indian context are identification of hookworm species existing in India using molecular tools, without need for laborious identification of adult worms at postmortem or post anthelmintic purging, the factors responsible for skin penetration in dogs as well as human beings, development of standard protocol for control of hookworms as it has complex life cycle and control of stray dog population. Public health awareness at school level, registration of pet dogs by municipalities and proper disposal of faeces of pet dogs are other areas where work can be initiated which will help in control of other zoonotic diseases of dog-borne parasitic origin.Dewormers should be incorporated in government supported measures for control of stray dog population. Veterinary services for companion animals should be upgraded. Research, surveillance and control of diseases in companion animals should be given priority.

References

Agnihotri, R.K., Sharma, D. and Sharma, Y. (2008). Incidence of gastrointestinal helminthes in dogs of Himachal Pradesh.*J. Vet.Parasitol.*, 22(1): 67-68.

Aiello, S.E. and Mays, A. (1998).The Merck Veterinary Manual. 8th ed., Merck and Co. Inc., NJ, USA, pp. 2305.

Aijaz, P. (2010). Prevalence of gastrointestinal helminthes in dogs of Jammu. M.V.Sc. thesis submitted to Sher-e-Kashmir University of Agricultural Sciences and Technology of Jammu.

Andresiuk, V., Sardella, N. and Denegri, G. (2007). Seasonal fluctuations in prevalence of dog intestinal parasites in public squares of Mar del Plata city, Argentina and its risk for humans.*Revista Argentiana de Microbiologia*, 39: 221-224.

Asati, A.K., Sisodia, R.S. and Shukla, P.C. (1999).Faecal prevalence of eggs of gastrointestinal helminthes of dogs in Malwa region of Madhya Pradesh.*Indian Vet. Med. J.*, 23 (9): 237: 238.

Balasubrmaniam, G.A.,Rao, G.V.S.,Balchandran, C., George,V.T. and Vairamuthu,S. (2001).Incidence of parasitic diseases among domestic animals in Nammakal district of Tamilnadu.*Indian J. Anim.Sci.*, 71: 340-341.

Baruah, N. and Gogoi, H.R. (1989). Incidence of different helminthes in dogs in Guwahati (Assam). *J. Vet.Parasitol.*, 3:155-156.

Bethony, J., Loukas, A., Smout, M., Brooker, S., Mendez, S., Plieskatt, J., Goud, G., Bottazzi, M.E., Zhan, B., Wang, Y., Williamson, A., Lustigman, S., Correa-Oliveira, R., Xiao ShuHua and Hotez, P.J. (2005). Antibodies against a secreted protein from hookworm larvae reduce the intensity of hookworm infection in humans and vaccinated laboratory animals. *FASEB J.*, 19: 1743-1745.

Bhatia, B.B., Chouhan, P.P.S., Agarwal, R.D. and Katra, R.P. (1988). Incidence of parasitic infection amongst stray dogs in Mathura (Uttar Pradesh). *Vet. Res. J.*, 3:120-123.

Bhutia, N.T., Tamang, R.K., Rai, M.K. and Sen, G.P. (1995).Incidence of hookworm infection in dogs at Gangtok, Sikkim.*Indian Vet. J.*, 72(11): 1206-1207.

Blagburn, Lindsay, D.S., Vaughan, J.L., Rippey, N.S., Wright, J.C., Lynn, R.C., Kelch, W.J., Ritchie, G.C. and Hepler, D.I. (1996). Prevalence of canine parasites based on faecal floatation. *Comp. Contin. Educ. Vet. Pract.*, 18: 483-509.

Bowman, D.D. (2009).Georgi's Parasitology for veterinarians.9th ed., Saunders Elsevier Publication.

Boag, P.R..,Parsons, J.C.,Presidente, P.J.A.,Spithill, T.W. andSexton, J.L.(2003).Characterization of humoral immune responses in dogs vaccinated with irradiated *Ancylostoma caninum. Vet.Immunol.Immunopathol.*, 92: 87-94.

Burke, T.M. and Roberson, E.L.(1983).Fenbendazole treatment of pregnant bitches to reduce prenatal and lactogenic infections of *Toxocara canis* and *Ancylostoma caninum* in pups.*Am. Vet. Med. Assoc.*,83: 198.

Chakravarty, A.K. and Roychoudhury, R.K. (1971).Epizootiology and canine ancylostomiasis (Studies on incidence in dogs in Guwahati area from 1966 to 1971).*Vetecol J.College Vet. Sci., Assam Agri. Uni.*: 12: 64-67.

Chhabra, M.B. and Mahajan, R.C. (1978).A not on the prevalence of *Toxocara canis* and other intestinal parasites of dogs on Chandigarh.*Indian J. Anim. Sci.*, 48(12): 929-931.

Coggins, J.R. (1998). Effect of season, sex and age on the prevalence of parasitism in dogs from Southeastern Wisconsin.*J.Helminthol. Soc. Washington*, 65: 219-224.

Das, S.S., Kumar, D., Sreekrishan, R. and Ganesan, R. (2009).Gastrointestinal parasitic infections in dogs of Puducherry.*J. Vet.Parasitol.*, 23(1): 77-79.

DasGupta, C.K., Ray, S. and Banerjee, K.N. (1973). Incidence of gastrointestinal parasites in dogs studied at Calcutta. *Indian J. Anim. Hlth.*, 12(1): 109-110.

Deka, D.K., Islam, S., Borkakoty, M.,Saleque, A., Hussain, I. and Nath, K. (2008). Prevalence of *Echinococcus granulosus* in dogs and hydatidosis in herbivores of certain North Eastern states of India. *J. Parasitol.*, 22(1): 27-30.

Deka,D.K.,Choudhary,S. and Chakraborty,A. (1995). Parasites of domestic animals and birds in Lakhimpur (Assam).*J. Vet.Parasitol.*,9:21-25.

D'souza, P.E.,Dhanlakshmi,H. and Jagannath,M.S. (2002).Soil contamination with canine hookworm and roundworm ova in Bangalore.*J.Parasit. Dis.*, 26:107-108.

Eguia-Aguilar, P., Cruz-Reyes, A. and Martinez-Maya, J.J. (2005). Ecological analysis and description of the intestinal helminths present in dogs in Mexico City. *Vet.Parasitol.*, 127: 139-146.

Fujiwara, R.T.,Loukas, A.,Mendez, S.,Williamson, A.L.,Bueno, L.L.,Wang, Y.,Samuel, A.,Zhan, B.,Bottazzi, M.E.,Hotez, P.J.and Bethony, J.M. (2006).Vaccination with irradiated *Ancylostoma caninum* third stage larvae induces a Th2 protective response in dogs.*Vaccine*, 24: 501-509.

Godara, R., Sharma, R.L., Sharma, S.C. and Sharma, D.K. (2010).Parasitic infection in dogs in semi-arid Jaipur (Rajasthan).*J. Vet.Parasitol.*, 24(1): 83-86.

Gokak, A.G. (1990). Study on the incidence of hookworm disease (ancylostomiasis) in dogs at Belgaum. *Pashudhan*, 5:5.

Georgi, J.R.,LeJambre,L.F. and Ractliffe,L.H. (1969).*Ancylostoma caninum* burden in relationship to erythrocyte loss in dogs.*J. Parasitol.*, 55:1205-1211.

Hazarika,G.C. and Roychoudhary,G.K. (1985). Serum protein in dogs infected with *Ancylostoma caninum*. *Indian J. Vet. Med.*, 5:40-41.

Hedge, K.S. and Jagannath, M.S. (1974). Survey of parasites of digestive tract of dogs in Bangalore.*Mysore J. Agri. Sci.*, 8(4): 597-601.

Jacob, L. and Pillai, K.M. (1991). Influence of parasitic infection in dogs in Thrissur, Kerala. *J. Vet. Anim. Sci.*, 22: 149-150.

Jani,R.G. (2004).Epidemiological study of diarrhoea in dogs in Gujarat state.*J. Vet. Parasitol* 18: 200-202.

Jani, R.G., Jani, B.M. and Dave, M.R. (1995).Prevalence of intestinal parasites in dogs at Anand (Gujarat).*J. Vet. Parasitol.*, 9: 51-53.

Kalkofen,U.P. (1987). Hookworms of dogs and cats.Veterinary Clinics of North America.*Small Anim. Pract.*, 17:1341-54.

Kachhawaha, S. andTanwar, R.K. (2007).Prevalence of worm infestations in stray dogs in and around Jodhpur.*J. Vet. Parasitol.*, 21(2): 171-172.

Katoch, R., Yadav, A., Panda, A.K. Agnihotri, R.K. and Katoch, M. (2006). Prevalence of gastrointestinal parasites in dogs of north western Himalayan region.Presented in V annual conference of IVPHS held at CSKHPKV, Palampur. 12th - 14th October, 2006.

Katoch, R., Yadav, A., Vohra, S., Khajuria, J.K. and Katoch, M. (2007).Status of endoparasites in dogs of Jammu and their zoonotic importance. Presented in 18th NCVP held at SKUAST-J, Jammu, 7th - 9th September, 2006.

Khante, G.S., Khan, L.A., Bodkhe, A.M., Suryawanshi, P.R., Majed, M.A., Suradkar, U.S. and Gaikwad, S.S. (2009). Epidemiological survey of gastrointestinal parasites of non-descript dogs in Nagpur city. Vet. World, 2:22-23.

Kumar,G.M. and Sahai,B.N. (1972). A note on the incidence of helminthic infections in dogs at Patna, Bihar. *Indian Vet.J.* 49:737.

Lappin, M.R. (2002). Pet ownership by immunocompromised people, Bayer Zoonosis Symposium, North American Veterinary Conference, 24(5): 16-25.

Little, M.D. (1978).Dormant *Ancylostoma caninum* larvae in muscle as a source of subsequent patent infection in the dog.In Fifty-Third Annual Meeting of the American Society of Parasitology, Chicago.

Lorenzini, G., Tasca, T. and Carli, G. (2007). Prevalence of intestinal parasites in dogs and cats under veterinary care in PoretoAlegre, Rio Grande do Sul, Brazil. *Brazilian J. Vet. Res. Anim. Sci.*, 44(2): 137-145.

Loukas,A.,Bethony,J.M.,Mendez,S.,Fujiwara,R.T., Goud,G.N.,Ranjit,N.,Zhan,B., Jones,K.,Bottazzi, M.E. and Hotez (2005).Vaccination with recombinant aspartic hemoglobinase reduces parasite load and blood loss after hookworm infection in dogs. *PLOS Medicine*, 2:10pp e295.

Mamatha, G.S., D'Souza, P.E. and Bhat, M.N. (2005).Gastrointestinal parasitism in dogs and cats in Bangalore.*Intas Polivet*, 6(2): 152-153.

McCoy, O.R. (1930). The influence of temperature, hydrogen-ion concentration and oxygen tension on the development of the eggs and larvae of the dog hookworm *Ancylostoma caninum*.*Am. J. Hyg.*, 11: 413-446.

Migasema, S., Gilles, H.M. and Maegraith, B.G. (1972).Studies in *A. caninum* infection in dogs.Absorption from small intestine of amino acids, carbohydrates and fat.*Ann. Trop. Med. Parasitol.*, 66(1): 107-128.

Miller,T.A. (1966).Blood loss during hookworm infection, determined by erythrocyte labeling with radioactive 51-chromium.II.Pathogenesis of *Ancylostoma braziliense* infection in dogs and cats.*J. Vet.Parasitol.*, 52: 856-65.

Miller, J.A. (1970). Prenatal colostral infection of pups with *A. caninum*.*J. Parasitol.*, 56(11): 239.

Miller, T.A. (1978). Industrial development and field use of the canine hookworm vaccine. *Adv. Parasitol.*, 16: 333-342.

Mishra, U.K., Das, R.K., Panda, M.R. and Swain, P. (1994). Histopathological and haematological studies and mixed helminthic infection of stray dogs. *Indian J. Vet. Res.*, 3(2): 38-41.

Mitra, K., Ghost, A., Ghosh, G.L., Mitra, S., Chaudhuri, S. and Biswas, G. (1990). Ancylostomiasis in pet dogs: A note. *Indian Vet.Med. J.*, 14(3): 215-217.

Mittra, S. and Sasmal, N.K. (1985). A study of the haemogram of dogs infected with *A. caninum* through different routes. *Indian Vet. Med. J.*, 9(1): 31-35.

MohanKumar, O.R. (1984).Incidence of hookworm disease (Ancylostomiasis) in dogs in Guntur.*Livestock Adviser*, 11: 43-48.

Murleedharan,L.,Ziauddin,K.S., Hussain,P.M., Puttabyattappa,B. and Seshadri, S.J. (1994).Prevalence of parasitic infectionamong small domestic animals.*Karnataka J. Agri. Sci.*, 7:64-68.

Nath,S., Das,G. and Roy,B. (2011).Incidence of gastrointestinal parasitic infection in stray dogs in and around Jabalpur (Madhya Pradesh).*Indian J Field Veterinarians*, 7:49-51.

Oge, S. and Oge, H. (2001). Prevalence of *Toxocara* spp. eggs in the soil of public parks in Ankara. Turkey. *Deutsch TierarztiWschr*,107: 72-75.

Oliveira-Sequeira, T.C.,Amarante, A.F., Ferrari, T.B. and Nunes, L.C. (2002).Prevalence of intestinal parasites in dogs from Sao Paulo State, Brazil. *Vet.Parasitol.*,103: 19-27.

Pal, M., Nair,R.P.N. and Dube,G.D. (1979).Prevalence of helminth parasite in the pet dogs of Delhi Metropolitan area.*Livestock Advisor*, 4:25-28.

Pierangeli, N.B.,Giayetto, A.L., Manacorda, A.M., Barbieri, L.M., Soriano, S.V. andVeronesi, A.(2003). Estacionalidad de parasites intestinales en suelosperiurbanos de lascludad de Neuquen, Patagonia, Argentina.*Trop. Med. Int.*, 259-263.

Prociv, P. and Croese, J. (1996). Human enteric infection with *Ancylostoma caninum*: hookworms reappraised in the light of a new zoonosis. *Acta Trop.*, 62: 23-44.

Qadir, S., Dixit,A.K., Dixit,P. and Sharma,R.L. (2011). Intestinal helminths induce haematological changes in dogs from Jabalpur, India. *J.Helminthol.*, 85: 401-403.

Rao,B.T. (2002). Prevalence of *Ancylostoma caninum* infection in companion dogs at Kakinda, Andhra Pradesh. *Intas Polivet*, 3:286-287.

Saravanan,M.,Nagarajan,B. and Kavitha,S. (2011).Endoscopic retrieval of *Ancylostoma caninum* from duodenum of a dog.*Intas Polivet*, 12:102-103.

Sandhu, S.S. (1995). Studies on the incidence, haematology, biochemical changes and treatment of ancylostomiasis in dogs. M.V.Sc Thesis, Punjab Agricultural University, Ludhiana.

Sandhu, S.S., Surinder, S., Jasmir, S., Singh, S. and Singh, J. (1997). A note on hookworm infection in dogs in Ludhiana (Punjab).*J. Vet. Parasitol.*, 11(2): 201-203.

Sharma, S.K., Sinha, S.R.P., Sinha, S., Kumar, L. and Mehta, R.K. (2006). Gastrointestinal helminthic parasites and treatment in different breeds of dogs.*Indian Vet. J.*, 83: 834-836.

Singh, H., Singh,R.P. and Bali,M.K. (1977). Prevalence of hookworm infection in dogs in the state of Haryana and Delhi. *HAU J. Res.*, 7:155-161.

Singh,H., Haque,M., Jyoti,Singh,N.K. and Rath,S.S. (2012).Occurrence of parasitic infection in dogs in and around Ludhiana.*App. Biol. Sci.*, 14:108-110.

Singh, L.A. and Das,S.C. (2004). Observations on the soil contamination with the zoonotic-canine gastrointestinal parasite in selected rural areas of Tezpur, Assam, India.*J.Parasit. Dis.*, 28:121-123.

Sushma Chhabra, Khabra, S.S., Nauriya, D.C. and Chhabra, S. (2001). On the prevalence and treatment of helminth parasites of dogs.*J. Vet.Parasitol.*, 15(2): 129-131.

Shan Qiang; Zhan Bin,Xiao ShuHua,FengZheng,Hotez, P.,Hawdon, J.M. (2000).Variation between ASP-1 molecules from *Ancylostoma caninum* in China and the United States. *J. Parasitol.*, 86: 181-185.

Steves, F.E., Baker, J.D., Hein, V.D. and Miller, T.A. (1973). Efficacy of a hookworm (*Ancylostoma caninum*) vaccine for dog.*J. Am. Vet. Med. Assoc.*, 163: 231-235.

Tegan, A.D., Malcolm, K.J., Danielle, S., Peter O' Donoghue, Peter, H. and Alex, L. (2004). A pore forming haemolysin from the hookworm*A. caninum.Int. J. Parasitol.*, 34: 1029-1035.

Traub, R.J., Robertson, I.D., Irwin, P., Mencke, N. and Thompson, R.C. (2002). Humans, dogs and parasitic zoonoses- unraveling the relationships in a remote endemic community in northeast India using molecular tools. *Parasitol. Res.*, 90 (Suppl3): 258-260.

Varshney, J.P. and Sharma, R.L. (2003). Caninediseases caused by helminths. In: Helminthology in India(ed. M.L. Sood), International Book Distributors, Dehra Dun, pp. 197-214.

Vatsya, S.,Garg, R., Kumar, R.R., Yadav, C.L. and Banerjee, P.S. (2010). Retrospective study on the incidence of gastrointestinal and blood parasite in dogs at Pantnagar and their public health significance. *Indian J. Public Hlth.*, 8:29-32.

Yadav, A.K. and Tandon, V. (1989). Prevalence of nematode eggs in the urban area of the city of Shillong, India. *Hlth.Hyg.*, 10:158-161.

Zhan, B., Wang, Y., Liu, Y.Y., Williamson, A., Loukas, A., Hawdon, J.M., Xue HaeChou, Xiao ShuHua and Hotez, P.J. (2004). *Ac*-SAA-1, an mmunodominant 16 kDa surface-associated antigen of infective larvae and adults of *Ancylostoma caninum.Int. J. Parasitol.*, 34: 1037-1045.

Zhan, B.; Gupta, R.; Wong, S. P. Y.; Bier, S.; Jiang, D. S.; Goud, G.; Hotez, P.(2008) Molecular cloning and characterization of *Ac*-TMP-2, a tissue inhibitor of metalloproteinase secreted by adult *Ancylostoma caninum. Molecular Bioch. Parasitol.*, 162: 142-148

Zhan, B.,Liu, S.,Perally, S.,XueJian,Fujiwara, R.,Brophy, P.,Xiao ShuHua,Liu, Y.Y.,Feng, J.J.,Williamson, A.,Wang, Y.,Bueno, L.L.,Mendez, S.,Goud, G.,Bethony, J.M.,Hawdon, J.M., Loukas, A.,Jones, K. andHotez, P.J.(2005).Biochemical characterization and vaccine potential of a heme-binding glutathione transferase from the adult hookworm *Ancylostoma caninum.Infect. Imm.*, 73: 6903-6911.

□□□

Chapter 3

Anthelmintic Resistance in Nematodes of Small Ruminants

C.P. Swarnkar and D. Singh
Division of Animal Health, Central Sheep and Wool Research Institute, Avikanagar (Rajasthan)

Introduction

With an ever expanding world population the ability to meet the demand for resources, whilst maintaining socio-political and economic stability, has become a very real and major issue for our society. An exhaustive review commissioned by an international donor consortium (WHO, OIE, FAO) to prioritise animal health research for poverty reduction in the developing world concluded that gastrointestinal parasitism (GIP), an important production limiting diseases of livestock had the highest global index as an animal health constraint to the poor. Gastrointestinal nematodes (GINs) are ubiquitous parasites of livestock. The highly pathogenic nematode parasite of small ruminants, *H. contortus,* was singled out as being of overwhelming importance (Perry *et al.*, 2002). The importance of haemonchosis may be explained by the parasite's ability to produce large numbers of eggs which results in extensive pasture contamination; the blood-sucking nature of the nematode that causes variable degrees of anaemia, loss of production and mortality in situations where few or inefficient control measures are used; and its ability to survive adverse climatic conditions through hypobiosis. *H. contortus* is known to produce calcium and a clotting factor binding substance known as calreticulin (Suchitra and Joshi, 2005), enabling the parasite to feed easily on host blood and in so doing, cause haemorrhagic lesions. Since long, the control of this menace is mainly through the use of anthelmintics. The anthelmintic use is mainly tactical and the animals are treated when found positive on faecal examination. This has led to indiscriminate use of anthelmintics resulting in emergence of resistant strains of parasites. Thus, the sustainability of this approach has now become threatened by the widespread emergence of resistance against anthelmintics. The problem becomes even more severe if new generation anthelmintics with unique mode of action are not developed and/or replaced in the coming future. There is a paradigm shift in the way to deal with parasites–away from flock control and the chemical 'big hit' approach to something more akin to parasite management i.e. "living with worms". The following are the three strong reasons for looking at reducing the use of anthelmintics for adult sheep.

- In the adult sheep, the level of immunity to most worms is high, apart from during the peri-parturient period. This means the ewes maintains a relatively low population of parasites so that any anthelmintic treatment will exert a very high selection pressure. On this basis, we should be advising against unnecessary treatment of ewes.
- There is a need to maintain a population of parasites within the overall population in refugia. This means they are not exposed to any selection pressure from an anthelmintic and as such provide a source of susceptible alleles within the population in a flock. Adult sheep are the obvious candidates for the maintenance of a population of parasites in refugia, because their immune system controls the number of worms, leaving them with a relatively small burden.
- Nutrition both in terms of current levels of nutrient intake and past nutritional level, as indicated, was seen as a vital component in the need to treat ewes. An assessment of the adequacy of nutrition (body condition scores) could, therefore be used as a guide to the need for anthelmintic treatment.

Due to the ever-accelerating global failure of anthelmintics, there has been a radical revision of previous worm control strategies and assumptions. This has caused a dramatic change in many of the "accepted wisdoms" that have governed expert advice to farmers for close to a century. For a start, we have had to abandon the underlying philosophy that internal parasites are an evil plague that should be maximally suppressed, or preferably totally eradicated. Nematodes are essentially challenge density dependant and thus, the primary aim of all prophylactic control strategies is simply to reduce challenge from pasture to an extent which does not compromise performance. We have had to learn to farm with the presence of parasites, trying to prevent only the unacceptable production losses while simultaneously breeding animals fit for the environment, rather than making the environment fit for the existing animals. By regarding parasites as part of the natural order of things, we will come to regard them simply as one of the many potential problems to be managed in order to achieve optimum productivity and profitability. Thus, research in this area has slowly shifted from simply recording its occurrence and using surveys to define the extent of the problem towards trying to understand the mechanisms involved and methods by which it may be managed. The way in which GI parasitic diseases are controlled has to be changed: since it is highly unlikely that GIPs can ever be eradicated (Le Jambre, 2006), animal producers must learn to 'live with worms' (Coles, 2005). The present communiqué provides an overview of the problem of Anthelmintic Resistance (AR) in GINs of livestock and its management.

Impact of GINs on productivity

Although specific parasites may be distributed throughout the world, they have different impact according to production system, management and agroclimatic conditions. In commercial/ industrialized/intensive production, the greatest impact is not through the loss of productivity but more likely through the cost of control, with considerable resources spent on anthelmintics. Depending upon the type of parasite, its location in the host's system, quantum of infection, susceptibility of host and environment, GIPs can exert their harmful effects through alteration in feed intake and its metabolism as well as through histopathological changes at tissue level in the body. The evident effects of parasitism are changes in the value of animals and their products (quantitative and qualitative), increased mortality and premature disposal through culling, reduced fertility and increased susceptibility to other diseases. These in turn can have effects on flock productivity, on the capacity to make genetic improvement of a flock, on human nutrition, on community development and on cultural issues relating to the use of livestock.

In parasitized animal the reduction in feed intake could be immunostimulatory or due to the fact that host may become more selective in their diet (Kyriazakis *et al.*, 1998). GINs decrease the livestock production by absorbing the host's blood and food, depressing the appetite, decreasing the digestion, increasing nitrogen losses, decreasing absorption of bone minerals and increasing requirement of protein at the expense of muscle growth. The cost of parasitism in small ruminants was determined either in term of losses caused by parasites or in term of cost involved in management of parasitism (Table 1).

Table 1: Reported estimates of economic losses caused by parasites in sheep and goats

Country	Magnitude of losses	Reference
Australia	Worm control cost in sheep : 222 - 500 million US$/yr	Emery and Wagland, 1991; McLeod, 1995
	Production loss in sheep and goats : 113 million US$/yr	McLeod, 2004
Indonesia	Production loss in sheep : 5.6 million US$ Goats : 7.1 million US$	McLeod, 2004
Pakistan	Economic loss : Rs. 19.7 millions /yr (Faisalabad)	Iqbal *et al.*, 1993
Kenya	Worm control cost : 26.0 US$/yr	McLeod, 2004
S. Africa	Worm control cost : 46.0 US$/yr	McLeod, 2004
	Cost of parasites : 45.0 million US$/yr	Nari *et al.*, 1997
Ethiopia	Looses due to helminths : 400 million US$/yr	Gezahegn, 1992
Uruguay	Cost of parasites : 41.8 million US$/yr	Nari *et al.*, 1997
Sumatra	Economic loss : 2.0 million US$/yr	Temaja, 1980
Chad	11.3% of total economic value of sheep and goats/yr	Graber, 1965
Nigeria	11.0% of total economic value of sheep and goats	Schillhorn van Veen, 1973
India	Production loss in sheep and goats: 103 million US$/yr	McLeod, 2004
	Losses in Rajasthan: Rs. 973.72 million/ yr in adult sheep and Rs 217.99 million/yr in yearling sheep	Swarnkar *et al.*, 2011 Singh *et al.*, 2011

Detailed economic evaluations repeatedly show that the major losses due to parasites are on animal production, rather than on mortality. In many instances, these costs exceed the costs of losses due to the major "killer" diseases due to viruses and bacteria (Anon, 1991). In Australia, internal parasites accounted for two-thirds of that cost of which 83% was due to wool production loss. Diarrhoea due to *Trichostrongylus* infections leads to accumulation of faecal material on the hindquarters of sheep, which lowers the value of the fleece and may lead to losses of up to $10 million in high rainfall regions in Australia (Larsen *et al.*, 1995). Worms cost the Australian sheep industry an estimated $369 million per annum, more than any other major sheep health issues (Holmes *et al.*, 2006).

In India, systematic study on economic losses caused by GINs in sheep was made at CSWRI, Avikanagar using partial farm budgeting approach and it was found that GINs in Rajasthan are responsible for causing an annual loss of Rs. 125.78/adult sheep. The pattern in quantum of losses revealed that maximum losses due to GINs was in mutton production (56.00%), followed by enhanced susceptibility for other diseases and resultant increased mortality (17.76%), increased premature culling (11.26%), reduced fertility (9.76%) and minimum losses due to wool production (5.22%). In yearling sheep, the overall loss due to GINs was Rs. 94.29. Among yearling sheep, maximum losses due to GINs was in mutton production (75.42%), followed by those due to enhanced susceptibility for other diseases and resultant increased mortality (11.25%), increased premature culling (11.23%) and minimum losses due to wool production (2.10%).

Stock management practices and anthelmintic resistance

Today, the question before us is whether farmers are administering the right product at the right time to right category of animals. Worm control practices for ruminants are well documented in England (Gettinby *et al.*, 1987), New Zealand (Scherrer *et al.*, 1990), Denmark (Maingi *et al.*, 1996), USA (Reinemeyer *et al.*, 1992) and India (Swarnkar and Singh, 2010a, b). Association between AR and risk factors in management which potentially contribute to its development has also been investigated on sheep farm in New Zealand (Kettle *et al.*, 1981), Australia (Riffkin *et al.*, 1984) and Denmark (Maingi *et al.*, 1996). Information on management of sheep flocks by farmers of Rajasthan indicated lack of knowledge about worm control strategies, anthelmintic use and the problem of AR among the majority of sheep farmers (Swarnkar and Singh, 2010a,b). There is great potential for improvement of control programme through utilizing epidemiological knowledge, grazing resources available and practices adopted by farmers and better targeting of anthelmintic treatments as opposed to the observed situation where most treatments are based on the availability of money and governed mainly by the chemists.

The mean number of anthelmintic treatments/year (2.57) recorded in Rajasthan were almost similar to that as reported in Australia (2.8) by Edwards *et al.* (1986b), in the USA (3.3-4.0) by Reinemeyer *et al.* (1992), in UK (2.44) by Gettinby *et al.* (1987) and in Denmark (2.3) by Maingi *et al.* (1996). The existing drench frequency is not justifiable and there is a high opportunity to harvest the benefits of agro-climatic conditions, grazing resources and practices in order to save money by avoiding unnecessary en-mass treatments in sheep flocks of Rajasthan. The use of anthelmintic was found to be dependent on the availability of money instead of on epidemiological need. The most commonly used occasion for drenching sheep was at the time of sale of wool after shearing. The anthelmintic treatment during climatic extreme (June and December/February) enhances the development of AR. It was found that in majority of flocks animals were under-dosed due to reliance on age and body confirmation through visual perception rather than weighing, use of faulty and non calibrated drenching device, use of sub-standard drugs and mixing of two drench types in some cases. AR was shown to be significantly greater on farms where sheep were treated according to perceived average weight of sheep in a flock than on farms where sheep were treated according to the weight of the heaviest sheep (Edwards *et al.*, 1986b).

Animals shared the same pasture sources particularly in monsoon and post-monsoon season, thus to prevent borrowing and probability of emergence of multiple resistance, there is a need to coordinate farmers in all management systems at a community or village level with respect to use of anthelmintic type for a particular year with greater involvement of researchers, pharmaceuticals, field veterinarian and extension workers. Mixed grazing with other species which is likely to reduce pasture infectivity due to host specificity of the predominant parasites was practiced by very few farmers, thus effect of reducing the worm population was therefore likely to be low (Maingi *et al.*, 1996a). Further rotation of flocks after drenching on harvested field or grazing only on top feed resulted in build up of resistant larvae on pasture in next favourable season with subsequent increase in the speed of emergence of AR. Treatment and movement of animals to clean pasture (dose and move strategy) has been an important strategy of worm control in order to prevent or reduce re-infection of the hosts. But, although this strategy is beneficial to control the infection with susceptible worms, it become highly dangerous when anthelmintic resistant worm appears with in the parasite population (Martin *et al.*, 1981; Mitchell *et al.*, 1991). This practice results in encouragement of the infection on pasture with eggs only from nematodes surviving the treatment (resistant worms) with simultaneous increased risk for selection for AR in worm population.

Anthelmintics and mechanism of resistance

Since the early 1960's there have been only three major classes of broad-spectrum anthelmintics (benzimidazoles/probenzimidazoles, tetrahydropyrimidines/ imidazothiazoles and the macrocyclic lactones or avermectins/mylbemycins) commercially released for the control of GINs of ruminants. Although there are novel classes of anthelmintic drugs that have been discovered (e.g. parahequamide, cyclooctadepsipeptides), possibly the greatest constraint in their commercial development are the enormous costs involved (Waller, 1997). Based on apparent mode of action, structure, spectrum of activity and efficacy against worm population, the anthelmintics are classified into five groups.

(a) Benzimidazole (BZ)/Probenzimidazole : These compounds act through disintegration of cytoskeletal tubulin-microtubule complex. These anthelmintics prevent polymerization of tubulin diamers to microtubules and thus causing the disassembly of existing cytoplasmic microtubule structure. Lubega and Prichard (1991a, b) showed that in H. contortus, BZ-resistance is associated with a decrease in affinity to tubulin. An alteration in β-tubulin also seems to be associated with BZ-resistance.

(b) Levamisole (LEV)/Morantel (MT) : These drugs act as cholinergic agonists, causing depolarization of nematode muscle bag membrane with an outflow of Na^+. Resistance to these drugs was due to reduction either in the number of cholinergic receptors or in the affinity of these receptors for drugs (Sangster, 1990).

(c) Ivermectins (IVM)/Macrocyclic Lactones : These compounds act by opening glutamate dependent Cl- channels of neuromuscular membrane of nematodes. IVM is known to paralyze the somatic musculature of nematodes and to inhibit feeding of adult worms. Compared with susceptible worms, feeding in IVM-resistant H. contortus is less sensitive to IVM, suggesting that pharynx is an important target of these drugs (Sangster and Gill, 1999). Genetic analysis of IVM resistance in an Australian H. contortus isolate has traced to be due to an autosomal complete dominant trait in the larvae, whose expression is sex-influenced (Le Jambre *et al.*, 2000).

(d) Salicylanilides/Substituted Nitrophenols : These proton ionopheres are narrow spectrum and act by uncoupling the oxidative phosphorylation leading to depletion of energy.

(e) Organophosphates (OP) : These are thought to interrupt neurotransmission in nematodes by inhibiting acetylcholine esterase, thus allowing a build-up of acetylcholine and continuous stimulation of nerve endings leading to spastic paralysis of worms.

GINs have a number of genetic characteristics that promote the development of AR. Among most important of these features are:

- Rapid rates of nucleotide sequence evolution and extremely large reproducing population that have given these nematodes an exceptionally high level of genetic diversity.
- A population characteristic consistent with high level of gene flow, suggesting that host environment is an important determinant of nematode population genetic structure.

AR in nematodes is thought to be a pre-adaptive phenomenon. While studying the molecular basis for the resistance of ovine *H. contortus* to the benzimidazole (BZ), Ross *et al.* (1990) observed reduction in the number of ß-tubulin probe reactive DNA fragments from 5 to 1 and concluded that genes conferring BZ resistance were present in *H. contortus* populations before BZ came in the market, and could explain the fast selection for BZ resistance in the field. The worms possess not only the genetic potential to respond successfully to chemical attack but also the means to assure dissemination of their resistant genes via host movement from farm to farm. The rapid onset and wide spread occurrence of resistance support the contention that selection by treatment, not mutation, is the driving force in the establishment of resistance (Smith *et al.*, 1999). The decline in susceptibility of parasite is caused by an increase in frequency of allele of resistant gene that results by selection through the repeated use of anthelmintics. BZ resistance is known to be inherited as an incomplete dominant/incomplete recessive trait. Therefore, heterozygotes were not fully resistant, but do have a survival advantage in the face of drug treatment, especially if drug levels are sub-optimal. Likewise, ivermectin, moxidectin and levamisole resistance are believed to be multi-genetic traits and worms possess only a subset of resistant alleles leaving them still susceptible to the drug, but able to tolerate higher doses than worms that are fully susceptible.

The development of AR is a multi-stage phenomenon as described under:

- Prior to drenching a few individual parasites on farm carry genes for resistance (R) to a particular anthelmintic type(s). Most parasites carry genes that make them susceptible (S) to an anthelmintic.
- Ruminants ingest a mixture of these R and S parasites as larvae with pasture.
- Effective anthelmintics kill most of these ingested parasites. Those that survive are usually resistant parasites and lay mostly R eggs on pasture.
- Resistant eggs continue to be shed until a new population of susceptible parasites establishes within the grazing ruminants.
- If environmental conditions are favourable for translation of R eggs and the developed larvae are ingested by suitable, non-immune stock like lambs/kids, then the proportion of R to S larvae increases on the pasture.
- As this cycle is repeated, the proportion of anthelmintic resistant individuals within the population of a parasite species grows.

The problem of AR has been described as multi-dimensional as it is a physiological or biological property, its inheritance is genetic, development of genetic strain is evolutionary and finally the evolution of resistance depends on ecological factors. Individual worms that tolerate recommended anthelmintic treatment are likely to have biological characteristics, which render them resistant to the toxic effect of the drug. These characteristics may be transmitted to off springs,

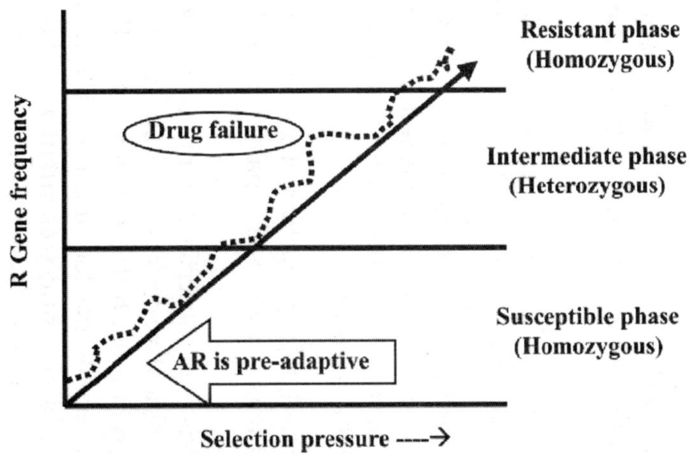

Susceptibility phase: Where the frequency of resistant individuals within the population is low and occurs when the drug was used initially.

Intermediate phase: It develops following continued exposure to a drug where the frequency of heterozygous resistant individuals within the population increases.

Resistant phase: It is an outcome of sustained selection pressure where homozygous resistant individuals predominate within the population.

Fig. 1 : Intrinsic phases in the selection process for anthelmintic resistance in worms (Singh and Swarnkar, 2008)

thus repeated treatment can select for an increasing proportion of resistant individuals. There are following three intrinsic phases in the selection process (Fig. 1) which are linked to the accumulation of resistant alleles:

The current knowledge on the mechanism of AR based on molecular studies has been reviewed by Wolstenholme *et al.* (2004). BZ resistance in nematodes had shown to be correlated with changes in the gene coding for the BZ target, β-tubulin. Two distinct single nucleotide polymorphisms leading to changes in the amino acid sequence from phenylalanine to tyrosine at position 167 and 200 appears to play a major role in the mechanism of BZ resistance.

The genetics of AR resistance is complex as the number of genes involved and whether they are dominant or recessive, affects the rate at which resistance develops (Leathwick *et al.*, 2001). Gene dominance refers to the ability of heterozygotes to survive a particular drug. If a drug kills the same high percentage of heterozygotes as the susceptible heterozygotes, the resistance gene is recessive. If the heterozygous genotype has equivalent ability to survive the resistant homozygote, the resistance gene is dominant. Different anthelmintics and different species of parasites develop different genetic forms of resistance. BZ resistance in *H. contortus* and *T. colubriformis* and other strongylids appears partly recessive trait (Roos, 1997). With *T. colubriformis,* LEV resistance is inherited as a sex-linked recessive trait, controlled either by a single gene or a cluster of tightly linked genes (Martin and McKenzie, 1990). In contrast LEV resistance in *H. contortus* is inherited as a recessive trait that is sex-linked (Dobson *et al.,* 1996). This difference probably accounts for the common occurrence of LEV resistance in *T. colubriformis* and rare occurrence in *H. contortus* (Sangster, 1999). Resistance to macrocyclic lactones in *H. contortus* appears to be inherited as a completely dominant trait but its expression is influenced by sex in that efficacy against heterozygous female is lower than against heterozygous male (Le Jambre *et al.*, 2000). Ivermectin resistance in *O. circumcincta* may be inherited as a completely dominant trait (Leathwick *et al.*, 2001) while in *T. colubriformis* may be inherited as a partially dominant trait, not under the control of a single trait (Gopal *et al.*, 1999).

Head Selection : It occurs when worms already within the animal survive the initial dose of anthelmintic. When an anthelmintic is administered, resistant worms are left behind in the animal. These resistant parasites are only contributors to the pasture contamination by way of egg output in faeces. Thus they have reproductive advantages over susceptible worms till new infection establishes. Drenches with high potency will allow fewer worms to survive treatment and it will take longer for resistance to that anthelmintic to develop to high levels within the population. When the treatment interval is close to the pre-patent period of the nematode species involved, non-resistant worms do not have an opportunity to contribute to the population, and resistance can develop rapidly. Drought conditions can also increase mortality amongst the free living stages thus reducing the size of *refugia*. Treatments given under these circumstances can thus select more strongly for resistance (Papadopoulos *et al.*, 2001). Strategic control programs based on the seasonal absence of worm larvae on pasture results in high levels of AR (Besier and Love, 2003).

Tail Selection : It occurs where worm larvae successfully infect the animal following treatment, despite the presence of the anthelmintic. Resistant worms can establish in the animal sooner and therefore have a competitive advantage over susceptible worms. Anthelmintics with persistent activity (e.g. moxidectin, avermectin, closantel) are particularly likely to select for resistance in this way. These anthelmintics with persistent activity provide protection for longer period. Thus the reproductive advantage enjoyed by surviving resistant worms is much longer. Moreover, during this period only resistant worms can establish in the host and contribute to pasture contamination with resistant genotype.

Factors affecting rate of selection for anthelmintic resistance

The rate of development of AR is influenced by genetic, biological, environmental or operational factors.

Worm biology : Worm characteristics like the method of inheritance of AR, life cycle and biotic potential of worm species are known to be important factors affecting development of AR. In trichostrongylid species with a low biotic potential, the progeny of worms surviving treatment are diluted by free-living population, resulting in slower development of resistance while in parasitic spp. having high biotic potential (like *H. contortus*), rate of development of resistance is faster.

Host-parasite relationship : Frequent treatments are instituted to control highly pathogenic worms subjecting them to higher selection pressure resulting in quick emergence of AR. Similarly, hypobiotic worms escape the exposure of drug and contribute greatly to *refugia* population.

Environmental factors : Climatic conditions determine the type and intensity of parasites prevalent in a particular area. Climate also governs the size of *refugia.* If treatment is carried out when all the worms are in the host (as during summer), then selection pressure will be high as all next generations are offspring of resistant worms. On the other hand, when worms in *refugia* are numerous (as during monsoon) than those in host the selection pressure on whole population is low.

Operational factors : Following operational/managemental factors are found responsible for emergence of AR at higher rate.

Drench frequency : The reasons for increased drench frequency in a flock are adoption of unplanned deworming schedule due to lack of proper epidemiological knowledge, failure to consider the epidemiology and ecology of parasites while devising worm control programme, strong liaison between chemist and sheep breeder, poor turn out of farmers at hospitals (Swarnkar *et al.,* 2004) and good productive response of broad-spectrum anthelmintics when used initially. In a state-wide survey in Rajasthan, it was observed that that emergence of BZ and TEM resistance in *H. contortus* was significantly influenced by drench frequency and had positive correlation (Singh and Swarnkar, 2008). There is a direct relationship between emergence of resistance in parasites and frequency of anthelmintic treatment, preferably at interval close to prepatent period (Donald, 1983). This is because the resistant genotypes not affected by the treatment, continue to reproduce, while the susceptible populations acquired from pasture are killed before they can reproduce any offspring. An increase in the rate of development occurred on continuous use of anthelmintics having similar mode of action. Suppressive treatment regimes inevitably favour the selection of a parasitic population, which contain mostly resistant phenotype(s).

Dose rate and drug selection : Underdosing enables survival of the heterozygous worms and thus, plays a key role by influencing the rate of development. In field situation, under-dosing of sheep with anthelmintics is probably common because weight of the sheep is never taken in to consideration while dose calculation, dosing devices (e.g. use of glass vials) are faulty and use of spurious/sub-standard anthelmintics. There is a wide gap of communication between veterinarians and sheep breeders, which makes chemist as primary source of anthelmintics. Both BZ and TEM groups are in use in field flocks of the same locality, the parasite population in *refugia* as well as in host were comprised of both susceptible and resistant to different anthelmintic. Thus, it could be the reason behind such results that flocks in which BZ was never used showed high prevalence of BZ resistant strains of parasite (Swarnkar and Singh, 2010a). Like-wise in flocks never drenched with TEM indicated prevalence of TEM resistance strains of parasites. Failure to make proper or pre-planned rotation of drug classes on an annual basis may lead to an increase in selection pressure for resistance to multiple drug classes.

Timing of drench : Treatment at the beginning and end of dry season as well as during climatic extremes when there is no worm population on pasture will lead to selection of resistant worms. Any management systems that markedly reduce larvae on pasture will, if used in conjunction with anthelmintics, select for resistance. The most dramatic reduction in pasture larval burden comes either through draught or where grasses are grown as a rotational crop between other crops. In Australia, treatment of animals before draught was recommended as a very effective method of worm control but it is also an excellent way of selecting for resistance which will explain why AR is worse in the southern hemisphere than in western Europe (Coles, 2005). In field it was observed that in order to accomplish the targets, the organization of health camps (with predominant activity of anthelmintic drenching to small ruminants) takes place in haphazard manner without taking in account of epidemiology of parasites, environmental condition, status of *refugia* and efficacy of anthelmintics. Such practices are further responsible for reducing the size of *refugia* and increased selection pressure for resistance.

Continuous use of drug with similar mode of action : For years, it is considered as one of the factors enhancing the rate of resistance. This statement is supported by surveys in New Zealand (Scherrer *et al.*, 1990), South Africa (van Wyk *et al.*, 1999), UK (Hong *et al.*, 1996), Australia (Edwards *et al.*, 1986b) and India (Swarnkar and Singh, 2010a, b). However, Elard *et al.* (1998) demonstrated that a strategy of alteration has no effect on resistant worms if their fitness is similar to that of susceptible ones.

Grazing management : Le Jambre (1978) demonstrated that moving the animals on safe pasture after anthelmintic treatment enhanced the selection of resistant alleles in parasitic population because the next generation of parasite constituted mainly of the progeny of the worms which survived the treatment. Control programmes that involved little or no anthelmintic treatment such as the cattle grazed on the pasture earlier grazed by the sheep, are ideal for maintaining anthelmintic susceptibility.

Physiology of animals and anthelmintic pharmacology

Both, drug metabolism and host physiology influence the rate of development of resistance in parasites. The pharmacology of an anthelmintic is a crucial determinant of selection for resistance in a parasite population. There are many examples, how the behavior of drug in the host influences the selection process in a parasitic population (Hennessy, 1994). For instance, underdosing which can occur through faulty administration of drugs, type of animals like goats, which are capable of rapidly metabolizing the drug, and prolonged drug persistence can favour selection for resistance. The systemic availability of anthelmintics is likely to be affected by following factors:

(a) *Route of administration* : It has an important role in the bioavailability of anthelmintics and their metabolites. In ruminants, oral administration of drug can stimulate the closure of oesophageal groove leading to diversion of drug to abomasum, decreased bioavailability of metabolites of BZ anthelmintics and decreased efficacy resulting in enhanced rate of development/ selection of resistant worms (Swarnkar *et al.*, 1998).

(b) *Quality and quantity of feed* : Retention time of drug in the rumen and the rate of its outflow are dependent on flow of digesta. Larger feed intake particularly with higher water content was found to increase the rate of digesta flow, reduced period for absorption and recycling of drug (Singh *et al.*, 1999).

(c) *Host species* : In India, dose rate set in native animals is translated in animals having anatomical similarity without considering the host physiology. For anthelmintic treatment sheep and goats, cattle and buffalo are grouped together and recommended similar dose rate. The most pronounced host related differences in the kinetic disposition of BZ have been observed between sheep and goat (Sanyal and Godke, 1996) and between cattle and buffalo (Sanyal and Singh, 1992). Now it is well established that metabolism of BZ is faster in goats compared to sheep. Similarly in buffaloes, high metabolic rate of BZ reduces the efficacy of anthelmintic at doses similar to cattle. Thus, use of sheep dose in goats and cattle dose in buffaloes may pose risk of selection for resistance in nematodes.

Borrowing of resistance : AR may be introduced from one farm to another through animal purchase or by grazing on pastures shared by flocks from several farms. Hertzberg *et al.* (2000) suggested that frequent movement of small ruminants most likely contributed to spreading resistant nematodes between flocks.

Influx of pharmaceuticals : Unfortunately trends in marketing of anthelmintics for sheep flocks reveal that there are strong nexuses between farmers and chemist with a very limited role of veterinarian in selection and use of anthelmintics. Further, the marketing of anthelmintics to farmers has not taken into account the best option in formulation, duration of effect and dose rate to slow the development of AR, but rather to maximize chemical sales in an environment where resistance and demise of chemical classes is considered inevitable.

Detection of anthelmintic resistance

AR is first suspected by poor clinical response to anthelmintic treatments. Often resistance is not diagnosed and continued use of same anthelmintic group increases the frequency of resistant individuals in parasitic population until there is a major failure of control. On the other hand, a lack of response to an anthelmintic treatment may, sometimes, be misinterpreted for resistance when it is due to other causes viz. ill-thrift due to non-parasitic causes such as malnutrition, rapid reinfection, wrong choice of drug, faulty administration, under dosing and presence of developing or arrested larvae. The growing importance of AR has led to an increased demand for reliable and efficient detection methods (Coles *et al.*, 2006). AR can be detected by a number of *in vivo* and *in vitro* techniques. In general, *in vivo* methods are bio- or parasitological assays suited for all types of anthelmintics inspite of being time consuming, expensive, labour intensive and characterized by poor quality data with low precision and reproducibility due to inter-animal variation and drug pharmacodynamics in the host. *In vitro* techniques offer rapid, sensitive and considerably more economic methods of screening, being parasitological, biochemical or genetic in nature but suffer from certain limitations (Taylor and Hunt, 1989). In *in vitro* assays removal of the host as the primary source of data greatly improves the precision of resistance estimates. These techniques can be considered as pharmacological or biochemical or molecular in nature.

(A) *In-vivo* techniques

Faecal Egg Count Reduction Test (FECRT) : The test provides an estimate of anthelmintic efficacy by comparing worm egg counts from animals before and after treatment and does not necessarily relate to worm numbers because it only measures the effect on adult female worms. The efficacy of test is doubtful when the proportion of the resistant worms in population is less than 25%. A standardized protocol for the FECRT was recommended by WAAVP for the detection of AR in nematodes (Coles *et al.*, 1992). The interval between treatment and sampling is also critical because if the interval is short, a temporarily suppression of egg production by gravid female may occur giving a false high efficacy. Conversely, if the interval is long, new patent infection may be acquired, giving a false low efficacy. To overcome these problems, it was recommended to collect faecal samples 10–14 days post-treatment in case of BZ, 7 days after for LEV and 14 days after for IVM (Coles *et al.*, 2006). The % FECR could be calculated either by using post-treatment FECs (Method 1) or by using pre- and post-treatment FECs (Method 2, 3 and 4) as described below:

Method 1 (Coles et al., 1992) : In this method only post-treatment faecal egg counts for treated and control groups are utilized for calculation of % FECR by arithmetic means as% FECR = 100 × [1-(T/C)], where T and C represents mean post-treatment FEC in treated and control group, respectively. The resistance is declared when FECR was <95 %.

Method 2 (Presidente, 1985) : In this method both pre-treatment and post-treatment FEC are utilized to calculate % FECR through geometric means as% FECR = 100 × [1 – (T_2 × C_1)/ (T_1 × C_2)], where C_1 and T_2 represents mean pre-treatment FEC in control and treated group while C_2 and T_2 represents mean post-treatment FEC in control and treated group. The strain of parasites having less than 90% FECR was considered as resistant.

Method 3 (Dash et al., 1988) : It is similar to the method as described by Presidente (1985) except that in this arithmetic means were used instead of geometric means without transforming the faecal egg count data.

Method 4 (Kochapakdee et al., 1995) : Using arithmetic means % FECR is calculated as: 100 × [1 – (T_2/ T_1)], where T_1 and T2 represents mean pre and post-treatment FEC in treated group. Less than 90% reduction in FEC was considered as the state of AR.

Use of any of the methods has likely to influence the decision taken concerning the resistant status on a farm. Maharshi *et al.* (2009) compared the status of AR using all the four calculation method and found that the proportion of flocks revealing BZ resistance in strongyle worms varied from 81.82 % (Method 3) to 86.36 % (Methods 1, 2 and 4). Like-wise the extent of TEM resistant strongyle worm in flocks ranged from 31.81 % (Method 2) to 41.91 % (Method 3). High concordance was found between Methods 1 and 2 for BZ resistance and between Methods 2 and 3 for TEM resistance. Further, Mejia *et al.* (2003) reported that there might be disagreement in the presentation of the results calculated from different FECR methods depending on whether they were based on the use of the arithmetic mean or geometric mean for FEC. Similarly, inclusion of the FEC at pre-treatment stage or in control group for the calculation of % FECR could influence the determination of resistance. By comparing the arithmetic and geometric means, Dash *et al.* (1988) concluded that the arithmetic mean was the most appropriate statistics to use in the FECRT. Estimates of reduction in the FEC derived from geometric mean tend to be higher than those obtained using arithmetic mean and may also vary according to the transformation used (McKenna, 1990). Moreover, unlike the arithmetic mean, which is directly proportional to the total egg output of the group, the magnitude of geometric mean may be greatly influenced by the distribution of the individual. Arithmetic mean is simpler to calculate, better suited to comparative purpose and provides a more conservative and truer measure of anthelmintic efficacy than geometric mean.

Critical Anthelmintic Test : It is based on the collection of faeces from animals for at least 4 days after treatment, from which the number of expelled worms are estimated. A residual worm burden if any is then estimated by post-slaughter examination of GI tract. The % efficacy of drug is calculated as per the method of Gordon (1950). It is costly, labour intensive, time consuming and unsuitable for animal worms which undergo digestion during passage through intestinal tract.

Controlled Test : Wood *et al.* (1995) described the detailed guidelines to conduct this test and considered it as the most reliable method to confirm the anthelmintic efficacy. However, it is time consuming and costly in terms of animal and labour required. It compares the worm burdens of animals post-treatment which have been experimentally infected with susceptible or suspected resistant isolate of nematodes.

The test can also be used to determine the anthelmintic activity against all stages of development of nematode by slaughtering at varying interval after infection.

(B) *In-vitro* techniques

Egg Hatch Assay (EHA) : It is based on the ovicidal property of BZ, which prevents egg embryonation and hatching. In this assay eggs are incubated with serially diluted BZ (pure thiabendazole as reference drug) for predetermined time and the proportion, which fail to embryonate or hatch determined. It is found to be inexpensive, sensitive, less time consuming and repeatable, but requirement of fresh eggs is essential. Taylor and Hunt (1989) described anaerobic storage of faeces to overcome this difficulty. Johansen (1989) described several intrinsic variables of EHA viz. single or mixed species, fresh or embryonated eggs, pure or commercial drug, drug dilutions or fixed drug concentration, incubation temperature and time, larvae plus embryonated eggs or larvae which affect the result and make its objective assessment difficult to interpret.

Larval Development Assay : It is the only *in-vitro* test that allows the detection of resistance against all drug types irrespective of their mode of action. Lacey *et al.* (1990) and Hubert and Kerboeuf (1992) developed this test system in which nematode eggs are added to agar matrix containing drug and developed through to infective L_3 in the presence of nutritive medium. This test assay gave excellent dose-response curve with all types of anthelmintic classes. The test is based on the assumption that (1) sites of action of drug that exit in the developing larvae are similar to that of the adult parasites, (2) role of site of action in maintaining viability in developing larvae and adult is either unchanged or comparable, (3) a free equilibrium of the drug between the agar matrix and larvae is maintained and (4) the active constituent *in vivo* is the drug used *in vitro*. LDA marketed as DrenchRite® kit (Horizon Tech, Australia) claimed as most suitable *in vitro* test to detect AR among all major broad-spectrum anthelmintics. It is more sensitive than FECRT and EHA and detects AR when about 10% of the worm population carries resistance genes.

Larval Paralysis Test : Martin and Le Jambre (1979) described a test for detecting MT resistance by comparing the proportion of paralyzed L_3 over a range of drug concentrations for discrimination between resistant and susceptible strains of nematodes. The limitation of the test was that the assay could not facilitate counting at later time and objective assessment of paralyzed L_3 was difficult to make. To overcome these problems, Dobson *et al.* (1986) developed an assay, which was based on paralysis of first stage larvae within the eggs, with the index of response being the occurrence of hatching. The assay could be preserved for counting at a convenient time. However, time of adding the drug in the test system was critical and made the assay count complicated.

Some more tests have been developed for detecting AR in nematodes. Folz *et al.* (1987) used micromotility meter to differentiate resistant and susceptible isolates and found that resistant parasites were motile compared to susceptible one (larval motility assay). Stringfellow (1988) described an adult development test for detection of BZ-resistance of *in-vitro* cultured adult *H. contortus*. Petersen *et al.* (2000) described adult migration inhibition test with the limitation that animals have to be sacrificed for the collection of adult worms. Sutherland and Lee (1989) described a biochemical assay based on the comparison between the non-specific esterase and acetylcholinesterase of susceptible and resistant strains of parasites, measured by isoelectric focusing or calorimetric technique. Lacey and Prichard (1986) developed tubulin binding assay based on differential binding of BZ to tubulin prepared from susceptible and resistant nematodes.

Molecular assays

Above mentioned assays are relatively less sensitive and efforts are underway to develop appropriate molecular assays. These assays detect the mutation at the codon 200 of the β-tubulin isotype 1 gene that is linked to the BZ resistance in nematodes. The mutation (TTC to TAC) leads to a change in the amino acid from phenylalanine to tyrosine. Allele specific-PCR (AS-PCR) technique was used successfully to detect the BZ resistance in nematode species (Elard *et al.*, 1999; Garg and Yadav, 2009; Maharshi *et al.*, 2011b). Kwa *et al.* (1993) carried out RFLP analysis in *H. contortus* probe and observed different RFLP patterns between susceptible and resistant parasites. Tiwari *et al.* (2006) describe a new PCR based RFLP technique for detection of BZ resistance in *H. contortus*, which is easy, reproducible and less expensive. RFLP-PCR can successfully be used to identify the mutation at 200 codon in β-tubulin gene of *H. contortus*. With PCR, 1% level of resistant individuals can be detected within a susceptible worm population (Ross *et al.*, 1995). However, the emergence of BZ resistance has also been reported due to mutation at 167 codon (Phe to Tyr) in the β-tubulin isotype 1 or 2 gene (Prichard, 2001). Real time PCR for the diagnosis of BZ resistance in trichostrongylids of sheep is found to be more sensitive, rapid and less expensive. Real time PCR offers the opportunity to analyze allele frequencies based on samples of pooled larvae, however, this technique has not yet been used on mixed species or field samples and thus, remains to be seen what extent further optimization will be required.

Extent of anthelmintic resistance

When one considers in retrospective, the problem of AR is though five decades old and the literature is rather exhaustive. Therefore, only literature pertinent to the most commonly used anthelmintics viz. BZ and TEM/LEV are reviewed here. First time the occurrence of resistance to phenothiazine was reported in *H. contortus* from sheep in USA (Drudge *et al.*, 1957).

World scenario

Resistance to BZ : Following introduction of thiabendazole (TBZ) in 1961, the emergence of TBZ resistance in *H. contortus* strain was occurred very soon (Drudge *et al.*, 1964). In a survey, in New South Wales, Australia, it was observed that 45% of the flocks showed reduced efficacy of the TBZ to a level where the drug had no perceptible chemotherapeutic activity (Webb *et al.*, 1979). At a farm in southern Germany, Bauer *et al.* (1987) observed presence of large number of *H. contortus* in abomasum following treatment with BZ. In Sri Lanka, van Aken *et al.* (1989) confirmed BZ resistance by observing only 79.4% reduction in FEC in goats infected with *H. contortus* and treated with TBZ. In Malaysia, Dorny *et al.* (1993) reported emergence of BZ resistance in *H. contortus* from goats first time. An outbreak of haemonchosis associated with AR was recorded in 1995 in a flock of Dorper sheep from Nairobi, Kenya (Waruiru *et al.*, 1998).

In addition to *H. contortus*, more and more cases of BZ resistance in other nematodes have been reported. Other GINs reported 1st time to have BZ resistance were *T. colubriformis* (Hotson *et al.*, 1970), *O. circumcincta* (Hall *et al.*, 1979), *T. vitrinus* (Prichard *et al.*, 1980), *N. spathiger* (Middleberg and Mckenna, 1983), *C. curticei* (Borgsteed, 1986), *O. venulosum* and *Strongyloides* spp. (McKenna, 1989), *O. trifurcata, T. axei, N. abnormalis and N. filicolis* (Beveridge *et al.*, 1990).

Epidemiological investigations on emergence of AR have been made throughout the world involving a large scale survey on sheep farms. The reports on systematic screening for AR that merit a mention are from Brazil (Vieira *et al.*, 1992), France (Kerboeuf and Hubert, 1985), Germany (Duwel *et al.*, 1987), Kenya (Waruiru *et al.*, 1991), Netherlands (Boersema *et al.*, 1987), South Africa (van Wyk and Malan, 1988), Sri Lanka (van Aken *et al.*, 1989) and UK (Hong *et al.*, 1992). Hertzberg *et al.* (2000) examined 20 sheep and goat farms in Switzerland and detected BZ resistance in 15 farms. In New Zealand, McKenna (1989) observed AR in southern north Island, with a prevalence of 21-45%. In lower North Island, Hughes *et al.* (2005) reported oxfendazole resistance in 43% sheep farms. Prevalence of AR ranged from 62.5 to 85.0% in different regions of Australia (Overend *et al.*, 1994). In France, Kerboeuf *et al.* (1988) observed resistant strains of strongyle worms in 20% of 26 flocks. In America, the prevalence of BZ resistance was 39% in Rio Grande do Sul (Echevarria and Pinheiro, 1989), 86% in Uruguay, 73% in Paraguay, 90% in Brazil, 100% in Londrina-Parana region of Brazil (Cunha-Filho *et al.*, 1998) and 90% in Argentina (Romero *et al.*, 1998). In Zimbabwe, Boersema and Pandey (1997) obtained FECR between 0 to 80% for FBZ in ten commercial sheep farms of Highveld region, predominantly infected with *H. contortus*.

Resistance to imidazothiazoles : Le Jambre *et al.* (1976) detected first time the resistance to this group of anthelmintic in *H. contortus* of sheep in Australia. Later on, resistance to LEV or MT was recorded in other species of ovine nematodes *viz. O. circumcincta* and *O. trifurcata* (Le Jambre *et al.*, 1978), *T. colubriformis* (Sangster *et al.*, 1979), *Nematodirus* spp. (Edwards *et al.*, 1986a) and *T. vitrinus* (Beveridge *et al.*, 1990). The study conducted by Waller *et al.* (1995) showed alarming and critical situation, where LEV resistance was found to the tune of 70%, 68%, 84% and 22% in Uruguay, Paraguay, Brazil and Argentina, respectively.

The emergence of TEM resistance was slow to occur than against BZ group of anthelmintics. Prevalence of BZ resistance was >60% in majority of countries (45.94%) while TEM resistance remained between 20-40% in 35.71% of countries. The pattern of average prevalence exhibited that there was a linear rise in the magnitude of existence of BZ resistance in nematodes at farms throughout the world. The declining trends in number of surveys and extent of BZ resistance after 2001 are suggestive of shifting of investigator's interest throughout the world from routine survey to other aspects (like mechanism, diagnostic methods, management) of AR.

Indian scenario

Compared to world scenario, the reports of AR from India are meagre and available reports are mainly from organized farms. The extent of problem of AR and related aspects in Indian prospective has reviewed by Singh *et al.* (2002) and by Yadav and Garg (2005, 2007). Following the first report of AR in *H. contortus* to phenothiazine and TZB in sheep from Pashulok, Rishikesh, UP by Varshney and Singh (1976), there were no documented reports of AR till 1990. From 1990 onwards, there has been a renewed interest on this aspect and since then a considerable number of reports of AR in GINs of small ruminants are pouring in from various parts of the country.

In northern India, at Sheep Breeding Farm, Makku (UP) resistance to FBZ and TEM was reported following heavy mortality in flocks (Srivastava *et al.*, 1995). Following, the failure of anthelmintic treatment to control GINs in a mixed flock of sheep and goats, Yadav *et al.* (1996) observed 65 and 39% reduction in FEC for FBZ and TP, respectively. Laha *et al.* (1999) reported multiple AR, involving FBZ and IVM resistant *H. contortus*, in pashmina producing goats, while Hira Ram *et al.* (2004) reported resistance to ABZ and RFX in *H. contortus* of goats from temperate zone of Uttarkhand. Sankar (2003, 2007) reported extent of BZ resistance in strongyle worms of small ruminants from UP and Uttarkhand by using EHA and AS-PCR. Garg *et al.* (2007) reported BZ, imidazothiazole and salicylanide resistance in *H. contortus* at an organized sheep farm in Uttarakhand. Molecular assay (AS-PCR) was used to investigate the BZ resistance in strongyle worms of sheep from UP and Uttarkhand (Garg and Yadav, 2009). Yadav and Uppal (1992) reported LEV resistance in *H. contortus* of goats. Further, multiple AR in *H. contortus* from goats has been reported involving BZ, LEV, MT and TP by Uppal *et al.* (1992). An outbreak of ovine haemonchosis associated with strains of *H. contortus*, resistant to FBZ and MT has reported by Yadav *et al.* (1993). On extensive survey of sheep farms in Haryana, Kumar and Yadav (1994) found that none of the traditionally managed sheep flocks had BZ resistant *H. contortus*, but 19 (out of 32) intensively managed sheep flocks tend to have BZ resistance. Multiple AR in *H. contortus* on a sheep farm in western part of Haryana, using BZ, LEV and MT was confirmed by Yadav *et al.* (1995). Chaudhri *et al.* (1997) observed resistance in *H. contortus* of sheep to a new substitute methyl benzimidazole carbamate compound. Chaudhri (2000) reported TEM resistance in *H. contortus* from sheep in Hisar. Gupta *et al.* (2003) reported CLS resistance in *H. contortus* in sheep from western Haryana. Das and Singh (2005) observed moderate to severe level of AR on all sheep and goat farms in Hisar with multiple AR on one farm. Recently, Chaudhri *et al.* (2007) conducted a survey on status of AR in sheep flocks in two different regions (eastern and western) of Haryana and observed resistance in *H. contortus* to FBZ, TEM and MT in 76.9, 66.7 and 83.3% flocks, respectively. In Himachal Pradesh, Singh *et al.* (1992) identified a TBZ resistant *H. contortus* strain of sheep.

In western India, AR in sheep has been reported from Rajasthan and Gujarat. Failure of anthelmintic treatment at CSWRI, Avikanagar was noticed during early 90's (Swarnkar *et al.*, 1993). On FECRT, resistance to ABZ (Singh *et al.*, 1995) and RFX (Singh *et al.*, 1996) was detected in *H. contortus*. In a national wide survey, Gill (1996) reported resistance to ABZ and LEV in GINs of sheep maintained at ARC, CSWRI, Bikaner and sheep farm at Dantiwada (Gujarat). Later on, Swarnkar *et al.* (1999b) conducted a study in animals from ARC, Bikaner and found that both FBZ and LEV were 100% effective in reducing the FEC in sheep naturally infected with *H. contortus* and ED_{50} value on EHA was 0.074±0.015 μg TBZ ml^{-1}. The investigations on status of AR in *H. contortus* at SBF, Fatehpur, (Rajasthan), confirmed emergence of BZ and LEV resistant *H. contortus* strains (Swarnkar *et al.*, 1999a). Monitoring of AR in strongyle nematodes by FECRT and LDA, Swarnkar *et al.* (2001) observed emergence of resistance to BZ (53-93% FECR) and RFX (69-80% FECR) and a potential risk of the development of LEV resistance on an organized sheep farm in the semi arid area of Rajasthan. On extensive survey in Rajasthan, Swarnkar and Singh (2010a) observed high (86.4%) and moderate (55.7%) prevalence of BZ and TEM resistance, respectively. There was distinct regional variation in prevalence of AR with higher magnitude of resistance in semi-arid compared to arid Rajasthan (Swarnkar *et al.*, 2004). Maharshi *et al.* (2011a) reported emergence of BZ resistance in *H. contortus* of sheep 100% of farm and field flocks except in field flocks from north-eastern Rajasthan where 66.7% flocks possessed BZ resistant *H. contortus*. Resistance to TEM in *H. contortus* was observed in farm flock of north-eastern region whereas among field flocks it ranged from 33.33% (north region) to 83.33% (eastern region). A high agreement (86.4%) with poor linear correlation (r = 0.087) was observed between results of both FECRT and EHA for BZ resistance. The poor correlation between FECR and ED_{50} values as well as variation in ED_{50} value during patent period might be due to fact that the anthelmintic activity of BZ in host is not necessarily in a linear relationship with the ovicidal effect of BZ anthelmintics as measured by EHA. Makvana and Singh (2009) reported multiple AR in strongyle worms of sheep from Gujarat.

Using molecular approaches, Tiwari *et al.* (2006, 2007) observed significantly higher proportion of BZ homozygous resistant adult male *H. contortus* in with overall 86% prevalence of BZ resistant alleles. The study conducted on the seasonal variation in different genotypes of adult *H. contortus* (w.r.t. BZ-resistance) revealed that sheep harbour more number of BZ-susceptible worms during monsoon and winter compared to summer (Swarnkar *et al.*, 2006). For BZ-resistance the overall annual frequency of rr, rS and SS types of *H. contortus* larvae was 86.38, 13.19 and 0.43%, respectively in semi-arid farms of Rajasthan. Seasonal analysis exhibited that following deworming in mid-September the proportion of rr, rS and SS genotypes was 40.0, 55.0 and 5.0%, respectively. In succeeding months when environment is not favourable for dissemination of pre-parasitic stages of parasite with minimal chances of re-infection, the ratio of different genotypes in suprapopulation returned to previous level with>95% of rr genotypes. In arid farm the overall annual frequency of rr type of *H. contortus* larvae was 59.41% and varied from 49.50% (winter) to 73.56% (summer). The relatively higher proportion of rr genotype in suprapopulation during the period from March to July indicates existence of unsuitable climate for larval dissemination as well as meagre chances of re-infection from pasture. The proportion of rr genotype of *H. contortus* larvae from field flocks of semi-arid Rajasthan found to contribute to gene pool of suprapopulation on pasture was 97.58, 88.57 and 96.43%, respectively during summer, monsoon and winter seasons. It has been observed that in pre-drench gene pool the frequency of rr genotype was 92.5% which decreased slightly to 75.0% in October indicating that smaller proportion of susceptible genotypes able to disseminate in later half of monsoon and dilute the gene population on pasture. Similarly in arid field, the proportion of rr genotype of *H. contortus* larvae found to contribute to gene pool of supra-population on pasture was 85.62, 86.54 and 92.13%, respectively during summer, monsoon and winter season. Similar to semi-arid region, it has been observed that in pre-drench gene pool the frequency of rr genotype was around 90.0% which reduced to 40.0% in October but reached to pre-drench level thereafter. Thus, deworming in later half of monsoon is helpful in increasing the efficacy of anthelmintics by increasing the size of *refugia* (Swarnkar *et al.*, 2012). Rising trend in prevalence of rr genotype from November onwards might reflect the role of migration and unplanned grazing and anthelmintic use in field flocks in maintaining the high level of BZ-resistance (Singh and Swarnkar, 2008). On AS-PCR, Maharishi *et al.* (2011b) reported that frequency of BZ- resistance genotype in infective larvae of *H. contortus* ranged from 72.22% (north-eastern region) to 96.87% (eastern region) in farm flocks and from 61.79% (north-eastern region) to 95.83% (eastern region) in field flocks of Rajasthan. The phenotypic expression of BZ resistance on FECRT was evident with occurrence of >30% rr genotypes in population. Likewise presence of >30% r alleles in population were found to express the BZ resistance on EHA.

From southern India, resistance to ABZ and LEV was reported from organized sheep farms at Palamner (Andra Pradesh), Sanddynallah and Kattupakkam (Tamil Nadu) by Gill (1996). BZ resistance in GINs has been observed on 9 sheep farms situated in Karnataka (Dhanalaxmi *et al.*, 2003). From Tamil Nadu, Jayanthilakan *et al.* (2003) confirmed BZ resistance and suspected TEM resistance in *H. contortus* in sheep flocks, Arunachalam *et al.* (2005) observed resistance to FBZ, ABZ, LEV and MT in GINs from a flock of Mecheri sheep maintained at an organized farm. Sankar (2003, 2007) reported extent of BZ resistance in strongyle worms of small ruminants from Tamil Nadu using EHA and AS-PCR, while Easwaran *et al.* (2009) used FECRT and EHA to determine the extent of BZ and LEV resistance in sheep and reported multiple AR.

Management of anthelmintic resistance

As the saying goes, "if you can't beat them, join them", we are never going to achieve eradication of worms. It is AR worms which are our major concern and we need to keep worms susceptible to anthelmintics that we have, in order to have some control over them. So we need to think sideways and implement an additional strategy that will hinder the growth of the resistant worms in population. The development of methods to conserve efficacy of anthelmintics are, and will become, increasingly important as we seek to maintain and/or expand livestock production.

Refugia : One approach to conserving efficacy is to maintain parasite populations *in refugia* (Soulsby, 2007). In the case of AR the population *in refugia* can simply be defined as a population that is either unexposed to or, in certain circumstances, unaffected by an anthelmintic. Since AR is a heritable trait the expectation is also that the genetic structure of an exposed population will have been altered in some way. Initially AR management strategies were not specifically directed towards maintaining *refugia* but understandably, at a time when parasitism appeared to be an omnipresent threat, tended to be largely concerned with achieving effective control with fewer treatments (Dash, 1986), ways of maximising and extending efficacy (Hennessy *et al.*, 1991) and maintaining biosecurity (Dobson *et al.*, 2001).

More recently, attention has been given to maintaining a nematode population *in refugia* in an effort to maintain susceptibility within the suprapopulation. By maintaining the same proportion of larvae in *refugia* for 6 generations of parasites (a mixture of 5% thiabendazole-resistant and 95% non thiabendazole-resistant *H. contortus* larvae), Martin *et al.* (1981) observed that *refugia* delayed the development of resistance in *H. contortus*. Where none or small proportions of larvae were in *refugia*, a rapid increase in resistance occurred. With an increased proportion of larvae in *refugia*, resistance was slower to develop. In small ruminants, the urgent need to develop easily applicable refugia-based systems for resistance management has led to investigation of a variety of "targeted treatment" approaches for different nematodes, with the emphasis on easily-applied indicators for the need for treatment.

Sources of refugia : The infrapopulations in untreated hosts that provide *refugia* is refractory (but not resistant, e.g. histotropic larvae) to a particular drug treatment (Fleming *et al.*, 2006). In temperate areas, the majority (up to 95%) of the parasite population is usually on pasture and provides a relatively large reservoir of susceptibility while in tropical areas, this may not always be the case, since the extreme heat desiccates the free living worm stages on pasture within as short a period as 4 weeks. In some cases, stage specific differences in susceptibility to an antiparasitic compound that are not attributable to resistance may provide some *refugia* even in treated animals. For example, the immature stages of some *T. circumcincta* populations are refractory to LEV treatment and under these circumstances LEV treatments may inadvertently maintain *refugia*. In contrast, treatments with the macrocyclic lactones, which have efficacies approaching 100% against all developmental stages, result in negligible levels of *refugia*. Where environmental conditions promote the continual survival of worm larvae on pasture, a substantial pool of larvae in *refugia* is usually available on the farm.

Approaches to maintain *refugia*

Host based : These include reducing the numbers of treatments by targeting them effectively and/or selectively. Whenever anthelmintics are used it is important to consider not only the impact on the infrapopulation but also what is happening at that time to the free living stages. For example anthelmintic treatments that are administered when the suprapopulation size is drastically reduced, such as during dry periods or by the use of reseeded pastures, pose a considerable risk with regard to the selection of resistance. An understanding of this phenomenon has led to a move away from summer treatments in winter rainfall areas of Australia (Besier and Love, 2003) and recommendations not to dose animals onto clean grazing (Abbott *et al.*, 2004). Other important factors are the classes of animal to be treated, the nature of the anthelmintics used in the treatments, the biotic potential of the nematode species exposed to treatment and the treatment regimes being employed. Sharing of common grazing by groups of animals with different patterns of treatment may provide *refugia* and has been exploited in the management of resistance in Ethiopia (Sissay *et al.*, 2006) and believed to be an important factor in accounting for the lack of resistance recorded in studies on the Greek mainland (Papadopoulos *et al.*, 2001).

Attempting to modify AR status of the parasite populations either through reintroducing susceptible parasite species (community dilution approach) or by modifying resistance mechanisms has an intuitive appeal. Though studies in South Africa have shown that it is possible to reintroduce susceptible populations onto irrigated areas (Carmichael, 2002) but the practical difficulties of doing this on a large number of farms in temperate climates where a resistant suprapopulation can survive for many months on pasture are challenging. In addition, studies using parasitic nematodes have also shown that it is possible to reverse resistance using p glycoprotein or cytochrome P_{450} inhibitors (Prichard and Roulet, 2007). However, identification of the most appropriate inhibitors and then producing and registering these combinations represents a formidable scientific and commercial challenge.

Host-associated factors regulating the level of *refugia* also include the level of resilience to parasitic infection and the extent of the expression of immunity. The interaction between the immune status of the host and *refugia* may, at least in part, account for the differences in the rate of appearance of resistance and its prevalence in different ruminant species (Silvestre *et al.*, 2002). Resistance appears to develop most rapidly in goats where, because of their perceived lack of immunity, it is common practice to treat all age classes. In sheep, however the contribution to *refugia* is likely to be affected by temporal changes in both the species contributing to parasite challenge within a grazing season and the susceptibility of the host to each of those species. Species prevalence and host susceptibility are two important factors that need to be taken into account when managing *refugia* particularly when single species resistance is an issue. Resilient animals continue to perform whilst under parasite challenge and therefore require less anthelmintic treatments than non-resilient animals (Bisset *et al.*, 2001).

Parasite based : These includes the frequency of the resistant alleles in the parasite population, the biotic potential of the parasite and the longevity of both the supra and infrapopulations. The frequency of resistant genes influences the rate at which homozygous resistant parasites appear in the population. If the proportion of resistance genes is high, then there is an increased probability that heterozygotes will have the opportunity to mate and produce homozygous resistant offspring. The degree of biotic potential of a parasite species determines the numbers of individuals of that species required to provide a given level of *refugia*. For example, species with high biotic potential, e.g. *H. contortus*, can provide a high degree of pasture contamination from relatively few individuals and therefore, effective refugia can, assuming successful completion of the lifecycle, be maintained by leaving a relatively small proportion of the host population unexposed to treatment. In other species with lower biotic potential, e.g. *T. circumcincta*, a greater proportion of the host population would need to be left unexposed to treatment to provide the same level of *refugia*.

Climate and management based : Environmental conditions and management practices that influence the development of eggs and larvae on pasture can also had impact upon the maintenance of *refugia*. For example, control programs that leave relatively low or no parasites in *refugia*, i.e. spring treatments against a parasite species that overwinters poorly or dose and move to clean pasture, select strongly for resistance (Abbott *et al.*, 2004).

Strategies for application of *refugia* concept

The importance of refugia can be illustrated by looking at the difference in development of resistance in Australia compared to New Zealand. In New Zealand, where the climate is wet, up to 75% of the *H. contortus* population are larval stages on the pasture, which is considerably higher than in the more dry climate in Australia. In spite of the fact that the BZ and LEV have been used over the same period of time, the resistance to these drugs was detected much later in New Zealand (Kettle *et al.*, 1981). In the Nordic countries parasites which do not over-winter on the pasture, such as *H. contortus* have only a small proportion in *refugia* and hence have a greater selection pressure when animals are treated in this period than in species where larval stages over-winter on pasture (Ihler, 2010).

Community dilution strategy : Once AR has been identified to a particular drug on a farm it may be possible to substitute the resistant parasite community for a susceptible one. To date, several studies have been conducted to examine the feasibility of replacing BZ resistant *H. contortus* (van Wyk and van Schalkwyk, 1990) or *T. circumcincta* (Moussavou-Boussougou *et al.*, 2007), or multi-drug resistant nematodes (Sissay *et al.*, 2006) with susceptible nematodes on pasture.

Similarly, Singh and Swarnkar (2010) observed that inadvertently community dilution strategy helped in reversion to susceptibility for BZ at SBF, Fatehpur. In this farm BZ resistance was first confirmed in 1998 as 0.00% FECR for BZ (Swarnkar *et al.*, 1999a). On subsequent years there was gradual rise in % FECR whenever examined and with marginal rise in BZ susceptible alleles (Swarnkar *et al.*, 2004). On exploration the causes of these findings it was found that unwanted introduction of field animals infected with BZ susceptible strains of *H. contortus* (Anon, 2004) for grazing on pasture area of farm led to dilution of resistant population in *refugia* with resultant increase in anthelmintic efficacy at farm. The correlated response between genotypic frequency of homozygous BZ-resistant larvae and BZ-efficacy exhibited that a marginal rise in the proportion of BZ-susceptible alleles during September to November resulted in increased efficacy of BZ anthelmintics as well as reduces the proportion of flocks harbouring BZ-resistant *H. contortus*. It is clear from the molecular analysis that community dilution strategy for reversion of susceptibility to BZ in *H. contortus* could be feasible in farm condition. Under prevailing managemental and grazing practices in field flocks the variation in genotypic frequency could not be recorded. The period from September to November in semi-arid and from June to February in arid Rajasthan was found appropriate in increasing the frequency of BZ-susceptible alleles in the *refugia* (Singh and Swarnkar, 2008).

These studies have shown that it is possible to reintroduce susceptible nematodes either by reducing the resistant parasites to negligible levels on pasture and infecting either entire flocks or seeder lambs with susceptible parasites to re-contaminate pastures or by reducing resistant nematodes to very low levels in the hosts and transferring the hosts to pastures with high levels of nematodes in natural *refugia*. Although this approach has the potential to reduce the prevalence of resistant parasites on a given area, there are practical limitations which may prevent its widespread use, e.g. the availability of large numbers of pathogen-free susceptible larvae with which to infect seeder animals and the ability to reduce pasture contamination to negligible levels.

Targeted treatment (TT) : It means whole flock treatments given at the most appropriate times bearing in mind the need to maintain *refugia*. These treatments differ from strategic treatments which are generally given prophylactically on the basis of epidemiology in a given area and are used to protect animals and prevent disease over a substantial period. The TT approach serves to reduce the numbers of anthelmintic treatments and thus minimise pasture contamination with resistant genotypes. Effective targeting should also lead to an increased interval between treatments, allowing susceptible genotypes a better opportunity to establish on pasture and so reduce the risk of heterozygotes mating and producing homozygous resistant offspring. Examples of the use of TT approach include studies conducted in western Australia (Besier and Love, 2003) and Italy (Cringoli *et al.*, 2008) where treatments were stopped during summer months when few parasites were present on pasture and given instead at other times when more parasites were present in *refugia*.

Targeted selective treatment (TST) : It involves selective treatment of only those animals that will most benefit from treatment, leaving the rest of the flock untreated. GI parasite populations in small ruminants are highly aggregated and over-dispersed within the host, with around 80% of the worms found in only 20-30% of the host, whilst the vast majority of hosts posses low worm burden (Hoste *et al.*,

2002). The detailed epidemiological studies in sheep flocks of Rajasthan revealed that even during favourable monsoon season (July–September) around 20-30% and 50% of animals in field and farm conditions, respectively had FECs to the tune of >1000 epg. Other wise in rest of seasons, majority of animals had either < 200 epg or free of infection (Swarnkar *et al.*, 2008). This phenomenon of over-distribution of worm burdens in host populations could be utilised for reducing selection for AR by applying TST approach. TST exploit both epidemiologically appropriate treatment times and treat only those animals that would benefit from treatment.

Markers/indicators for TST : An ideal indicator for use in TST would be cost-effective, simple to use, require minimal operator training and allow treatment decisions to be made "sheep side". For application of TST, markers as indicators range from visually identifying the animals to treat, to using parasite-based like FECs or patho-physiological markers such as anaemia, dag scores or performance based indicators such as live body weight gain, milk yield and efficiency of nutrient utilization. In South Africa, FAMACHA© method was devised and evaluated for TST (Malan *et al.*, 2001). FAMACHA© assesses the colour of the conjunctival mucous membrane, on a five-point scale, to estimate the degree of anaemia caused by *H. contortus*. Anaemic animals falling in the category 4 or 5 are at the risk of haemonchosis and are treated. This system has been used with success in many countries such as USA (Burke *et al.*, 2007) and Kenya (Ejlersten *et al.*, 2006). Hoste *et al.* (2002) compared effectiveness of selective and systematic treatments in goats and observed that anthelmintic treatments restricted to 50-60% of the flock allowed a control of GIPs similar to that achieved with systematic administration.

In eastern Ethiopia, Sissay *et al.* (2006) found that the preservation of anthelmintic susceptibility amongst the nematode parasites population in the sheep flocks, in contrast to the high level of multiple resistance in the goat flock is mainly attributed to differences in *refugia*. In Brazil, Molento *et al.* (2009) compared reproductive performance of sheep under selective and suppressive anthelmintic treatment and observed almost similar lambing rate, lamb weight and lamb mortality in both the strategy. The study demonstrated that the FAMACHA method allowed a large number of naturally infected ewes to be raised with reduced anthelmintic intervention without a negative impact on their reproductive potential. FAMACHA strategy showed a reduction of 77.8% in the use of anthelmintics when compared to the routine strategic anthelmintic intervention. In South Africa, a decrease in between 38 and 96% was observed with an average reduction of 58% in costs of anthelmintic after implementation of FAMACHA in 13 flocks (Bath and van Wyk, 2001). Considerable improvement in susceptibility of *H. contortus* population at sheep farm in South Africa was observed through genetic dilution of worm population using FAMACH© system and maintained improved level of efficacy over the ensuing 8 years with the use of TST (van Wyk, 2008).

In India, attempt to formulate a mechanism for TST approach was made at CSWRI, Avikanagar and a colour chart based on ocular mucous membrane, microhaematocrit and intensity of infection was developed (Plate 1) and implement to test its effectiveness in sheep flock. The relation between FEC and degree of anaemia (eye colour) was strongly positive only in wormy season. The mean FEC remained significantly higher (around 3 times) in visually anaemic group compared to visually normal group during wormy season (August-November). However, in non-wormy season (December-March) the intensity of strongyle infection remained at acceptable level (< 500 epg) in both the groups. The FEC pattern and clinical anaemia exhibited that anthelmintic intervention is required only in anaemic group during wormy season. The application of TST approach exhibited that the monthly proportion of animals fall under category 4 or 5 (anaemic) varied from 0.81% (Nov) to 17.35% (Sep) and the number of anthelmintic treatment were reduced to only 0.23/head/year compared to 1.0/head/year under strategic drenching schedule. In addition there was reduction in the cost of anthelmintics for worm management from Rs. 7.00/sheep/year to Rs. 0.81/head/year. Thus, application of TST in our situation is feasible and effective not only in managing the haemonchosis but also help in increasing the size of *refugia* which may ultimately resulted into both maintenance of drug efficacy against parasites and sizeable reduction in the cost of worm management (Swarnkar and Singh, 2010c; Singh and Swarnkar, 2012).

The impact of TST could also be influenced by both the composition of parasite population and farm management. Thus, the studies in different range of production system are required to determine the proportion of treated and untreated animals necessary to maintain effective *refugia*. It is also crucial that end-users are made aware not only of the cost benefits and potential losses resulting from TST but also those associated with extreme multi-drug resistance. Although the system is labour intensive and is suitable for the identification of infection by haematophagous parasites only, the benefits include the ability to make the decision to treat 'sheep – side', it is low cost and require low levels of expertise and training for implementation. The benefit of avoiding expensive whole-flock treatment is likely to have additional appeal, especially to resource-poor farmers. As with all new approaches to AR management, a goal of current research will be to translate the targeted treatment concept into practical and effective recommendations before new anthelmintics arrive to tempt livestock owners back to chemical-based solutions (Singh and Swarnkar, 2008). TST particularly aims at treating only those animals unable to withstand current worm challenges, is not only exceptionally affordable in relation to other conventional control programmes, but will also help to delay selection for AR (Sanyal, 2009), reduced selection pressure, lower drug residues in animal products and lower costs of worm management. Further, while applying TST, one should not ignore other important parasite infestations that may or may not be accompanied by detectable anaemia.

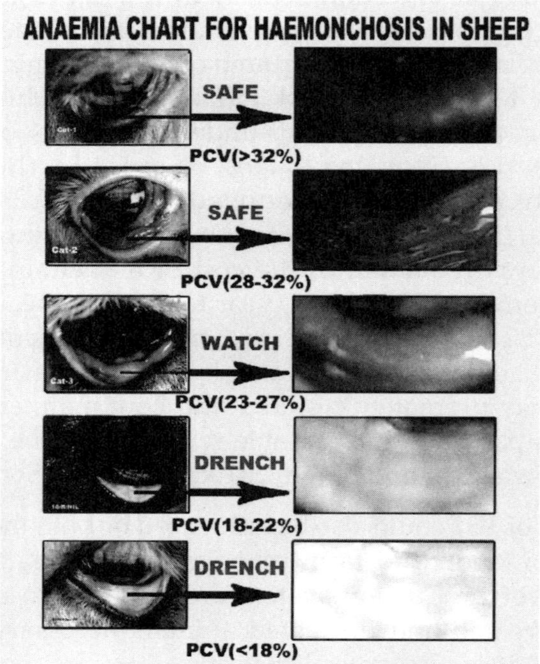

Plate 1: Showing colour chart based on ocular mucous membrane, microhaematocrit and intensity of infection

Factors working against implementation

There are many reasons why farmers do not accept or implement much of the currently advocated holistic and sustainable advice on internal parasite control.

- Farmers like simple and quick solutions even though these may be unsustainable in the longer term. This largely comes down to the fact that controlling worms by management is more complicated than a standard treatment programme and therefore, a "treat and forget" approach seems to be preferable for most farmers. It is also clear that farmers are generally more willing to pay for drugs than for advice. Advice not paid for is often advice ignored.
- Advisors and researchers cannot escape some blame for the reluctant implementation of holistic worm management. Most of the researchers who develop worm control systems are parasitologists who tend to be worm-centred, and not sheep production or farmer profitability oriented in their thinking and their advice is added on independently. Unfortunately, unrealistic advice by parasitologists may be based on perfect worm control and not on the economics or practicalities of the situation. Equally important, if on-farm veterinary advisors are also selling the drugs, there is a potential clash of interests. This can occur particularly when private veterinarians fill both roles, as there will be a temptation to sell drugs on financial grounds and not primarily for the benefit of farmers.
- Pharmaceutical companies and distributors must also accept a share of the blame. Major drug companies have huge advertising budgets and field forces and can therefore exert a significant influence on farmer thinking and behaviour when it comes to parasite control. This can apply to the thinking and advice of veterinarians in the field as well. The driving force in these firms is sales volume, usually related to projected targets and budgets. Therefore, they continue to advocate and encourage reliance on drugs, blanket treatments and excessive treatments which are certainly good for short-term profits but are not sustainable in the long-term.

Future strategy

There is a burgeoning of generic anthelmintic products in the market because patent protection of all the currently available broad-spectrum anthelmintics has lapsed. In most instances, freeing-up the anthelmintic market in the tropics/subtropics has not been in the farmer's best interests. As poor quality products assume a significant market share, then not only do the farmers waste their money, by failing to control parasites in their animals, but they hasten the selection process for AR. Therefore, strategies need to be adopted at different levels are.

Immediate strategies

- *Reduction in stocking density* : Most farms where these problems have been reported have high stocking density. A reduction in stocking density on pasture would provide more ease and flexibility to undertake the recommended strategy in addition to provide opportunities for dilution of pasture infectivity through higher growth of pasture coupled with decrease contamination rate.
- *Removal of existing worm infection* : Though this may be a difficult task, however effective drugs with different mode of action should be tried for removal of existing AR strains of parasites. Dobson *et al.* (2001) stated that older drugs like napthalophos, phenothiazine etc. may now play an important role in the management of multiple, high level resistance in nematode parasites.
- *Interrupting the life cycle of parasites* : The life cycle of strongyle worms can be broken either by adopting stall feeding (commercial flocks) for at least two months (implementation of cut and carry practice for fodder) or by adopting pasture resting strategy. Ecological studies in the wet tropics have shown that survival of the free-living stages of *H. contortus* is very short, with the majority of infective larvae disappearing from pasture within 4-6 weeks (Banks *et al.,* 1990).

Short term strategies

- *Adoption of rotational grazing* : At farm level, this requires the subdivision of available pastures into small plots. Animals are then moved around these pastures in quick succession (3-4 days grazing only on each plot), followed by returning to their original plot after 30-40 days.

- *Regular monitoring for FEC and AR :* It should be a regular phenomenon before selecting anthelmintic type.
- *Application of part-flock treatment :* Flock should be screened for anaemia by visual appearance of gradation in conjunctiva using colour chart and treat only those animals which are anaemic particularly during wormy season.
- *Improve nutritional status (Resilience) :* Introduce molasses/mineral feed blocks to improve the general nutrition of the animals.
- *Use of long-term low-level medication strategy :* Knox (1996) demonstrated restoration of BZ efficacy by adopting long-term low-level medication (through medicated feed block) instead of oral drench in locations where BZ resistance has developed.

Long term strategies

- *Breeding for disease resistance* : In order to lessen the dependence on anthelmintics, where appropriate and as a long-term priority, attempt to change the genotype of the sheep to those which have been shown to have natural resistance to *H. contortus* infections. Further, resistant line within existing breed can be developed by selective breeding for resistant or resilience to infection.

Conclusions

Being ubiquitous nature of GI parasites and omnipresence in small ruminants, management/control of these, presents a particularly difficult challenge following wide-spread emergence of AR, further complicated by recent and radical changes in approach to worm management. Research on the management of *refugia* is currently hampered by our limited understanding of the molecular mechanisms of resistance, particularly to macrocyclic lactones and imidazothiazole families, and the lack of sensitive genotyping tools. It has been suggested that there are several AR mechanisms that operate at the molecular level (Wolstenholme *et al.*, 2004). Firstly, there may be changes at the target site or amplification of target genes which render the drug ineffective. Secondly, there may be changes in the metabolism that affect drug activation or removal. Finally, there may be changes in the distribution of the drug in the organism which limit its access to the site of action. It is only when we understand the relative importance of these mechanisms that we will be able to develop sensitive DNA based technologies using SNPs/mutations and/or gene expression to determine both species and AR status of field material. Advances being made in diagnostic technologies, such as metabolimics, real time PCR and pyrosequencing, all have the potential to be used with pooled material to provide the sensitive and affordable monitoring capacity that is needed for managing *refugia.*

The veterinary advisors and parasitologists are the groups that have to take on the primary role. The advisors in particular, with their regular contact with farmers and the position of trust they have earned, have to make a sustained effort to make farmers aware of the need for change by giving frequent warnings of the dangers inherent in a drug-dominated worm control strategy and by encouraging them to adopt an incremental approach of holistic internal parasite management. Moreover, there should be regular camps, ghosti/meetings, seminars and visits in rural areas by qualified veterinarians. Parasitologists need to establish and then emphasize the relative economic importance of different worm species in each area. They should certainly continue to research practical alternatives to chemical control as experience has shown that nothing is static and the worms too will adapt to changed circumstances. The advice that is given must be simplified and practical, and should be fully integrated with other priorities and realities and not stand-alone or contradict economic imperatives.

The pharmaceutical industry must also accept its responsibilities beyond short-term profit. Pharmaceutical firms need to acknowledge that it is in their interest to advocate sustainable anthelmintic use to prolong the useful life of their products. Unfortunately, this will go against current commercial practice. Drug testing legislation also needs to be revised. Testing of drugs should be done not only against "tame" laboratory worms, but rather on existing field strains. The efficacy of generics also needs stricter evaluation before acceptance of them as equivalent to other products.

References

Abbott, K.A., Taylor, M.A. and Stubbings, L.A. (2004). Anthelmintic resistance management in sheep. *Vet. Rec.*, 154: 735-736

Anon (1991). Report of the FAO Expert Consultation of the Helminth Infections of Livestock in Developing Countries. FAO, Rome, AGA 815, Sep. 23-27, pp. 32.

Anon (2004). Annual progress report on "All India Network Program on Gastrointestinal Parasitism". CSWRI, Avikanagar, pp. 1-45

Arunachalam, K., Raman, M., Jayathilakan, N. and Karunanidhi, K. (2005). Multiple anthelmintic resistance in gastrointestinal nematodes from Mecheri sheep in an organized farm in Tamil Nadu. *Indian J. Anim. Sci.*, 75: 203-205

Banks, D.J.D., Singh, R., Barger, I.A., Pratap, B. and Le Jambre, L.F. (1990). Development and survival of infective larvae of *H. contortus* and *T. colubriformis* in a tropical environment. *Int. J. Parasitol.*, 20: 155-160

Bath, G.F. and van Wyk, J.A. (2001). Using the FAMACHA© system on commercial sheep farms in South Africa. In: *Int. Sheep Vet. Cong.*, 10 Cape Town, pp. 29-41

Bauer, C., Ullrich, D., Fiege, N., Konig, D., Luft, W. and Burger, H.J. (1987). Benzimidazole resistant *H. contortus* in einer suddeutschen schafherde. *Dt. Tierarztl. Wschr.*, 94: 205-206

Besier, R.B. and Love, S.C.J. (2003). Anthelmintic resistance in sheep nematodes in Australia: the need for new approaches. *Aust. J. Exp. Agric.*, 43: 1383-1391

Beveridge, I., Ellis, N.J.S., Riley, M.J. and Brown, T.H. (1990). Prevalence of resistance in sheep nematode populations to benzimidazole and levamisole anthelmintics in the high rainfall areas of South Australia. *Aust. Vet. J.*, 67: 413-415

Bisset, S.A., Morris, C.A., McEwan, J.C. and Vlassoff, A. (2001). Breeding sheep in New Zealand that are less reliant on anthelmintics to maintain health and productivity. *New Zealand Vet. J.*, 49: 236–246

Boersema, J.H. and Pandey, V.S. (1997). Anthelmintic resistance of trichostrongylids in sheep in the highveld of Zimbabwe. *Vet. Parasito.*, 68: 383-388

Boersema, J.H., Borgsteede, F.H.M., Eysker, M., Hendrikx, W.M.L., Jansen, J. and Smith-Buys, C.M.C. (1987). Prevalence of benzimidazole resistance of nematodes in sheep in the Netherlands. *Res. Vet. Sci.*, 43: 18-21

Borgsteede, F.H.M. (1986). Resistance of *C. curticei* against fenbendazole. *Res. Vet. Sci.*, 41: 423-424

Burke, J.M., Kaplan, R.M., Miller, J.E., Terrill, T.H., Getz, W.R., Mobini, S., Valencia, E., Williams, M.J., Williamson, L.H. and Vatta, L.F. (2007). Accuracy of the FAMACHA system for on-farm use by sheep and goat producers in the southeastern US. *Vet. Parasitol.*, 147: 89-95

Carmichael, I.H. (2002). Influences on internal parasitism of sheep in south-east Australia: Studies of (1) internal parasite control on pivot irrigation systems and (2) cobalt nutrition and internal parasite interactions. *Wool Tech. Sheep Breed.*, 50: 518-533

Chaudhri, S.S. (2000). Reduced responsiveness of oxyclozanide and tetramisole hydrochloride combinations to gastrointestinal parasites of sheep. *Indian J. Anim. Sci.*, 70: 396-398

Chaudhri, S.S., Yadav, C.L. and Gupta, R.P. (1997). Resistance in *H. contortus* of sheep to a new substituted methyl benzimidazole carbamate compound. *Indian J. Anim. Sci.*, 67: 974-975

Chaudhri, S.S., Gupta, S.K. and Bisla, R.S. (2007). Resistance to gastrointestinal nematodes to tetramisole hydrochloride, morantel tartrate and fenbendazole in sheep of Haryana. *J. Vet. Parasitol.*, 21: 113-115

Coles, G.C. (2005). Anthelmintic resistance - looking to the future: a UK perspective. *Res. Vet. Sci.*, 78: 99-108

Coles, G.C., Bauer, C., Borgsteede, F.H.M., Greats, S., Klei, T.R. and Taylor, M.A. (1992). WAAVP methods for the detection of anthelmintic resistance in nematodes of veterinary importance. *Vet. Parasitol.*, 44: 35-44

Coles, G.C., Jackson, F., Pomroy, W.E., Prichard, R.K., von Samson-Himmelstjerna, G., Sivestre, A., Taylor, M.A. and Vercruysse, J. (2006). The detection of anthelmintic resistance in nematodes of veterinary importance. *Vet. Parasitol.*, 44: 35-44

Cringoli, G., Veneziano, V., Jackson, F., Vercruysse, J., Greer, A.W., Fedele, V., Mezzino, L. and Rinaldi, L. (2008). Effects of targeted anthelmintic treatments on the milk production of dairy cattle naturally infected by gastrointestinal strongyles. *Vet. Parasitol.*, 156: 340-345

Cunha-Filho, L.C. da, Luz-Pereira, A.B. da and Yamamura, M.H. (1998). Anthelmintic resistance in sheep in the region of Londrina - Parana - Brazil. *Semina Londrina*, 19: 31-37

Dash, K.M. (1986). Control of helminthosis in lambs by strategic treatment with closantel and broad-spectrum anthelmintics. *Aust. Vet. J.*, 63: 4-7

Dash, K.M., Hall, E. and Barger, I.A. (1988). The role of arithmetic and geometric mean worm egg count reduction test and in monitoring strategic drenching programme in sheep. *Aust. Vet. J.*, 65: 66-68

Das, M. and Singh, S. (2005). Anthelmintic resistance to nematodes in sheep and goat farms in Hisar. *J. Vet. Parasitol.*, 19: 103-106

Dhanalakshmi, H., Jagannath, M.S. and Placid, E.D. (2003). Multiple anthelmintic resistance in gastrointestinal nematodes of sheep. *J. Vet. Parasitol.*, 17: 89-91.

Dobson, R.J., Donald, A.D., Waller, P.J. and Snowdown, K.L. (1986). An egg hatch assay for resistance to levamisole in trichostrongyloid nematode parasites. *Vet. Parasitol.*, 19: 77-84

Dobson, R.J., Le Jambre, L.F. and Gill, J.H. (1996). Management of anthelmintic resistance and selection with persistant drugs. *Int. J. Parasitol.*, 26: 993-1000

Dobson, R.J., Besier, R.B., Barnes, E.H., Love, S.C.J., Vizard, A., Bell, K. and Le Jambre, L.F. (2001). Principles for the use of macrocyclic lactones to minimise selection for resistance. *Aust. Vet. J.*, 79: 756-761

Donald, A.D. (1983). The development of anthelmintic resistance in nematodes of grazing animals. In: *Facts and Reflection* IV. *Resistance of Parasite to Anthelmintics.* (eds. F.H.M. Borgsteede, S.A. Henriksen and H.J. Over). Central Veterinary Institute, Lelystad, pp. 15-28

Dorny, P., Claerebout, E., Vercruysse, J., Jalila, A. and Sani, R. (1993). Benzimidazole resistance in *H. contortus* in goats in Malaysia. *Vet. Rec.*, 133: 423-424

Drudge, J.H., Leland, S.E. and Wyant, Z.N. (1957). Strain variation in the response of sheep nematodes to the action of phenothiazine. I. Studies of mixed infections in experimental animals. *Am. J. Vet. Res.*, 18: 133-41

Drudge, J.H., Szanto, J., Wyant, Z.N. and Elam, G. (1964). Field studies on parasite control in sheep: comparision of thibendazole, ruelene and phenothiazine. *Am. J. Vet. Res.*, 25: 1512-18

Duwel, D., Scmid, K. and Bechmann, C. (1987). Benzimidazole resistant *H. contortus* in sheep in Federal Republic of Germany. *Berliner and Munchener Tierarztiliche Wochenschrift*, 100: 120

Easwaran, C., Harikrishnan, T.J. and Raman, M. (2009). Multiple anthelmintic resistance in gastrointestinal nematodes of sheep in southern India. *Veterinarski Arhiv*, 79: 611-620

Echevarria, F.A.M. and Pinheiro, A.C. (1989). Evaluation of anthelmintic resistance in sheep flocks in the municipality of Bage, Rio Grande do Sui. *Pesquisa Veterinaria Brasileira*, 9: 69-71

Edwards, J.R., Wroth, R., De Chaneet, G.C., Besier, R.B., Karlsson, J., Morcombe, P.W., Dalton-Morgan, G. and Roberts, D. (1986a). Survey of anthelmintic resistance in Western Australian sheep flocks. I. Prevalence. *Aust. Vet. J.*, 6(3): 135-38

Edwards, J.R., Wroth, L., de Chaneet, G.C., Brasie, R.B., Karlson, J., Mercombes, P.W., Parton-Morgan, G. and Robert, D. (1986b). Survey for anthelmintic resistance in Australian sheep flocks. 2. Relationship with sheep management and parasite control practices. *Aust. Vet. J.*, 63: 139-143

Ejlersten, M., Githiquia, S.M., Otieno, R.O. and Thamsborg, S.M. (2006). Accuracy of an anaemia scouring chart applied on goats in sub-humid Kenya and its potential for control of *H. contortus* infections. *Vet. Parasitol.*, 141: 291-301

Elard, L., Sauve, C. and Humbert, J.F. (1998). Fitness of benzimidazole-resistant and susceptible worms of *T. circumcincta,* a nematode parasite of small ruminants. *Parasitol.,* 117: 571-578

Elard, L., Cabaret, J. and Humbert, J.F. (1999). PCR diagnosis of benzimidazole-susceptibility or -resistance in natural populations of the small ruminant parasite- *T. circumcincta. Vet. Parasitol.,* 80: 231–237

Emery, D.L. and Wagland, B.M. (1991). Vaccines against gastrointestinal nematode parasites of ruminants. *Parasitol. Today,* 7: 347-349

Fleming, S.A., Craig, T., Kaplan, R.M., Miller, J.E., Navarre, C. and Rings, M. (2006). Anthelmintic resistance of gastrointestinal parasites in small ruminants. *J. Vet. Int. Med.,* 20: 435-444

Folz, S.D., Pax, R.A., Thomas, E.M., Benett, J.L., Lee, B.L. and Conder, G.A. (1987). Detecting *in-vitro* anthelmintic effects with a micromotility meter. *Vet. Parasitol.,* 24: 241-250

Garg, R. and Yadav, C.L. (2009). Genotyping of benzimidazole susceptible and resistant alleles in different populations of *H. contortus* from Himalayan and sub-Himalayan regions of North-West India. *Trop. Anim. Hlth. Prod.,* 41: 1127-1131

Garg, R., Kumar, R.R., Yadav, C.L. and Banerjee, P.S. (2007). Duration of anthelmintic effect of three formulations of ivermectin (oral, inject able and pour-on) against multiple anthelmintic-resistant *H. contortus* in sheep. *Vet. Res. Comm.,* 31: 749-755

Gettinby, E., Armour, J., Bairden, K. and Plenderleith, R.W.J. (1987). A survey by questionnaire of parasitic worm control in cattle and sheep at the Glasgow University Lanark practise. *Vet. Rec.,* 121: 487-490

Gezahegn, L. (1992). Report to the Ministry of Agriculture, Addis Ababa, Ethiopia, pp. 28

Gill, B.S. (1996). Anthelmintic resistance in India. *Vet. Parasitol.,* 63: 173-176

Gopal, R.M., Pomray, W.E. and West, D.M. (1999). Resistance of field isolates of *T. colubriformis* and *O. circumcincta* to ivermectin. *Int. J. Parasitol.,* 29: 781-786

Gordon, H.M. (1950). Some aspects of parasitic gastroenteritis. *Aust. Vet. J.,* 26: 65-72

Graber, M. (1965). Helminthes and helminthiosis faisant obstacle a al ameleration de la production ovine en republique de Chad. *Int. J. Parasitol.,* 7: 435-442

Gupta, S.K., Chaudhri, S.S. and Poonia, J.S. (2003). Preliminary report of closantel resistance against *H. contortus* in sheep in western Haryana. *Indian J. Anim. Sci.,* 73: 1024-1026

Hall, C.A., Campbell, N.J. and Carroll, S.N. (1979). Resistance to thiabendazole in a field population of *O. circumcincta* from sheep. *Aust. Vet. J.*, 55: 229-231

Hennessy, D.R. (1994). The disposition of antiparasitic drugs in relation to the development of resistance by parasites of livestock. *Acta Trop.*, 56: 125-141

Hennessy, D.R., Ali, D.N. and Steel, J.W. (1991). The pharmacodynamic relationship of oxfendazole with feed intake in sheep. *Acta Vet. Scand.*, 87: 389-391

Hertzberg, H., Rossmann, J., Kohler, L. and Willi, U. (2000). Benzimidazole-resistance in gastrointestinal nematodes of sheep and goats in Switzerland. *Wiener Tierarztliche Monatsschrift*, 87: 3-9

Hira Ram, Ram Naresh, Singh, S.K. and Sharma, A.K. (2004). Comparative efficacy of albendazole plus rafoxanide and ivermectin against gastrointestinal nematodes in Pashmina goats 15th NCVP, GBPUAT, Pantnagar, Oct. 25-27

Holmes, P., Sackett, D., Abbott, K., Jephcott, S. and Barber, M. (2006). Assessing the economic cost of endemic disease on the profitability of Australian beef cattle and sheep producers. Meat and Livestock Australia Project No. AHW 087

Hong, C., Hunt, K.R., Harris, T.J., Coles, G.C., Grimshaw, E.T.R. and McMullin, P.F. (1992). A survey of benzimidazole resistance in sheep in three counties of southern England. *Vet. Rec.*, 131: 5-7

Hong, C., Hunt, K.R. and Coles, G.C. (1996). Occurrence of anthelmintic resistant nematodes on sheep farms in England and goat farms in England and Wales. *Vet. Rec.*, 139: 83-86

Hoste, H., Chartier, C. and Le Frileux, Y. (2002). Control of gastrointestinal parasitism with nematodes in dairy goats by treating the host category at risk. *Vet. Res.*, 33: 531-545

Hotson, I.K., Campbell, N.J. and Smeal, M.G. (1970). Anthelmintic resistance in *T. colubriformis*. *Aust. Vet. J.*, 46: 356-60

Hubert, J. and Kerboeuf, D. (1992). A microlarval development assay for the detection of anthelmintic resistance in sheep nematode. *Vet. Rec.*, 130: 442-446

Hughes, P.L., McKenna, P.B. and Dowling, A.F. (2005). A survey of the prevalence of emerging macrocyclic lactone resistance and of benzimidazole resistance in sheep nematodes in the lower North Island of New Zealand. *New Zealand Vet. J.*, 53: 87-90

Ihler, C.F. (2010). Anthelmintic resistance. An overview of the situation in the Nordic countries. *Acta Vet. Scand.*, 52 (Suppl. 1): S24

Iqbal, Z., Akhtar, M., Khan, M.N. and Riaz, M. (1993). Prevalence and economic significance of haemonchosis in sheep and goat slaughtered at Faisalabad. *Pakistan J. Agri. Sci.*, 30: 51-53

Jayathilakan, N., Radha, G., Gomthinayagam, S. and John, L. (2003). Emergence of anthelmintic resistance in nematodes of sheep in Tamil Nadu. *J. Vet. Parasitol.*, 17: 159-160

Johansen, M.V. (1989). An evaluation of techniques used for the detection of anthelmintic resistance in nematode parasites of domestic livestock. *Vet. Res. Comm.*, 13: 455-466

Kerboeuf, D. and Hubert, J. (1985). Benzimidazole resistance in field strains of nematodes from goats in France. *Vet. Rec.*, 116: 133

Kerboeuf, D., Beaumont-Schwartz, C., Hubert, J. and Maillon, M. (1988). Anthelmintic resistance of gastrointestinal helminths in small ruminants. Results of a survey in Val de Loire, France. *Recueil de Medecine Veterinaire*, 164: 1001-1006

Kettle, P.R., Vlassoff, A., Lukies, J.M., Ayling, J.M. and McMurtry, L.W. (1981). A survey of nematode control measures used by sheep farmers and of anthelmintic resistance on their farms. Part I. North Island and the Nelson region of the South Island. *New Zealand Vet. J.*, 29: 81-83

Knox, M.R. (1996). Integrated control programs using medicated blocks. In: *Sustainable Parasite Control in Small Ruminants.* (eds. L.F. Le Jambre and M.R. Knox). ACIAR Proc. No. 74. Canberra, Australia, pp. 141-145

Kochapakdee, S., Pandey, V.S., Pralomkarn, W., Choldumrongkul, S., Ngampongsai, W. and Lawpetchara, A. (1995). Anthelmintic resistance in goats in southern Thailand. *Vet. Rec.*, 137: 124-125

Kyriazakis, I., Tolkamp, B.J. and Hutching, M.R. (1998). Towards a functional explanation for the occurrence of anorexia during parasitic infection. *Anim. Behaviour*, 56: 265-274

Kumar, R. and Yadav, C.L. (1994). Prevalence of fenbendazole resistance in ovine nematodes in North West India. *Trop. Anim. Hlth. Prod.*, 26: 230-234

Kwa, M.S., Veenstra, J.G. and Roos, M.H. (1993). Molecular characterisation of b-tubulin genes present in benzimidazole resistant population of *H. contortus. Mol. Bioch. Parasitol.*, 60: 133-144

Lacey, E. and Prichard, R.K. (1986). Interactions of benzimidazoles (BZ) with tubulin from BZ-sensitive and BZ-resistant isolates of *H. contortus. Mol. Bioch. Parasitol.*, 19: 171-181

Lacey, E., Redwin, J.M., Gill, J.H., Dermarghesiti, V.M. and Waller, P.J. (1990). A larval development assay for simultaneous detection of broad-spectrum anthelmintic resistance. In: *Resistance of Parasites to Antiparasitic Drugs* (eds.

J.C. Boray, P.J. Martin and R.T. Rouch), MSD AGVET, Rahway, New Jersey, pp. 177-184

Laha, R., Hemaprasanth and Harbola, P.C. (1999). Anthelmintic resistance in Pashmina (cashmere) producing goats in India. *Vet. Res. Comm.*, 23: 187-189

Larsen, J.W., Vizard, A.L. and Anderson, N. (1995). Production losses in Merino ewes and financial penalties caused by trichostrongylid infections during winter and spring. *Aust. Vet. J.*, 72: 58-63

Leathwick, D.M., Pomroy, W. and Heath, A.C.G. (2001). Anthelmintic resistance in New Zealand. *New Zealand Vet. J.*, 49: 227-235

Le Jambre, L.F. (1978). The epidemiology and control of gastrointestinal parasites of sheep in Australia. CSIRO, Division of Animal Health, Melbourne, pp. 109

Le Jambre, L.F. (2006). Eradication of targeted species of internal parasites. *Vet. Parasitol.*, 139: 360-370

Le Jambre, L.F., Southcott, W.H. and Dash, K.M. (1976). Resistance of selected lines of *H. contortus* to thiabendazole, morantel tartrate and levamisole. *Int. J. Parasitol.*, 6: 217-222

Le Jambre, L.F., Southcott, W.H. and Dash, K.M. (1978). Development of simultaneous resistance in *O. circumcincta* to thiabendazole, morantel tartrate and levamisole. *Int. J. Parasitol.*, 8: 443-447

Le Jambre, L.F., Gill, J.H., Lenane, I.J. and Baker, P. (2000). Inheritance of avermectin resistance in *H. contortus*. *Int. J. Parasitol.*, 30: 105-111

Lubega, G.W. and Prichard, R.K. (1991a). Specific interaction of benzimidazole anthelmintics with tubulin: high affinity binding and benzimidazole resistance in *H. contortus*. *Mol. Bioch. Parasitol.*, 38: 221-32

Lubega, G.W. and Prichard, R.K. (1991b). Interaction of benzimidazole anthelmintics with *H. contortus* tubulin: binding affinity and anthelmintic efficacy. *Exp. Parasitol.*, 73: 203-213

Maharshi, A.K., Swarnkar, C.P., Singh, D. and Manohar, G.S. (2009). Comparative evaluation of different methods of calculation for faecal egg count reduction. *Indian J. Small. Rum.*, 15: 205-211

Maharshi, A.K., Swarnkar, C.P., Singh, D., Manohar, G.S. and Ayub, M. (2011a). Status of anthelmintic resistance in gastrointestinal nematodes of sheep in Rajasthan. *Indian J. Anim. Sci.*, 81: 105-109

Maharshi, A.K., Swarnkar, C.P., Singh, D. and Manohar, G.S. (2011b). Correlation between status of benzimidazole resistance in *H. contortus* on bio and molecular assays. *Indian J. Anim. Sci.*, 81: 110-115

Maingi, N., Bjorn, H., Dangolla, A. and Kyvsgaard, N.C. (1996). A questionnaire survey of nematode parasite control practices on goat farms in Denmark. *Vet. Parasitol.*, 66: 25-37

Makvana, V.N. and Singh, V. (2009). Emergence of anthelmintic resistance in nematode parasites of sheep at an organized farm in Gujarat. *J. Vet. Parasitol.*, 23: 43-46

Malan, F.S., van Wyk, J.A. and Wessels, C.D. (2001). Clinical evaluation of anaemia in sheep: early trials. *Onderstepoort J. Vet. Res.*, 68: 165-147

Martin, P.J. and Le Jambre, L.F. (1979). Larval paralysis as an *in-vitro* assay of levamisole and morantel tartrate resistance in *Ostertagia. Vet. Sci. Comm.*, 3: 159-164

Martin, P.J. and McKenzie, J.A. (1990). Levamisole resistance in *T. colubriformis*: a sex-linked recessive character. *Int. J. Parasitol.*, 20: 867-872

Martin, P.J., Le Jambre, L.F. and Claxton, J.H. (1981). The impact of *refugia* on the development of thiabendazole resistance in *H. contortus. Int. J. Parasitol.*, 11: 35-41

McKenna, P.B. (1989). Multigeneric resistance to benzimidazole anthelmintics in sheep. *New Zealand Vet. J.*, 37: 62-64

McKenna, P.B. (1990). The detection of anthelmintic resistance by the faecal egg count reduction test: an examination of some of the factors affecting performance and interpretation. *New Zealand Vet. J.*, 38: 142-147

McLeod, R.S. (1995). Costs of major parasites to the Australian livestock industries. *Int. J. Parasitol.*, 25: 1363-1367

McLeod, R.S. (2004). The economic impact of worm infections in small ruminants of Southeast Asia, India and Australia. In: *Worm Control for Small Ruminants in Tropical Asia*, (eds. R.A. Sani, G.D. Gray and R.L. Baker), ACIAR Monograph 113, Australia, pp. 23-33

Mejia, M.E., Fernandez-Igartua, B.M., Schmidt, E.E. and Cabaret, J. (2003). Multi-species and multiple anthelmintic resistance on cattle nematodes in a farm in Argentina: the beginning of high resistance? *Vet. Res.*, 34: 461-467

Middelberg, A. and McKenna, P.B. (1983). Oxfendazole resistance in *N. spathiger. New Zealand Vet. J.*, 31: 65-66

Mitchell, G.B.B., Jackson, F. and Coop, R.L. (1991). Anthelmintic resistance in Scotland. *Vet. Rec.*, 129: 58

Molento, M.B., Gaviao, A.A., Depner, R.A. and Pires, C.C. (2009). Frequency of treatment and production performance using the FAMACHA method compared with preventive control in ewes. *Vet. Parasitol.*, 162: 314-319

Moussavou-Boussougou, M.N., Silvestre, A., Cortet, J., Sauve, C. and Cabaret, J. (2007). Substitution of benzimidazole-resistant nematodes for susceptible nematodes in grazing lambs. *Parasitol.*, 134: 553-560

Nari, A., Salles, J., Castell, D. and Hansen, J.W. (1997). Control of gastrointestinal nematodes in farming systems of Uruguay. In: *Biological Control Workshop.* (eds. J.W. Hansen and P.J. Waller), FAO Technical Series Report No. 141, pp. 89-94

Overend, D.J., Phillips, M.L., Poulton, A.L. and Foster, C.E.D. (1994). Anthelmintic resistance in Australian sheep nematode populations. *Aust. Vet. J.*, 71: 117-121

Papadopoulos, E., Himonas, C. and Coles, G.C. (2001). Drought and flock isolation may enhance the development of anthelmintic resistance in nematodes. *Vet. Parasitol.*, 97: 253-259

Perry, B.D., Randolph, T.F., McDermott, J.J., Sones, K.R. and Thornton, P.K. (2002). Investing in animal health research to alleviate poverty. ILRI, Nairobi, Kenya, pp. 148

Petersen, M.B., Craven, J., Bjorn, H. and Nansen, P. (2000). Use of a migration assay for the separation of adult pyrantel-susceptible and resistant *O. dentatun. Vet. Parasitol.*, 91: 141-145

Presidente, P.J.A. (1985). Methods for detection of nematode resistance to anthelmintics. In: *Resistance in nematodes to anthelmintic drugs.* (eds. N. Anderson and P.J. Waller), Division of animal health and Australian wool corporation, CSIRO, Sydney, pp. 13-28

Prichard, R. (2001). Genetic variability following selection of *H. contortus* with anthelmintics. *Trends Parasitol.*, 17: 445-453

Prichard, R.K. and Roulet, A. (2007). ABC transporters and beta-tubulin in macrocyclic lactone resistance: prospects for marker development. *Parasitol.*, 134: 1123-1132

Prichard, R.K., Hall, C.A., Kelly, J.D., Martin, I.C.A. and Donald, A.D. (1980). The problem of anthelmintic resistance in nematodes. *Aust. Vet. J.*, 56: 239-251

Reinemeyer, C.R., Rohrbach, B.W., Grant, V.M. and Radde, G.L. (1992). A survey of ovine parasite control practices in Tennessee. *Vet. Parasitol.*, 42: 111-122

Riffkin, G.C., Callinan, A.P.C., Freemantle, A.M., Wescott, J.M., Napthine, D.V. and O'Connor, A.J. (1984). Anthelmintic resistance and sheep management practices in South-western Victoria. *Aust. Vet. J.*, 61: 248-251

Romero, J., Boero, C., Vazquez, R., Aristizabal, M.T. and Baldo, A. (1998). Study of anthelmintic resistance in sheep flocks in Argentine Mesopotamia. *Revista de Medicina Veterinaria Buenos Aires*, 79: 342-346

Roos, M.N. (1997). The role of drugs in the control of parasitic nematode infections: must we do without? *Parasitol.*, 14: 137-144

Roos, M.H., Boersema, J.H., Borgsteede, F.H., Cornelissen, J., Taylor, M. and Ruitenberg, E.J. (1990). Molecular analysis of selection for benzimidazole resistance in the sheep parasite *H. contortus*. *Mol. Bioch. Parasitol.*, 43: 77-88

Roos, M.H., Kwa, M.S. and Grant, W.N. (1995). New genetic and practical implications of selection for anthelmintic resistance in parasitic nematodes. *Parasitol. Today*, 1: 148-150

Sangster, N.C. (1990). Biochemical diagnosis of anthelmintic resistance. In: *Resistance of Parasites to Antiparasitic Drugs* (eds: J.C. Boray, P.J. Martin and R.T. Rouch), MSD AGVET, Rahway, NJ., pp. 171-176

Sangster, N.C. (1999). Anthelmintic resistance: past, present and future. *Int. J. Parasitol.*, 29: 115-124

Sangster, N.C. and Gill, J. (1999). Pharmacology of anthelmintic resistance. *Parasitol. Today*, 15: 141-146

Sangster, N.C., Whitlock, H.V., Russ, I.G., Gunawan, M., Griffin, D.L. and Kelly, J.D. (1979). *T. colubriformis* and *O. circumcincta* resistant to levamisole, morantel tartrate and thiabendazole: occurrence of field strains. *Res. Vet. Sci.*, 27: 106-110

Sankar, M. (2003). Studies on benzimidazole resistance in *H. contortus* in sheep, MVSc thesis, Deemed University, IVRI, Izatnagar

Sankar, M. (2007). Molecular characterization of â-tubulin gene in benzimidazole resistant and susceptible populations of common gastrointestinal nematodes in small ruminants, PhD thesis, Deemed University, IVRI, Izatnagar

Sanyal, P.K. (2009). Automated technology transfer for sustainable control of parasitic gastroenteritis in small ruminants: A review. *Indian J. Small Rum.*, 15: 134-155

Sanyal, P.K. and Godke, Y. (1996). The influence of species and sub clinical parasitism on the kinetic disposition of fenbendazole in domestic small ruminants. *Indian Vet. J.*, 73: 392-395

Sanyal, P.K. and Singh, D.K. (1992). Plasma oxfendazole profile in buffalo and cattle: A marker of pharmacokinetics of fenbendazole. *Buff. J.*, 8: 157-61

Scherrer, A.M., Pomroy, W.E. and Charleston, W.A.G. (1990). Anthelmintic usages on goat farms in New Zealand: Results of a postal survey. *New Zealand Vet. J.*, 38: 133-135

Schillhorn van Veen, T.W. (1973). Small ruminant health problems in northern Nigeria with emphasis on the helminthiasis. *Nigerian Vet. J.*, 2: 26-31

Silvestre, A., Leignel, V., Berrag, B., Gasnier, N., Humbert, J.F., Chartier, C. and Cabaret, J. (2002). Sheep and goat nematode resistance to anthelmintics: pro and cons among breeding management factors. *Vet. Res.*, 33: 465-480

Singh, D. and Swarnkar, C.P. (2008). Role of *refugia* in management of anthelmintic resistance in nematodes of small ruminants- A review. *Indian J. Small Rum.* 14: 141-180

Singh, D. and Swarnkar, C.P. (2010). Harnessing the advantages of over-dispersion in faecal egg counts through targeted selective treatment and breeding for diseases resistance, 20th NCVP, CCS HAU, Hisar, Haryana, Feb. 18-20

Singh, D. and Swarnkar, C.P. (2012). Evalution of targeted selective treatment strategy in sheep form of Rajasthan. *Indian J. Anim. Sci.*, 82: 679-686.

Singh, D., Gulyani, R. and Bhasin, V. (1992). Occurrence of thiabendazole resistance strain of *H. contortus* in sheep. *Indian Vet. Med. J.*, 16: 139-141

Singh, D., Swarnkar, C.P., Khan, F.A., Srivastava, C.P. and Bhagwan, P.S.K. (1995). Resistance to albendazole in gastrointestinal nematodes of sheep. *J. Vet. Parasitol.*, 9: 95-98

Singh, D., Swarnkar, C.P., Srivastava, C.P., Bhagwan, P.S.K. and Dimri, U. (1996). *H. contortus* resistant to rafoxanide in sheep. *J. Vet. Parasitol.*, 10: 53-56

Singh, D., Sanyal, P.K., Swarnkar, C.P., Khan, F.A. and Bhagwan, P.S.K. (1999). Influence of diet type and pre treatment fasting on the disposition kinetics of albendazole in sheep. *Vet. Res. Comm.*, 23: 229-40

Singh, D., Swarnkar, C.P. and Khan, F.A. (2002). Anthelmintic resistance in gastrointestinal nematodes of livestock in India. *J. Vet. Parasitol.*, 16: 115-130

Singh, D. Swarnkar, C.P., Prince, L.L.L. and Pathak, K.M.L. (2011). Economic analysis and impact of gastrointestinal nematodes on sheep production in Rajasthan. Directorate of Knowledge Management in Agriculture, ICAR. New Delhi. pp. 1-84.

Sissay, M.M., Asefa, A., Uggla, A. and Waller, P.J. (2006). Anthelmintic resistance of nematode parasites of small ruminants in eastern Ethiopia: exploitation of *refugia* to restore anthelmintic efficacy. *Vet. Parasitol.*, 135: 337-346

Smith, G., Greenfall, B.T., Isham, V. and Corneu, S. (1999). Anthelmintic resistance revisited: under-dosing, chemoprophylactic strategies and matting probabilities. *Int. J. Parasitol.*, 29: 77-91

Soulsby, E.J.L. (2007). New concepts in strongyle control and anthelmintic resistance: the role of refugia. *Vet. J.*, 174: 6-7

Srivastava, V.K., Kumar, P.N., Khanna, P.N. and Singh, M. (1995). Gastrointestinal nematodiasis and drug resistance in sheep. *Indian Vet. J.*, 72: 14-16

Stringfellow, F. (1988). An *in-vitro* test for drug resistance in *Haemonchus contortus. Proc. Helminthol. Soc. Washington*, 55: 19-23

Suchitra, S. and Joshi, P. (2005). Characterisation of *H. contortus* calerticulin suggests its role in feeding and immune evasion by the parasite. *Biochimica et Biophysica Acta*, 1722: 293-303

Sutherland, I.A. and Lee, D.L. (1989). Colorimetric assay for detection of benzimidazole resistance in trichostrongylides. *Res. Vet. Sci.*, 46: 363-366

Swarnkar, C.P. and Singh, D. (2010a). Worm control practices, anthelmintic use and its implication on anthelmintic resistance in gastrointestinal nematodes of sheep in Rajasthan. *Indian J. Anim. Sci.*, 80: 593-600

Swarnkar, C.P. and Singh, D. (2010b). Questionnaire Survey on sheep husbandry and worm management practices adopted by farmers in Rajasthan. *Indian J. Small Rum.*, 16: 199-209

Swarnkar, C.P. and Singh, D. (2010c). Targeted selective treatment for management of haemonchosis in sheep flocks. In: *National Seminar on Stress Management in Small Ruminants Production and Product Processing*, ISSGPU, Jaipur, Jan. 29-31

Swarnkar, C.P., Khurana, K.L., Srivastava, C.P., Dimri, U., Bhagwan, P.S.K. and Lonkar, P.S. (1993). Evaluation of anthelmintic resistance in ovine haemonchosis in an organised sheep farm, Vth NCVP, Udgir, April 21-23

Swarnkar, C.P., Sanyal, P.K., Singh, D., Khan, F.A. and Bhagwan, P.S.K. (1998). Comparative disposition kinetics of albendazole in sheep following oral and intraruminal administration. *Vet. Res. Comm.*, 22: 545-551

Swarnkar, C.P., Singh, D., Khan, F.A. and Bhagwan, P.S.K. (1999a). Multiple anthelmintic resistance in *H. contortus* of sheep in arid Rajasthan. *Indian J. Anim. Sci.*, 69: 547-549

Swarnkar, C.P., Khan, F.A., Singh, D. and Bhagwan, P.S.K. (1999b). Further studies on anthelmintic resistance in sheep at an organised farm in arid region of Rajasthan. *Vet. Parasitol.*, 82: 83-84

Swarnkar, C.P., Sanyal, P.K., Singh, D., Khan, F.A. and Bhagwan, P.S.K. (2001). Anthelmintic resistance in an organised sheep farm in India. *Trop. Anim. Hlth. Prod.*, 33: 305-312

Swarnkar, C.P., Singh, D., Khan, F.A., Tiwari, R. and Dubey, S.C. (2004). Prevalence of anthelmintic resistance and seasonal variation in efficacy of anthelmintic in sheep, 15th NCVP, GBPUAT, Pantnagar, Oct. 25-27

Swarnkar, C.P., Singh, D., Kumar, S., Khan, F.A. and Tiwari, J. (2006). Investigations on the seasonal pattern of strongyle infection in sheep and interaction between genotypes of *H. contortus* in *refugia* and benzimidazole resistance in Rajasthan, 17th NCVP, RGCVS, Puducherry, Nov. 15-17

Swarnkar, C.P., Singh, D., Lal Krishna and Khan, F.A. (2008). Epidemiology and Management of Gastrointestinal Parasites of Sheep in Rajasthan, CSWRI, Avikanagar, pp. 1-145

Swarnkar, C.P., Singh, D., Price, L.L.L. and Paswan, C. (2011). Estimation of economic losses due to natural strongyle infection in adult sheep of Rajasthan. XXI NCVP, Bombay Veterinary College, Mumbai, Maharashtra, Jan. 5-7

Swarnkar, C.P., Singh, D. and Kumar, Satish, (2012). Prevalence of benzimidozole resistant β-tubulin alleles in *H. contortus* larvae from sheep of Rajasthan. *Indian J. Anim. Sec.* 82: 1477-1481.

Taylor, M.A. and Hunt, K.R. (1989). Anthelmintic drug resistance in UK. *Vet. Rec.*, 125: 143-147

Temaja, T.T.G.N. (1980). Redoma Pengendalian Penyakit Menular. Jilid-II, Direktorat Keschatan Hewan. Direktorat Jenderal Penernakan, Jakarta, pp. 83-89

Tiwari, J., Kumar, S., Kolte, A.P., Swarnkar, C.P., Singh, D. and Pathak, K.M.L. (2006). Detection of benzimidazole resistance in *H. contortus* using RFLP-PCR technique. *Vet. Parasitol.*, 138: 301-307

Tiwari, J., Kolte, A.P., Kumar, S., Swarnkar, C.P., Singh, D. and Pathak, K.M.L. (2007). Diagnosis of benzimidazole resistance in *H. contortus* of sheep by allele specific PCR. *Asian-Australian J. Anim. Sci.*, 20: 7–11

Uppal, R.P., Yadav, C.L., Godara, P. and Rana, J.S. (1992). Multiple anthelmintic resistance in a field strain of *H. contortus* in goats. *Vet. Res. Comm.*, 16: 195-198

van Aken, D., De Bont, J. and Vercruysse, J. (1989). Benzimidazole resistance in a field population of *H. contortus* from goats in Sri Lanka. *Small Rum. Res.*, 2: 281-287

van Wyk, J.A. (2008). Production trials involving use of the FAMACHA© system for haemonchosis in sheep: preliminary results. *Onderstepoort J. Vet. Res.*, 75: 331-345

van Wyk, J.A. and Malan, F.S. (1988). Resistance of field strains of *H. contortus* to ivermectin, closantel, rafoxanide and benzimidazole in South Africa. *Vet. Rec.*, 123: 226-228

van Wyk, J.A. and van Schalkwyk, P.C. (1990). A novel approach to the control of anthelmintic-resistant *H. contortus* in sheep. *Vet. Parasitol.*, 35: 61-69 van Wyk, J.A., Stenson, M.O., van der Merwe , J.S., Vorster, R.J. and Viljoen, P.G. (1999). Anthelmintic resistance in South Africa: survey indicates an extremely serious situation in sheep and goat farming. *Onderstepoort J. Vet. Res.*, 66: 273-284

Varshney, T.R. and Singh, Y.P. (1976). A note on development of resistance of *H. contortus* against phenothiazine and thiabendazole in sheep. *Indian J. Anim. Sci.*, 46: 666-668

Vieira, L.S., Berne, M.E.A., Cavalcante, A.C.R. and Costa, G.A.F. (1992). *H. contortus* resistance to ivermectin and netobimin in Brazilian sheep. *Vet. Parasitol.*, 45: 111-116

Waller, P.J. (1997). Anthelmintic resistance. *Vet. Parasitol.*, 72: 391-412

Waller, P.J., Dash, K.M., Berger, I.A., Le Jambre, L.F. and Plant, J. (1995). Anthelmintic resistance in nematode parasites of sheep: learning from Australian experience. *Vet. Rec.*, 136: 411-413

Waruiru, R.M., Maingi, N. and Gichanga, E.J. (1991). The prevalence of anthelmintic resistance in sheep in three districts of Kenya. *Bull. Anim. Hlth. Prod. Afr.*, 39: 423-428

Waruiru, R.M., Kogi, J.K., Weda, E.H. and Ngotho, J.W. (1998). Multiple anthelmintic resistance on a goat farm in Kenya. *Vet. Parasitol.*, 75: 191-197

Webb, R.F., McCully, C.H., Clarke, F.L., Greentree, P. and Honey, P. (1979b). The incidence of thiabendazole resistance in field populations of *H. contortus* on the northern Tablelands of New South Wales. *Aust. Vet. J.*, 55: 422-426

Wolstenholme, A.J., Fairweather, I., Pritchard, R., von Samson-Himmelstjerna, G. and Sangster, N.C. (2004). Drug resistance in veterinary helminths. *Trends Parasitol.*, 20: 469-476

Wood, I.B., Amaral, N.K., Bairden, K., Duncan, J.L., Kassai, T., Malone, J.B., Pankavich, J.A., Reinecke, R.K., Slocombe, O., Taylor, S.M. and Vercruysse, J. (1995). World Association for the Advancement of Veterinary Parasitology (WAAVP), 2nd edition of guidelines for evaluating the efficacy of anthelmintics in ruminants (bovine, ovine, caprine). *Vet. Parasitol.*, 58: 181-213

Yadav, C.L. and Garg, R. (2005). Status of anthelmintic resistance in gastrointestinal nematodes in India. In: *FAO Symposium on Integrated Animal Parasite Management: from academic interest to realty*. Dec. 8, pp. 9-22

Yadav, C.L. and Garg, R. (2007). Anthelmintic resistance in India: Current status and future directions. In: XVIII NCVP, SKUAT-J, Sept. 7-9, pp. 121-128

Yadav, C.L. and Uppal, R.P. (1992). Levamisole resistant *H. contortus* in goats. *Vet. Rec.*, 130: 228

Yadav, C.L., Uppal, R.P. and Kalra, S. (1993). Outbreak of haemonchosis associated with anthelmintic resistance in sheep. *Int. J. Parasitol.*, 23: 411-413

Yadav, C.L., Kumar, R., Uppal, R.P. and Verma, S.P. (1995). Multiple anthelmintic resistance in *H. contortus* on a sheep farm in India. *Vet. Parasitol.*, 60: 355-60

Yadav, C.L., Ghorui, S.K., Singh, B.P. and Sharma, M.C. (1996). Benzimidazole resistance in *H. contortus* of sheep and goats in Uttar Pradesh, *India. J. Vet. Parasitol.*, 10: 47-51.

□□□

Chapter 4

Cryptosporidiosis in Bovine and Human

Anish Yadav and M. Katoch*
Division of Veterinary Parasitology,
Faculty of Veterinary Sciences and Animal Husbandry, S.K. University of Agricultural Sciences and Technology, R.S. Pura, Jammu- 181102, India
* Indian Institute of Integrative Medicine (CSIR), Canal Road, Jammu

Introduction

Cryptosporidium, a coccidian, intracellular protozoan parasite of the phylum Apicomplexa once thought to be rare and host specific is now known to be ubiquitous and has multiple hosts (Navin and Juranek, 1984). It infects the gastrointestinal tract of both human and livestock and considered the third major cause of diarrhoea worldwide (Spano *et al.*, 2000). A variety of domestic and wild animals including calves, pigs, and wild rodents etc. appear to be important zoonotic reservoirs for *Cryptosporidium parvum* to man (Chalmers *et al.*, 1997). Among the entire animal hosts, calves are the most important from public health point of view, as they may serve as a source of human infection (O'Donoghue, 1995). In human, the infection in immunocompetent adult is generally acute and self-limiting, whereas immunocompromised individuals can develop chronic and potentially life threatening diarrhoea particularly in patients suffering from AIDS (Carraway *et al.*, 1996). Similar type of life threatening infection has been reported in neonatal animals suffering from malnutrition, hypovitaminosis and immunodeficiency syndromes (Fukushima and Helman, 1984). Attention to human cryptosporidiosis began with the emergence of chronic and life- threatening cryptosporidiosis with HIV/AIDS in early 1980s. The association with AIDS is so strong that cryptosporidiosis became one of the defining features of the syndrome before the discovery of causative virus (Tzpori and Widmer, 2008).

Cryptosporidiosis is considered as an emerging waterborne disease of public health significance because of the potential for environmental contamination with *Cryptosporidium* oocysts, although the actual cases have been under reported (Hunter and Nicholas, 2002). The chapter includes information on various aspects of cryptosporidiosis viz. epidemiology, clinical signs, diagnosis and treatment in bovines and humans (especially children and HIV positive patients). Literature pertaining to molecular and biological characterization of *Cryptosporidium* spp. as well as zoonotic potential of the same has also been incorporated.

Historical Perspective

Ernest Edward Tyzzer first recognized *Cryptosporidium* muris, from the gastric glands of laboratory mice (Tyzzer, 1907). Subsequently he recognized the multispecies nature of the parasite and proposed the genus *Cryptosporidium* with *C. muris* as the type species (Tyzzer, 1910). A few years later he described a second species *Cryptosporidium parvum*, also from laboratory mice (Tyzzer, 1912). *Cryptosporidium parvum* differed from the type species not only by infecting the small intestine rather than the stomach but also because the oocysts were smaller (Tyzzer, 1912; Upton and Current, 1985). Later many new species of *Cryptosporidium* were reported from different parts of the world (reviewed by Xiao, 2004). Following the initial discovery of *Cryptosporidium*, over 50 years elapsed during which *Cryptosporidium* spp. were regarded as commensals until their association with diarrhoea in young turkeys (*C. meleagridis*) in the 1950s, and with large outbreaks of diarrhoea in calves (*C. parvum*) in the 1970s. Infection by *Cryptosporidium* spp. in cattle was first reported in the 1971 (Panciera *et al.*, 1971). However, Tzipori *et al.* (1980) documented for the first time the role of *Cryptosporidium* spp. as primary enteropathogen associated with bovine neonatal diarrhoea. Attention to human cryptosporidiosis began with the emergence of chronic and life-threatening cryptosporidiosis with HIV/ AIDS in early 1980s.

The genus *Cryptosporidium* was classified under the family Cryptosporidiidae, suborder- Eimeriorina, Order- Eucoccidiorida, Subclass- Coccidiasina, Class- Sporozoasida. Phylum- Apicomplexa (Levine, 1985). Despite showing strong morphological similarities to the coccidian parasites and the presence of mitochondria like organelle, molecular data suggested that *Cryptosporidium* spp. was either more closely related to gregarines or Helicobacter bacteria (Striepen *et al.*,

2002). To date about 32 species of *Cryptosporidium* have been reported based on host specificity, but International Commission on Zoological Nomenclature (ICZN) has recognized only 19 species of these as valid (Xiao *et al.*, 2004). In recent years, molecular characterizations of *Cryptosporidium* have helped to clarify the confusion in *Cryptosporidium* taxonomy and validate the existence of multiple species in each vertebrate class. The discovery of sequence-based differences within various genes (ribosomal RNA[rRNA], *Cryptosporidium* heatshock protein 70, actin, *Cryptosporidium* oocyst wall protein [COWP], *Cryptosporidium* thrombospondin-related adhesive protein-1 and-2) and between individual isolates within a 'previously valid' species has resulted in revision of the taxonomy of the genus. Therefore, as for *Cryptosporidium* spp., the current classification of *Cryptosporidium* genotypes will be subject to change.

Life cycle

The first detailed description of the *Cryptosporidium* life cycle was published in 1910 (Tyzzer, 1910). The life cycle of *Cryptosporidium* is complex involving both sexual and asexual developmental stages. Sporulated oocysts are ingested or inhaled by a suitable host (Fayer and Unger, 1986). The sporulated oocyst is the only known exogenous stage, consisting of four sporozoites within an environmentally resistant oocyst wall. The endogenous part of the life cycle begins when the infectious oocyst is ingested. Once inhaled or ingested, oocysts excyst in the gastrointestinal or respiratory tract releasing infective sporozoites. The sporozoites rapidly invade the epithelial cells of the small intestine (mainly the ileum) and respiratory tract where the endogenous phase of the life cycle begins. Within the host cell, the sporozoite transforms into a circular stage known as a trophozoite. The trophozoite undergoes asexual proliferation by merogony (previously called schizogony) to form meronts which contain merozoites. Two types of meronts are formed. Type I meronts each form eight merozoites, which are liberated from the parasitophorous vacuoles when mature. It is believed that Type I merozoites have the ability to recycle indefinitely under suitable environmental conditions. Some type I merozoites penetrate host cells and form type II meronts containing four merozoites. Once liberated, Type II merozoites enter host cells and start the sexual phase in the life cycle. Once inside host cells, Type II merozoites either enlarge and form macrogametes (macrogametocyte), or undergo cellular fission forming microgametocytes contalning 14-16 non-flagellated microgametocytes. Microgametes rupture from microgametocytes and penetrate cells harbouring macrogametocytes, to form a zygote. A resistant oocyst wall is then formed around the zygote and sporozoites are formed by sporogony. The only exogenous stage of the *Cryptosporidium* life cycle is the sporulated, thick-walled oocyst, which is excreted in the faeces of an infected host. Fertilized macrogamonts develop into thick-walled oocysts (approximately 80%), which are excreted from the body, or into thin-walled oocysts (about 20%) responsible for repeated asexual and sexual multiplication (autoinfection) within the same host.

Pathogenesis

Cryptosporidium parvum causes acute self-limiting diarrhoea in cattle, humans and other mammals. From experimental infection studies, it has been observed that clinical signs occur within 2-7 days of challenge and a prepatent period of 7-21 days (Thompson *et al.*, 2005). Intestinal enterocytes are infected by sporozoites emerging from ingested thick-walled oocysts or from thin-walled oocysts emerging from infected cells where sexual and asexual reproduction has occurred. Attachment of the sporozoite leads to formation of parasitophorous vacuole on the epithelial surface.

After the initial infection, the endogenous forms are amplified within the gut leading to dissemination of infection throughout the small and large intestine. Occasionally, the gastric mucosa, bile duct, gall bladder and respiratory epithelium are also infected. The distribution of infection may determine the intensity of clinical signs as infection of the proximal small intestine frequently leads to severe watery diarrhoea, while infection localized to the distal ileum and large intestine are frequently asymptomatic. Infections of the pyloric region of the stomach or abomasum are usually asymptomatic. The invasion and colonization of the epithelial surface displaces the microvillus brush border and loss of surface epithelial cells. Villus shortening and fusion as well as crypt hyperplasia also occur as a result of epithelial damage. Colonization of the epithelial surface leads to decreased intestinal surface area, loss of membrane-bound digestive enzymes and impaired nutrient and electrolyte transport (Buret *et al.*, 2003). A putative enterotoxin has been proposed to lead to chloride secretion resulting in secretary diarrhoea (Guarino *et al.*, 1995). *Cryptosporidium* disrupt epithelial tight junctions that can lead to increased epithelial permeability (Buret *et al.*, 2003) and so, malabsorptive and secretary diarrhoea are noticed in cryptosporidiosis.

Bovine cryptosporidiosis

Molecular analysis of *Cryptosporidium* isolates from cattle has resulted in the identification of eight species viz. *C. parvum, C. bovis, C. andersoni C. ryanae, C. hominis, C. felis, C. canis, C. suis* and two genotypes (*C. suis* like genotype and *Cryptosporidium* pig genotype). Out of these, the first mentioned four species has been found most frequently (Fayer *et al.*, 2007). Buffaloes also harbor these four species.

Epidemiology

Cryptosporidiosis is considered to be an emerging disease in developing countries (Tzipori and Ward, 2002), which has greatest prevalence, although the actual cases have been under reported (Hunter and Nicholas, 2002).

In India, bovine cryptosporidiosis for the first time was reported by Nooruddin and Sarma (1987) and in later years many prevalence studies have been undertaken. These reports were based on acid fast staining methods, where in point prevalence was studied. The prevalence of *Cryptosporidium* spp. in different parts of India as reported in literature has been summarized in Table 1.

Table 1: Prevalence of *Cryptosporidium* spp. in animals in India

State	Host species	Prevalence (samples screened)	References
Uttar Pradesh	Cattle	12.9 (93)	Dubey *et al.* (1992)
	Buffalo	14.1 (78)	
	Cattle	33.3 (15)	Jeyabal and Ray (2005)
	Buffalo	53.3 (15)	
	Cattle	21.05 (38)	Maurya *et al.* (2012)
	Cattle and Buffalo	35.4 (291)	Paul *et al.* (2008)
West Bengal	Cattle and Buffalo	33.3 (66)	Roy *et al.* (2006)
Karanataka	Cattle and Buffalo	17.1 (35)	
Andhra Pradesh	Cattle and Buffalo	12.5 (32)	
Kerala	Cattle and Buffalo	9 (33)	

Uttar Pradesh	Cattle Buffalo	18.6 (97) 27 (111)	Pradeep (2008)
Karnataka and Kerala	Pig	22.2 (36)	
Uttar Pradesh, Uttarakhand, Bihar	Cattle and Buffalo Goat	18.7 (246) 1.6 (62)	Maurya (2011)
Jammu and Kashmir	Cattle Buffalo (Diarrhoeic) Non Diarrhoeic	28.1 (384) 11.94 (1440) 15.33 (515) 10.05 (925)	Yadav *et al.* (2010) Yadav *et al.* (2012)
West Bengal	Cattle Buffalo Dog	11.3 (159) 7.85 (51) 0 (50)	Chattopadhyay *et al.* (2000)
	Cattle	22.4 (210)	Das *et al.* (2004)
	Cattle	11.7 (180)	Khan *et al.* (2010)
	Cattle (Diarrhoiec) (Non-Diarrhoiec)	20.8 (149) 32.9 (79) 7.1 (70)	Das *et al.* (2011)
Puducherry	Cattle	25 (129)	Kumar *et al.* (2004)
Tamil Nadu	Cattle	9 (221)	Prakash *et al.* (2009)
Andhra Pradesh	Cattle	61.2	Shobhamani *et al.* (2006)
Karnataka	Cattle	5.7 (455)	Mallinath *et al.* (2009)
Tamil Nadu,	Cattle and Buffalo	11 (677)	Venu (2011)
Andhra Pradesh, Karnataka, Kerela, Puducherry	Cattle and Buffalo	39.65 (459)	Venu *et al.* (2012)
Chhattisgarh	Cattle and Buffalo	21.9 (306)	Sahu *et al.* (2010)

First PCR-based detection of bovine cryptosporidiosis in India was reported by Das *et al.* (2004). Roy *et al.* (2006) characterized the isolates of *Cryptosporidium* spp. from cattle from various parts of West Bengal and found *C. parvum* as the species responsible for bovine cryptosporidiosis. Paul *et al.* (2008) when examined 457 faecal samples of diarrhoeic and non- diarrhoeic neonatal bovine calves (0-3 months) from India using molecular methods detected *C. parvum* in 138 (30.2%) animals. Paul *et al.* (2009a) from India using PCR-RFLP reported 12.85% of the bovine calves (6-24 months of age) positive for *C. andersoni.* As per the findings of Khan *et al.* (2010) occurrence of *C. parvum, C. bovis, C. ryanae* and *C. andersoni* in cattle followed an age-related pattern. A *C.* suis like genotype was also detected in a calf. The study also revealed that farm workers were infected with *Cryptosporidium hominis, C. parvum* and a novel *C. bovis* genotype. These findings clearly suggest that there is a potential risk of zoonotic transmission of Cryptosporidium infections between cattle and humans on dairy farms in India. Venu *et al.* (2012) performed genotyping by PCR- RFLP of 64 samples of calves, where in 39 (60.94%) were classified as *C. andersoni,* 18 (28.13%) as *C. ryanae,* 4 (6.25%) as *C. parvum* and 3 (4.69%) were confirmed as *C. bovis.*

The prevalence of cryptosporidiosis in bovine has also been reported from many countries of the world. The result of prevalence varies widely depending on the sensitivity and specificity of the screening methods used. Conventional staining method like acid fast staining of *Cryptosporidium* spp. oocysts has been used in various prevalence studies. El- Rahim (1997) examined 168 newborn buffalo calves from a dairy herd in Upper Egypt by modified Ziehl-Neelsen and Giemsa staining techniques. The study revealed 38% calves positive for *Cryptosporidium* oocyst in their faeces. Clinical examination, of these 64 cases showed diarrhoea in 40 calves and subclinical positivity was in 24 cases. Naciri, *et al.* (1999) studied the importance of *C. parvum* in diarrhoea of neonatal calves and reported it as the major etiological agent responsible for neonatal diarrhoea as compared to *E. coli,* rotavirus, coronavirus, and *Salmonella.* de la Fuente *et al.* (1999) examined faecal samples from 218 diarrheic dairy calves in 65 dairy herds of 1 to 30-day-old age in Spain, for the presence of *Cryptosporidium* and concurrent infections with rotavirus, coronavirus, F5+ *E. coli* and *Salmonella* spp. *Cryptosporidium* infection was detected in 43.8%, 71.9%, 63.2% and 6.9% of the calves having 1–7, 8–14, 15–21 and 22–30 days of age respectively. *Cryptosporidium* was the only enteropathogen detected in 60 of the 114 (52.6%) diarrheic calves. Concurrent infections with other enteropathogen(s) were detected in 64.3%, 46.3%, 39.5% and 0% of the *Cryptosporidium*-infected calves in the age groups 1–7, 8–14, 15–21 and 22–30 days, respectively. Occurrence of *C. parvum* infection and the pattern of oocyst shedding in calves of Japan were studied by Uga *et al.* (2000). In the study 480 faecal samples from 30 calves (age, = 30 days) were examined by sucrose centrifugal floatation technique and it was observed that 93% calves were passing *Cryptosporidium* oocysts. Oocyst shedding was first detected on sixth day after birth, with 8% of the calves testing positive and reached approximately 80% by day 15. Oocyst shedding varied from 1 to 13 days, with a mean of 7 days. Calves infected with *C. parvum* had a significantly higher rate of diarrhoea (33%) than non-infected calves (8%). The mean number of oocysts excreted by calves (= 30 days old) was approximately 6×107 per gram of faeces. Kváè *et al.* (2006) examined 7021 faecal samples of calves by Sheather's floatation method and stained by aniline–carbol–methyl violet in South Bohemia (Czech Republic) and observed *Cryptosporidium* oocysts in 1814 (25.8%) samples. Based on oocysts morphology *C. parvum* was found in 561 samples (8%) and *C. andersoni* in 1253 (17.8%) calves. Pre-weaned dairy calves had higher infection levels of *C. parvum* than pre-weaned beef calves. The prevalence of *C. parvum* ranged from 1.4 to 56.5% on dairy farms. El-Khodery and Osman (2008) examined 458 fecal samples of buffalo calves (<3 month age) in 55 small scale herds in Middle Egypt by modified Ziehl- Neelsen staining technique and revealed 14.19% positivity for *Cryptosporidium* in calves. Calves of 1–15 days age were at the highest risk, and a significant relationship between season and infection was recorded. Further the study demonstrated the strong relation between infections by *Cryptosporidium* spp. and diarrhoea in buffalo calves. Del Coco *et al.* (2008) reported 48 calves positive for shedding of *Cryptosporidium* oocysts out of the 280 examined from dairy calves (= 30 days of age) of a rural area of Buenos Aires, Argentina using a modified Ziehl-Neelsen acid fast method. Prevalence was higher in =7 days calves (37.5%) as compared to =8 = 14 days calves (21.4%). Both normal and diarrhoeic faeces with blood were observed to be negative for *Cryptosporidium* spp. However 37.5% of diarrhoeic faeces without blood were found positive for *Cryptosporidium* oocysts. Faeces with mucus revealed 83.3% positivity. The relationship between intensity of infection and age group showed that 66.7% of positive samples from calves =7 days old, presented an average of >10 oocysts/field.

Cryptosporidium spp. infection has been recorded by using immunological techniques. Hamnes *et al.* (2006) reported 53% farms (72 out of 136) positive for *Cryptosporidium* in Norway using immunofluorescent staining. Out of 1386 faecal samples examined, 167 were found positive (12 %). Infection peaked in the age group of 2–3 months and the prevalence was higher during winter than summer. Increased herd prevalence was observed with increasing number of calves in the herd. Similarly Coklin *et al.* (2006) using same technique observed *Cryptosporidium* in 4 out of 11 farms examined in Prince Edward Island. Geurden *et al.* (2006) studied the prevalence of *Cryptosporidium* spp. in calves (< 3 months old) using copro-antigen ELISA kit in three different husbandry systems in Zambia. Examination of 250 samples collected from dairy farms, 238 from beef farms, and 256 from traditional husbandry farms, revealed *Cryptosporidium* infection in 42.8%, 8.0% and 6.3%, respectively. Rinaldi *et al.* (2007) examined 347 faecal samples of calves in Italy, using commercially available enzyme-linked immunosorbent assays and observed 63 (18.1%) buffalo calves (1-9 weeks age) positive for *C. parvum.* Among 90 farms screened 22 (24.4%) were found positive for *C. parvum.* Co-infection was observed only in ten (11.1%) farms with *Giardia duodenalis.*

In recent years, highly sensitive technique like PCR has been used for the prevalence studies. Becher *et al.* (2004) conducted a longitudinal study in Western Australia on calves from birth to weaning. *Cryptosporidium* was detected in 48% of animals and no significant association was observed between *Cryptosporidium* occurrence, season or management practices (housing). Calf-to-calf contact was the most common source of transmission. Molecular characterization of isolates revealed presence of *C. parvum.* Santín *et al.* (2004) observed 35.5% calves (345 of 971) to be positive irrespective of age for *Cryptosporidium* using PCR test in 15 dairy farms of seven states on east coast of US. Infection was 50.3% in pre-weaned calves of 5 days to 2 months (253 of 503) and 19.7% in post-weaned calves of 3–11 months (92 of 468). Genetic characterization of 278 positive specimens by gene sequencing revealed *C. parvum,* in 85% pre-weaned calves and 1% in post-weaned calves. The study recommended that persons handling or exposed to calves less than 2 months of age are at greater risk of zoonotic infection from *Cryptosporidium* as compared to person handling older calves.

Coklin *et al.* (2007) revealed *Cryptosporidium* spp. in 27.3% faecal samples of 143 animals from adults, heifers and calves collected from two dairy cattle farms in eastern Ontario, Canada. Molecular characterisation using18S rRNA gene and the heat-shock protein 70 (HSP-70) gene revealed *C. parvum* in 21.7%, and *C. bovis* in 1.4% animals. Geurden *et al.* (2007) observed the prevalence of *Cryptosporidium* in calves (<than 10 weeks) in a cross-sectional epidemiological study on 100 dairy and 50 beef farms in East Flanders (Belgium), using immunofluorescence assay. The prevalence of *Cryptosporidium* was 37% in dairy calves and 12% in beef calves. Santin *et al.* (2008) examined 30 calves from birth to 24 months of age in Maryland using immunofluorescence microscopy and PCR and reported shedding of oocysts of *Cryptosporidium* at some time by all calves during 24 months of the study. Highest prevalence was observed in calves of 2 weeks of age (29 out of 30). Pre-weaned calves (1–8 weeks of age) showed higher prevalence (45.8%) than post-weaned calves (3–12 months of age) 18.5% and lowest in heifers (12–24 months of age) 2.2%. Sequence data for 190 PCR-positive specimens revealed *C. parvum, C. bovis,* the *Cryptosporidium* deer-like genotype and *C. andersoni,* with cumulative prevalences of 100, 80, 60, and 3.3%, respectively. *C. parvum* constituted 97% of infections in pre-weaned calves but only 4% and 0% of infections in post-weaned calves and heifers, respectively. Brook *et al.* (2008) conducted a cross-sectional study for *Cryptosporidium* in young calves of 41 farms of North West England. Molecular diagnosis of 215 faecal samples by PCR of the 18S rRNA gene confirmed *Cryptosporidium* infection in 60 animals. The study suggested that intervention strategies should be targeted at calves under 21 days old as they represent a significant reservoir of infection on the farm and also pose a risk to public health. Keshavarz *et al.* (2009) examined faecal samples of 272 cattle from 15 dairy farms in Qazvin province, Iran. Further oocysts from 51 positive samples were analyzed using PCR assay of 18S SSU rRNA, restriction fragment length polymorphism (RFLP) and sequencing. It was observed that 72.6% of the positive samples were *C. parvum*, 17.7% as *C. andersoni*, 7.8% as *C. bovis* and 1.9% as novel genotype of *C. parvum* possessing a single mutation on MboII restriction. An infection rate of 19.5% of *C. parvum* among 174 pre-weaned calves was significantly higher than the 3.1% among 98 post-weaned calves. Silverlas *et al.* (2010) examined 1202 faecal samples collected from 50 cattle herds in Sweden and revealed 176 positive for *Cryptosporidium* spp. by FITC-labelled anti *Cryptosporidium* monoclonal antibody and PCR method. Molecular characterisation of 18S rRNA gene of *Cryptosporidium* revealed *C. bovis, C. parvum, C. ryanae* and *C. andersoni* in 83, 15, 10 and 2 samples,

respectively. An age related prevalence pattern in species distribution was seen and it was observed that *C. parvum* was detected only in calves younger than 6 weeks, and 11 of the 15 *C. parvum* positive calves were younger than 2 weeks.

Risk Factors for bovine cryptosporidiosis

There are various factors which determine the outcome of infection in livestock. Transmission can occur via any route by which material contaminated with viable oocysts excreted by infected individuals can be ingested. Practices likely to enhance the spread of cryptosporidiosis include indoor calving and feeding the neonates in groups, where young susceptible animals are in close contact with each other and the faeces of infected animals. Similarly, the disposal of faeces, farmyard manure or other contaminated waste in land-based dumps, when followed by periods of heavy rainfall or melting snow can lead to *C. parvum* oocyst contamination of water sources. These sources may be used as a source of drinking water for other animals and for potable water for human consumption. Numbers of studies have explained the effect of age as risk of shedding *Crvptospondium* spp. oocysts. Calves can begin shedding C. *parvum* oocysts as early as 2 days *of* age but the peak shedding occurs at approximately 14 days of age (Becher *et al.*, 2004). Typically, shedding is observed between 1 and 4 weeks of age with infection lasting for about 2 weeks. Similar findings have been reported from India by Kumar *et al.* (2004) , Shobhamani *et al.* (2006) and Paul *et al.* (2008).

Season has also an impact on the prevalence of cryptosporidiosis in bovine calves. The infection is more common in winter whereas lowest in summer (Tzipori 1983, El-Khodery and Osman 2008) which may be because of overcrowding of animals in the organized dairy farms. Paul *et al.* (2008) reported higher infection of *Cryptosporidium* infection in calves in the monsoon months in India (June to September). Higher incidence of cryptosporidiosis was also recorded during hot and humid monsoon months than dry and cooler months (Roy *et al.*, 2006). Gender has no effect on the prevalence of *Cryptosporidium* infection (El-Khodery and Osman, 2008). Higher prevalence of cryptosporidiosis was recorded in male calves than in the female calves (Paul *et al.*, 2008).

Types of floor also act as a risk factor for the infection. The infection is more in calves housed in pens with concrete floors than in those with earth floors (El-Khodery and Osman, 2008). On contrary, Castro-Hamida *et al.* (2002) found that cement floor had lower risk than straw/earth floor due to daily cleaning using water with pressure hose. Further it was observed that the use of straw and deep litter cause protection against *Cryptosporidium* infection or at least excretion (Maddox-Hyttel *et al.*, 2006). The frequency of cleaning (daily or weekly) had an effect on the risk of infection. Calves on herds where pens were cleaned once weekly had a higher prevalence than those pens cleaned daily. The depth of the bedding does play a role as risk factor for cryptosporidiosis. Brook *et al.* (2008) in a study carried on farm animals revealed that calves housed in bedding of 11-15 cm deep being at lower risk of infection than those on beds 0-5 cm deep. It may be because of fact that very scanty bedding is not sufficient to maintain hygienic conditions and may result in higher levels of environmental contamination than deeper bedding.

The water source also contributes to the disease prevalence. Calves drinking water from the wells or underground had higher infection than those were drinking from tap water. This may be attributed to pollution of underground water with drainage as *Cryptosporidium* oocysts have been demonstrated in runoff from agricultural areas (Fayer, 2004). On the other hand, Castro-Hamida *et al.* (2002) didn't record relationship between the source of water and the prevalence of cryptosporidiosis in bovine calves. Effect of the herd size on the occurrence of *Cryptosporidium* spp. infections has been studied. Castro-Hermida *et al.* (2002) found that the smaller numbers of adult cattle in the farm the greater prevalence of cryptosporidiosis. Whereas, it was stated that the higher the density of animals, the greater the number of infected calves and consequently higher prevalence (Mohammed *et al.*, 1999).

Colostrum antibodies and milk antibodies protect calves from developing severe clinical signs by blocking parasite invasion and immobilisation of gut luminal parasitic forms. Micronutrients may also play a significant role in the clinical outcome of cryptosporidiosis as severe clinical signs were observed in calves with selenium deficiency (McAllister *et al.*, 2005).

Clinical features of bovine cryptosporidiosis

Bovine cryptosporidiosis is predominantly a disease of young calves of less than 6 months of age and with the attainment of immunological maturity, the infection subsides in older cattle. The recovered animals become a carrier, thereby serving as a potential source of infection to susceptible population. Cryptosporidiosis in young calves is a costly disease to farmers because of its high prevalence and losses associated with mortalities, body weight loss, impaired body weight gain and costs of treatment.

Calves can begin shedding *C. parvum* oocysts as early as 2 days of age but the peak shedding occurs at approximately 14 days of age (Becher *et al.*, 2004). Typically, shedding is observed between 1 and 4 weeks of age with infection lasting for about 2 weeks. The disease is manifested by diarrhoea (varies from pale yellow with mucus to profuse watery diarrhoea), depression, anorexia and abdominal pain. Clinical signs can persist for 4-14 days and the severity and duration is highly variable. Occasionally dehydration, collapse and mortality rate of up to 35% were recorded due to *C. parvum* in calves less than 1 month of age from dairy animals of Punjab (Singh *et al.*, 2006). Shobhamani and Singari (2006) reported profuse watery faeces with some blood clots, mucus and undigested milk clots, accompanied by mild-fever, depression, lethargy and varying degree of emaciation in diarrhoeic calves affected with *C. parvum*, whereas non-diarrhoeic calves showed undigested food materials in faeces, reduced weight gain and progressive emaciation.

The pathogenesis of disease is frequently complicated by concurrent viral (rota virus, corona virus), bacterial (*E. coli, Salmonella*) and parasitic (*Giardia*) infections (Fayer *et al.*, 1998). Subclinical animals can remain infected and excrete oocysts that can be transmitted to other susceptible hosts. Calves can die from dehydration and cardiovascular collapse but cryptosporidiosis mortalities are highly variable. Colostrum antibodies and milk antibodies protect calves from developing severe clinical signs by blocking parasite invasion and immobilization of gut luminal parasitic forms. Micronutrients also play a significant role in the clinical outcome of cryptosporidiosis as severe clinical signs have been observed in calves with selenium deficiency (McAllister *et al.*, 2005). Calves that recover from *C. parvum* do not have recurrent cryptosporidiosis-associated diarrhoea and do not appear to shed oocysts for the rest of their life.

Cryptosporidium andersoni was named after Bruce Anderson, the finder of the parasite. It is associated with reduced milk production, infects abomasum of juvenile, post-weaned and mature cattle. The microvilli of peptic glands are destroyed by endogenous stages, which account for the elevated concentrations of plasma pepsinogen detected in infected hosts. Infected cattle do not develop diarrhoea, but can excrete oocysts for several months. *C. andersoni* can cause moderate-to-severe impairment of weight gain, decreased feed efficiency and reduced milk production (Ralston *et al.*, 2003). The mechanism of impaired performance is through inhibition of protein digestion by decreased gastric proteolytic function and increased gastric pH.

Cryptosporidium bovis (former bovine genotype B) was found to be the predominant species in 2-11 months old dairy calves but was not associated with overt clinical signs. *Cryptosporidium bovis* is a highly prevalent species that infects primarily post-weaned calves (Fayer *et al.*, 2005). *Cryptosporidium ryanae* (former deer-like genotype) has been reported from both pre-weaned and 2-11 month old calves, without associated signs of disease (Santin *et al.*, 2004).

Human cryptosporidiosis

Five *Cryptosporidium* species/genotypes are responsible for most human cryptosporidiosis cases, including *C. hominis*, *C. parvum*, *C. meleagridis*, *C. felis*, and *C. canis*. Among them, *C. hominis* and *C. parvum* are the most common, responsible for the majority of human infections. A few other *Cryptosporidium* spp. and genotypes are occasionally found in humans, including *C. muris*, *C. suis*, *C. andersoni* and *C. cervine*, horse, rabbit, skunk and chipmunk I genotypes (Robinson *et al.*, 2008). Transmission is through the faecal-oral route, following direct or indirect contact with *Cryptosporidium* oocysts via person-to-person, zoonotic, water borne, food borne or air borne contact (Fayer, 2004). Zoonotic transmission is probably responsible for cryptosporidiosis occurring in humans having direct contact with animals or water borne outbreaks due to contaminated surface water supplies. Person to person transmission is also probably common and responsible for the frequent occurrence of the infection in children attending day-care center and for the high prevalence in general, in preschool age children.

Epidemiology

Children : In India, 22% of total rural deaths and 12.3% of total urban deaths among children of <6 years of age are attributed to diarrhoea. *Cryptosporidium,* an enteric protozoon is one of the most common causative agents of diarrhoea and results in significant morbidity and mortality. In India, several studies have documented the prevalence of *Cryptosporidium* in pediatric diarrhoea (1.3 to 13.1%) from different parts of the country based on microscopic detection of oocysts in faecal specimens (Malla *et al.*, 1987; Saraswathi *et al.*, 1988). Subramanyam *et al.* (1989) from eastern India recorded *Cryptosporidium* infection in 14.3% children below the age of 2 years and also observed higher infection during rainy season as compared to other seasons. Nagamani *et al.* (2001) while examining stool samples of 202 children suffering from diarrhoea or other gastrointestinal symptoms recorded *C. parvum* oocysts in 2.99% of children by modified Ziehl Neelsen technique. Similarly Kaur *et al.* (2002) while examining stool specimens of 127 children in Delhi for intestinal parasites observed *Cryptosporidium* spp. in 24 (18.9%) patients. The study recommended that routine analysis of stool samples in diagnostic laboratories should consider *Cryptosporidium* spp. as an important causative agent of diarrhoea.

Earlier reports were based on microscopy by acid fast stains but later molecular techniques were used for *Cryptosporidium* spp. diagnosis in children of India. Das *et al.* (2006) carried out molecular characterization of 40 positive samples from Kolkata using PCR-RFLP and revealed that 35 samples were positive for *C. hominis* and 4 for *C. parvum* and 1 for *C. felis*. Nagamani *et al.* (2007) examined faecal samples from 681 children by microscopy and enzyme linked immunosorbent assay (ELISA). *Cryptosporidium* was found in 52 (7.6%) children. The prevalence of *Cryptosporidium* in children of six months to one year was 14.3%. PCR -RFLP revealed that of the 42 samples genotyped, 29 (69%) were *C. hominis* and 8 (19%) were *C. parvum* and 5 (11.9%) were mixed infection with the two species. Ajjampur *et al.* (2007) carried out genetic characterization of *Cryptosporidium* spp. by PCR-restriction fragment length polymorphism and spatial analysis of cases using Geographical Information Systems (GIS) technology for 53 children with cryptosporidial diarrhoea in an urban slum. Of the two most common species were *C. hominis* (81%) and *C. parvum* (12%). The other species identi?ed was *C. felis*. Five subgenotypes were identi?ed at the Cpgp40/15 locus. Subgenotype Ia predominated among *C. hominis* isolates, and all *C. parvum* isolates were subgenotype Ic.

Throughout the world, numerous prevalence reports of cryptosporidiosis in children have been documented. Bhattacharya *et al.* (1997) detected *Cryptosporidium* oocysts in the stools of 68 (3.5%)

of 1949 cases of acute diarrhoea in children (between the ages of birth to 59 month) examined in urban Bangladesh. *Cryptosporidium* was observed throughout the year, but was most frequent during April to October. Age below 2 years, non-breast feeding, and stunting were significantly associated with *Cryptosporidium* infection. *Cryptosporidium* oocysts were identi?ed more frequently in children with persistent diarrhoea (16.5%), than in those with acute (8.4%) or no (4.0%) diarrhoea. Low-birth-weight children and those living in densely crowded subdivisions were at greater risk for symptomatic infection. Nchito *et al.* (1998) reported 18% prevalence of cryptosporidiosis in stool samples of 222 children from four crowded townships of Lusaka, Zambia. The highest prevalence was observed in rainy season. It was concluded that cryptosporidiosis was not associated with keeping animals, nutritional status, or parental education, but was apparently more common in breast fed children. Xiao *et al.* (2001a) genotyped *Cryptosporidium* of 132 stool specimens received from 80 Peruvian children. Five types of *Cryptosporidium* were identi?ed as *C. parvum* human (67), bovine (8), and dog (2) genotypes, *C. meleagridis* (7), and *C. felis* (1) and observed no signi?cant difference in age, antecedent stunting, and percentage with diarrhoea. Duration of oocysts shedding was longer for human genotype than for zoonotic *Cryptosporidium*. Sulaiman *et al.* (2005) using PCR-RFLP genotyped 62 *Cryptosporidium* positive Kuwaiti children and observed that 94% children (58) to be positive for *C. parvum*, three (5%) for *C. hominis*, and one with both *C. parvum* and *C. hominis*. They further observed that 77% of infections occurred during the cool season of the year i.e. November to April. Gatei *et al.* (2006) analysed 4,899 faecal samples of children (<5 years of age) of Kenya and found 4% prevalence of cryptosporidiosis, which was highest between November to February. The prevalence of cryptosporidiosis was highest among children of 13–24 months of age (5.2%) and least among children of 48–60 months of age (2%). Cryptosporidiosis was significantly associated with persistent diarrhoea, vomiting, and abdominal swelling. Genotype analysis based PCR-RFLP of the 18S rRNA gene fragment showed that 87% of the *Cryptosporidium* isolates were *C. hominis*, 9% were *C. parvum*, and remaining 4% were *C. canis*, *C. felis*, *C. meleagridis*, and *C. muris*. In Brazil, Carvalho-Costa (2007) observed children with acute diarrhoea and found 9.3% positive for *Cryptosporidium* infection by safranin-methylene blue staining method. Bushen *et al.* (2007) identified *Cryptosporidium* in the stools of 58 of 157 children examined from birth to 5 years in an urban slum of northeast Brazil. Speciation of 42 samples further revealed 24 positive for *C. hominis* and 18 for *C. parvum*. Children with *C. hominis* shed more oocysts/ml of stool (3.5X106 vs. 1.7 X106) and oocysts counts were higher among symptomatic children. Molloy *et al.* (2010) conducted a longitudinal study in 1,636 children in Nigeria over one year and observed that *Cryptosporidium* prevalence ranged from 15.6% to 19.6%. PCR-RFLP technique revealed *C. hominis, C. parvum, C. parvum/C. hominis, C. meleagridis, Cryptosporidium* rabbit genotype, *Cryptosporidium* cervine genotype, and *C. canis* in 34, 25, 4, 5, 5, 3 and 1 children, respectively.

HIV infected individuals : Diarrhoea is a common complication of HIV positive patients inducing weight loss and cachexia. It occurs in almost 90% of AIDS patients in developing countries (Mukhopadya *et al.*, 1999). Diarrhoea due to *Cryptosporidium* infection has been reported as a defining feature of HIV infection in human. *Cryptosporidium* spp. cause chronic, fulminant (passage of more than 2 litres of stool/day; CD4 count less than 50/mm3), transient or relapsing diarrhoea which has even been associated with mortality (Manabe *et al.*, 1998) in untreated HIV infected patients.

The prevalence of cryptosporidiosis in HIV-infected individuals in India was first time reported from Chennai by Kumarasamy *et al.* (1995) and 16% prevalence was recorded by acid fast staining method. *Cryptosporidium* has been reported from different parts of the country with the prevalence ranging from as low as 0.7% (Becker *et al.*, 2007) to as high as 81% (Agarwal *et al.*, 1998). A high prevalence of 80% was reported from a study in Imphal (Agarwal *et al.*, 1998) and another in Maharashtra (Ghorpade *et al.*, 1996) but both had very small sample sizes. Most of these studies were done on HIV-infected adult patients and used modified acid-fast staining of concentrated stool samples. However, the data on prevalence are highly varied and could reflect geographical differences, as well as differences in the populations being studied especially with respect to socioeconomic status and access to potable water. A few recent studies that also did enzyme-linked immunosorbent assay (ELISA) and polymerase chain reaction (PCR) for detection (Jayalakshmi *et al.*, 2008; Kaushik *et al.*, 2008) found a higher sensitivity for PCR and lower for antigen detection ELISA compared with microscopy, which also contributed to variability in prevalence rates. Several studies in India have documented mean CD4 counts in these patients with most studies showing that symptomatic cases had CD4 counts <200 cells/cmm and asymptomatic cases had CD4 counts >300 cells/cmm, thus reinforcing the importance of CD4

T cells in mediating resistance to this pathogen (Muthusamy *et al.*, 2006). A study from Delhi that stratified patients based on their CD4 counts showed that *Cryptosporidium* was the commonest parasite seen in 46% of patients with counts<200 cells/cmm. The prevalence of cryptosporidial diarrhoea (56%) was also significantly higher when CD4 counts were<200 cells/cmm cowhen CD4 counts were<200 cells/cmm compared to patients with higher CD4 counts (40%).

Variable prevalence of cryptosporidiosis in HIV positive individuals in different parts of the world has been reported. Pedersen *et al.* (1996) studied epidemiology of cryptosporidiosis among 6548 European patients, from 52 centres in 17 European countries with AIDS. Cryptosporidiosis was diagnosed in 432 (6.6%) patients. The probability of being diagnosed with cryptosporidiosis at AIDS diagnosis was significantly lower for intravenous drug users (1.3%) than for homosexual men (4.1%). The probability was higher for patients from Central Europe compared with patients from South Europe (4.1% versus 2.5%, $p = 0.005$). Sorvillo *et al.* (1998) reported cryptosporidiosis in 5.3% HIV cases in Los Angeles County. The highest rates were observed in March to May and September-October. There was no difference in the rate of cryptosporidiosis for the periods of heaviest rainfall (December-March) and low rainfall (April-November). Infection rates were higher among males (1·59 per 100 person) than females (0·92) and lower in blacks (0·98) than other racial/ethnic groups (1·80). A significant trend of decreasing cryptosporidiosis was observed with increasing age, with the highest rate (2·34) in the 13-34 year age group. A strong association between cryptosporidiosis and CD4+ count was noted. It was found that the frequency of infection with Cryptosporidium in AIDS patients was 26.7% (20 cases) and recorded that the number of CD4 decreased in the patients, the probability of infection with opportunistic parasites increased. Ghimire *et al.* (2004) analysed 148 stool specimens (collected from 75 cases of HIV/ AIDS) using Kinyoun-modified acid fast staining from Nepal and recorded cryptosporidiosis in 10.7% cases. Four out of 62 (6.5%) HIV patients and four out of 13 (30.8%) AIDS patients were found infected with *C. parvum*. All infected cases were clinically diarrhoegenic. Certad *et al.* (2005) carried a cross-sectional study in Venezuelan HIV-infected patients to determine the prevalence of cryptosporidiosis and its clinical and laboratory pattern and observed *Cryptosporidium* spp. in 59 subjects (15%). They further reported the infection was strongly associated with acute and chronic diarrhoea, weight loss, older age in patients with leukopenia, and in persons with more than 5 stools per day when CD4+ counts were below 100 cells/ mm3.

The epidemiology based on molecular methods of *Cryptosporidium* isolates has proved useful in determining sources of infection. In USA, 13 strains of *Cryptosporidium* from people with AIDS were characterized and found that 10 were *C. parvum* type 1 (the human type) and 3 were *C. parvum* type 2 (the calf type) (McLauchlin *et al.*, 2000). Gatei *et al.* (2003) used 840-bp fragment of the 18S rRNA gene and RFLP technique to identify *Cryptosporidium* spp. recovered from human immunodeficiency virus (HIV)-infected patients from Kenya, Malawi, Brazil, United Kingdom, and Vietnam. Among 63 isolates analyzed, four genotypes of *Cryptosporidium* were identified *C. parvum* human genotype (75%), *C. parvum* bovine genotype (21.7%) of zoonotic potential, the *C. meleagridis* genotype (1.6% [one isolate]), and the *C. muris* genotype (1.6% [one case]). HIV-infected individuals were more likely to have zoonotic genotypes than the HIV-uninfected individuals. Gatei *et al.* (2008) recorded presence of *C. hominis, C. parvum, C. canis,* and *C. felis* in 25, 7, 1, and 1 HIV-positive persons from Jamaica, respectively; 1 person had both *C. hominis* and *C. felis.*

Clinical features of human cryptosporidiosis

Cryptosporidium primarily attacks intestinal tract. Although infection can be asymptomatic, most patients have profuse watery diarrhoea containing mucus, rarely blood or leukocytes. The duration and severity of clinical symptoms depend largely on the immune status of the infected person. In immunocompetent persons, the disease is usually either asymptomatic or self-limited. The three major clinical presentations in immunocompetent persons are asymptomatic carriage, acute diarrhoea, and persistent diarrhoea that may continue for several weeks (Farthing, 2000). After an incubation period of 7 to 10 days, more than 90 percent of infected patients present with acute watery diarrhoea that lasts approximately 2 weeks, accompanied by nausea, vomiting, fever and cramp-like abdominal pain. In the outbreak in Milwaukee, the mean duration of illness was 12 days, and the median maximal number of stools per day was 12. The clinical manifestations included watery diarrhoea (in 93% of patients), abdominal cramps (in 84%), fever (in 57%), vomiting (in 48%), and weight loss (in 75%) (MacKenzie *et al.*, 1994). Acute and chronic diarrhoea due to *C. parvum* in children in the developing world is associated with malnutrition and high morbidity and mortality rates (Farthing, 2000). The diarrhoea also has lasting adverse effects on weight and height.

The severity and duration of diarrhoea and the extra-enteric manifestations of the infection differ in immunocompetent and immunocompromised patients. Patients with AIDS who have cryptosporidiosis have a wide spectrum of disease, from asymptomatic shedding of cryptosporidial oocysts to a fulminant cholera-like illness, depending on the site of cryptosporidial infection and the CD4+ T-cell count. The four clinical patterns of disease in patients with AIDS are asymptomatic infection, in which patients have no change in bowel habits and pass fewer than three stools per day (4% of patients); transient infection, in which diarrhoea lasts for less than two months and is followed by a complete remission of symptoms and loss of *Cryptosporidium* from faecal specimens (29%); chronic diarrhoea lasting two months or more, with persistence of the parasites in stool or in biopsy specimens (60%); and fulminant infection, in which patients pass at least 2 litres of watery stool daily (8%) (Farthing, 2000). Fulminant infection occurs only in patients with a CD4+ T-cell count below 50 per cubic millimetre, whereas transient or asymptomatic infection is associated with higher CD4+ counts (Farthing, 2000). The diarrhoea in patients with AIDS is usually watery and the stools frequency can be up to 10 per day; these patients can have a 10% drop in body weight and usually have severe malabsorption (Farthing, 2000). Most patients never clear the infection, and they have a shorter survival than patients with AIDS who do not have cryptosporidiosis (Manabe *et al.*, 1998).

Extra-intestinal cryptosporidiosis has been reported principally in patients with AIDS. It may involve the lungs, middle ear, biliary tract, pancreas and stomach (Farthing, 2000). These sites probably represent extensions of a primary intestinal infection. Biliary cryptosporidiosis is the most common extraintestinal manifestation of infection. It has been described up to 26% in patients with AIDS and intestinal cryptosporidial infection in the era before highly active antiretroviral therapy (Farthing, 2000; Vakil *et al.*, 1996). The true frequency of this entity is difficult to determine, because invasive procedures are required for diagnosis. The clinical features include pain in the right upper quadrant, nausea, vomiting, and fever, usually accompanied by elevated serum alkaline phosphatase levels. Those with biliary symptoms have lower CD4+ T-cell counts (Farthing, 2000; Vakil *et al.*, 1996). A biliary reservoir of *Cryptosporidium* may contribute to the chronic nature of the infection and the inability of therapy to eradicate the organism. Although biliary cryptosporidiosis increases morbidity in patients with AIDS, it may not affect survival (Vakil *et al.*, 1996). Respiratory involvement is rare and is characterized by cough, dyspnoea, fever and thoracic pain (Farthing, 2000).

Detection of *Cryptosporidium* in the faecal samples

The diagnosis of cryptosporidiosis rests on the identi?cation of the 5 ìm spherical oocysts of *Cryptosporidium* (or oocyst components) in stool or the intracellular stages within biopsy specimens of human gastrointestinal mucosa. A variety of diagnostic options are available for the detection of *Cryptosporidium* in clinical stool samples. The particular assay used by a laboratory will depend on a number of factors, particularly cost containment and level of staff training. It is also likely that cryptosporidiosis is underdiagnosed as clinicians fail to consider this diagnosis in patients with diarrhoeal illnesses (particularly immunocompetent adults and children) and do not request stool analysis for *Cryptosporidium*, a test not normally included in routine stool analysis.

Microscopic staining method : Cryptosporidium is conventionally diagnosed by microscopic staining method. This methodology includes the concentration of oocysts and staining of faecal smears. The other supportive methods are the differential staining methods that include the safranin-methylene blue stain (Soave, 1983), the Ziehl-Neelsen (Henricksen and Pohlenz, 1981) and the DMSO-carbol fuchsin (Pohjola *et al.*, 1984). However, the differential staining method is time-consuming and its result depends on the sensitivity and specificity (Smith *et al.*, 1989). The fluorochrome staining method has a high sensitivity but is complicated. These staining methods are labour-intensive and require experienced microscopist for slide examination. The "gold standard" and most widely used staining technique for the detection of *Cryptosporidium* oocyst in stool was the modified acid-fast or Kinyoun stain (Fayer *et al.*, 2000). The detection limit of acid fast staining has been reported to be 50,000 oocyst per gram of faeces, whereas the detection limit was 5, 00,000 oocysts per gram faeces with flurochrome dye. Detection limit of modified Kinyoun technique was reported to be 1-5 x 10^4 oocysts per gram of faeces (Weber *et al.*, 1991).

Concentration techniques : The coprodiagnostic methods may fail to detect *Cryptosporidium* oocysts in stool specimens of infected patients. The concentration procedures provide excellent separation of parasites from stool debris and enhanced detection of *Cryptosporidium* oocysts in stool samples. Various procedures for concentration of *Cryptosporidium* oocyst from faeces namely formol-ether concentration, salt floatation, sucrose centrifugal floatation, zinc sulphate floatation were discussed in literature in which Sheather's sugar floatation was the most widely used and sensitive technique (Fayer *et al.*, 1997). Webster *et al.* (1996) reported detection limit of 4000 oocyst per gram of faeces by sugar floatation coupled with modified Ziehl-Neelsen staining/Auramine-phenol staining. Current *et al.* (1983) also reported modified Sheather's floatation technique to be highly sensitive for selective purification and recovery of oocysts from faeces.

Arrowood and Sterling (1987) reported up to 72% recovery of oocysts from crude faeces by discontinuous sucrose step-gradient centrifugation technique. This method was comparable to isopycnic percoll gradient centrifugation which yielded 79% recovery of oocysts from crude faeces. Caesium chloride (CsCl) step gradient centrifugation technique for oocyst recovery was reported highly efficient by Kilani and Sekla (1987). A further modification of the technique was done by Arrowood and Donaldsen (1996) to obtain higher concentration of oocysts. A modification of discontinuous sucrose step-gradient centrifugation with high sensitivity and threshold of detection up to 10 oocysts was reported by Ramirez and Sreevatsan (2006). Barwick *et al.* (2000) reported 93% sensitivity and 100% specificity of sucrose floatation method when a sample containing 1.5 x 103 oocysts was tested. Sodium chloride floatation method exhibited a detection limit of less than 40 oocysts per gm soil/faeces and efficiency of 61.6% for 1 gram faecal samples (Mawdsley *et al.*, 1996).

Among different density gradient methods, CsCl density gradient centrifugation was reported to be the most sensitive technique (Fayer *et al.*, 1997). A sophisticated procedure for concentration and purification of oocysts was immuno-magnetic separation (IMS) using magnetisible particles coated with antibodies. This method was used to obtain highly purified oocysts (Parker and Smith, 1994).

Immunological detection methods : Immunological-based techniques include polyclonal fluorescent antibody tests, latex agglutination reactions, immunofluorescence with monoclonal antibodies, enzyme linked immunosorbent assays, reverse passive haemagglutination, immunoserology using immunofluorescence detection and solid-phase qualitative immunochromatographic assays. The drawback of these methods is the non-specificity due to cross-reactivity with other genera and species.

The sensitivity and specificity of direct fluorescent antibody (DFA) test were reported to be 96-100% and 99.8-100%, respectively, and was equal to traditional examination of permanent smears prepared from concentrated stool specimens. A number of antigen capture ELISAs were reported with detection limit in the range of 3 x 10^5-10^6 oocysts per gram of faeces, which indicated that the assays did not appear to have superior sensitivity over microscopical methods (Anusz *et al.*, 1990). The antigen-capture ELISA exhibited 66.3% sensitivity and 99.8% specificity (Newman *et al.*, 1993) but both false positive and false-negative cases were recorded in the assay (Rosenblatt and Sloan, 1993). The monoclonal antibody based immunofluorescence test was found to be more efficient than modified Kinyoun technique (Alles *et al.*, 1995), whereas equal sensitivity and specificity of direct fluorescent antibody (DFA) test and modified Ziehl Neelsen staining (mZN) technique was reported by Kehl *et al.* (1995).

Enzyme immunoassay (EIA) was the most widely used antigen detection technique for *Cryptosporidium* spp. and exhibited sensitivity and specificity of 94-97% and 99-100%, respectively. However, false positive and false negative results had been reported. The Solid phase qualitative immune chromatographic assay (Garcia *et al.*, 2003) and immuno-chromatographic dip strip test (crypto-strip) used monoclonal antibody and a gold conjugate to give a sensitive and specific diagnosis (Llorente *et al.*, 2002).

Molecular techniques : PCR based detection of *Cryptosporidium* in clinical samples is attractive due to its extreme accuracy. A variety of PCR tests have been developed (Smith, 1998) which generate rapid, highly sensitive and accurate result. However, these techniques have several limitations in discriminating the wide range of different species or genotypes. False positives can result from naked nucleic acids, from non-viable microorganisms, laboratory contamination and also from the interference of some environmental contaminants. Carraway *et al.* (1996) used internal transcribed spacer-1(ITS-1) based PCR protocol and the assay reported to detect up to 100 oocysts per gm of faeces. Bonnin *et al.* (1996) used primers of random DNA sequences and reported threshold of detection of 20-100 oocysts in PCR. Spano *et al.*

(1997) recorded a threshold limit of up to 10 oocysts with a PCR assay using gene primer of *Cryptosporidium* oocyst wall protein (COWP) but the threshold level was decreased to 20 oocysts when a gene primer of thrombospondin related adhesive protein 1 (TRAP-C1) was used.

A threshold of detection of 50 oocysts per gm of faeces using gene primers of thrombospondin related adhesive protein 2 (TRAP-C2) was reported by Sulaiman *et al.* (1998.) Both dihydrofolate reductase (DHFR) based assay (Gibbons *et al.*, 1998) and the small sub-unit ribosomal RNA (18S ssu rRNA) based protocol (Xiao *et al.*, 1999) yielded threshold limit of up to 1 oocyst per gm of sample. Coupe *et al.* (2005) described another SSU rRNA based PCR protocol capable of amplifying DNA from a single oocyst. Balatbat *et al.* (1996) reported a *C. parvum* specific PCR assay which involved amplification of 194 bp DNA fragment and internal probing with enzyme linked chemiluminience system. A Nested PCR-RFLP protocol based on a 844 bp (Primary PCR) and 593 bp (secondary PCR) was described with 100% sensitivity for 10 oocysts per sample, 94% for 7 oocysts per sample, 92% for 5 oocysts per sample, 88% detection limit for sample containing 4 oocysts and 76% and 38% detection limit for samples containing 2 oocysts and 1 oocyst, respectively (Sturbaum *et al.*, 2001). Sulaiman *et al.* (2000) reported heat shock protein-70 (HSP-70) based PCR which was both sensitive and specific for detection of *Cryptosporidium* spp. Another HSP-70 based Nested PCR was reported having detection limits of 10-100 oocysts per sample (Lindergard *et al.*, 2003). Reverse-transcriptase PCR (RT-PCR) for detection of *C. parvum* oocysts after immunomagnetic separation was reported by Hallier and Guillot (2003). They used the HSP-70 heat shock induced mRNA and the threshold of detection was upto 10 oocysts per sample. Real-time PCR using Taq man probe was reported to be highly specific and sensitive for detection of *C. parvum* in faecal samples (Godiwala *et al.*, 2006). A PCR hybridization assay for detection of *C. parvum* oocysts in faecal samples was reported by Ramirez and Sreevatsan (2006).

Paul *et al.* (2009b) compared four conventional coprological techniques viz., direct faecal smear staining (DFSS), normal saline sedimentation staining (NSSS), Sheather's floatation (SF) and Sheather's floatation sedimentation staining (SFSS) with PCR directed against the 18S SSU rRNA gene as standard reference test for the diagnosis of cryptosporidiosis in bovines. Sheather's floatation sedimentation staining was found to be the most sensitive (82.6%)

and specific (98.76%) among the coprological techniques. As sample processing based cost analysis, DFSS was found to be the most economical method (15 cents) followed by NSSS (19.6 cents), SF (23.6 cents) and SFSS (33.9 cents). The time taken for complete processing and diagnosis varied between 70 and 100 min. PCR based diagnosis of a sample took about 7.5–8 h for completion and cost of diagnosis was estimated as approximately 7.604 US$ per sample. The study concluded that among the conventional coprological methods, SFSS provided the required sensitivity and specificity along with nominal cost for diagnosis on per sample basis, and may be considered as a viable diagnostic alternative when PCR is not an option for a particular laboratory setting, especially in developing countries.

Characterization of *Cryptosporidium* spp

Because of the difficulties associated with the taxonomy of *Cryptosporidium* spp., general guidelines were developed. The fourth edition of International Code of Zoological Nomenclature (International Commission on Zoological Nomenclature, 1999), which governs the taxonomy of protozoan parasites and other animals, took effect on 1 January 2000. According to ICZN four criteria are to be fulfilled for characterization of *Cryptosporidium*: (i) morphometric studies of oocysts; (ii) genetic characterization; (iii) demonstration of natural and whenever feasible, at least some experimental host specificity; (iv) compliance with ICZN (Xiao *et al.*, 2004).

Morphometric characterization : Although morphometry serves as the cornerstone of Apicomplexan taxonomy but in case of *Cryptosporidium* spp. it cannot differentiate the species of *Cryptosporidium* present if the oocysts fall within the range of 4-6 μm. Therefore, genetic and biological criteria were much important for proper characterization of *Cryptosporidium* spp. (OIE, 2008).

Genetic characterization : A host can be naturally infected with multiple *Cryptosporidium* spp. which frequently cannot be differentiated from each other on the basis of morphology and development. So, the genetic differences between species can play pivotal role in differentiating *Cryptosporidium* spp. (Xiao *et al.*, 2004). As reviewed by Xiao (2010) Various genetic loci like ssu rRNA, *Cryptosporidium* oocyst wall protein (COWP), thrombospondin related adhesive protein (TRAP-C1), TRAP-C2; dihydrofolate reductase (DHFR), Poly-T, internal transcribed spacer-1 (ITS-1), microsatellites, heat shock protein-70 (HSP-70) acetyl CoA, â-tubulin and glycoprotein 60 (GP-60) were used for molecular characterization of *Cryptosporidium* isolates from bovines.

A genotyping technique based on the SSU rRNA was developed by Xiao *et al.* (1999) which provided valuable information about sequence variation of different species of *Cryptosporidium* affecting bovines. The 18S ssu rRNA based nested PCR protocol was very sensitive as it amplified DNA from a single oocyst (Xiao *et al.*, 1999, 2004). The 834 bp nested product when digested by restriction enzymes Ssp1 and Vsp1 separately, provided specific diagnosis of the species of *Cryptosporidium* involved. *Cryptosporidium parvum* yielded 3 visible bands at 449, 267 and 108 bp with Ssp1 and 2 visible bands of 628 and 105 bp with Vsp1. *Cryptosporidium andersoni* yielded 2 bands of 448 and 397 bp with Ssp1 and 2 bands of 730 and 115 bp with Vsp1. *Cryptosporidium bovis* yielded 3 visible bands at 432, 267 and 103bp with Ssp1 and 2 visible bands 616 and 115 bp with Vsp1. Coupe *et al.* (2005) detected up to 95% of infection by *Cryptosporidium* spp. by amplifying the polymorphous region between nucleotides 179-271 of ssu rRNA gene. However, this was not able to differentiate between *C. andersoni* and some *C. parvum* genotypes. Feng *et al.* (2007) reported that single digestion of 834bp nested product with restriction enzyme MboII also differentiated the species of *Cryptosporidium*. *Cryptosporidium parvum* yielded 2 bands at 771 and 70 bp, *C. andersoni* yielded 2 bands of 769 and 76 bp and *C. bovis* yielded 3 bands at 485, 185 and 162 bp. In India Das *et al.* (2004) and Roy *et al.* (2006) used the 18S SSU rRNA nested PCR-RFLP and found *C. parvum* as the predominant species among bovines in India.

Sub typing tools have been used extensively in studies of the transmission of *C. hominis* in humans and *C. parvum* in humans and ruminants. One of the popular subtyping tools is the DNA sequence analysis of the 60 kDa glycoprotein (gp60, also called gp40/ 15). Sequence analysis of gp60 gene is widely used in *Cryptosporidium* subtyping because of its sequence heterogeneity and relevance to parasite biology. It is the most single polymorphic marker identified so far in the *Cryptosporidium* genome (Wielinga *et al.*, 2008). Unlike other subtyping targets, such as double stranded RNA, internal transcribed spacer-2 and traditional microsatellites and minisatellites, which are generally considered non-functional, gp60 is located on the surface of apical region of invasive stages of the parasite, and is one of the dominant targets for neutralizing antibody responses in humans

(O'Connor *et al.*, 2007). Thus, it is possible to link biologic characteristics of the parasites and clinical presentations with the subtype family identity. Some of the *C. parvum* subtype families, such as IIa and IId, are found in both humans and ruminants, responsible for zoonotic cryptosporidiosis.

Biological characterization : Small animal models such as neonatal mice have been successfully infected with *Cryptosporidium* (Meloni and Thompson, 1996). Extensive infection could be induced in 1-4 days old neonatal mice or by suppressing the immunity of adult mice with immunosuppressive drugs (Fayer *et al.*, 1997). Various routes of experimental infection namely oral, intra-uterine, intra-cervical, rectal and intra-gastric injection of oocysts were followed to infect mice (Fayer *et al.*, 1997). The dosage of oocysts varied with age of the animal and isolate of *C. parvum*. A technique for isolating purified oocysts from the gut of mice for further *in vitro* cultivation, molecular and biochemical studies has been successfully established (Current, 1990). Differences in the infectivity for laboratory animals also exist between *C. hominis* and *C. parvum* cattle genotype with the cattle genotype readily infecting mice and cattle, whereas C. *hominis* does not (Fayer *et al.*, 2006).

In experimentally infected mice, colony of *C. parvum* was detected in small intestine, caceum, colon, liver, lung and heart (Ernest *et al.*, 1986). Fayer *et al.* (1997) reported transient villous atrophy, crypt hyperplasia, inflammatory cell accumulations in distal small intestine and endogenous stages were found on brush border epithelium.

Zoonotic potential of bovine cryptosporidiosis

Human cryptosporidiosis is caused by *C. hominis* (previously known as *C. parvum* genotype I or human genotype) and *C. parvum* (genotype II or bovine genotype). *Cryptosporidium hominis* is found exclusively in humans, whereas *C. parvum* in domestic livestock, wild animals, and humans. In developing countries, the disease probably exerts most of its impact on pediatric health. In addition to the occurrence of diarrhoea, cryptosporidiosis has been attributed to malnutrition and stunted growth (Molbak *et al.*, 1997). In developed countries, water borne outbreaks of cryptosporidiosis have a signi?cant economic impact. A recent study estimates that the total illness-associated cost of 1993 Milwaukee water borne outbreak of cryptosporidiosis was $96.2 million: $31.7 million in medical costs and $64.6 million in productivity (Corso *et al.*, 2003).

Since 1976 (discovery of human infection with *Cryptosporidium*), considerable circumstantial evidence has been accumulated of zoonotic exposure associated with farms and farm animals, riding stables, animal manure and contaminated water. Early reports drew attention to the association of human infection with exposure to infected livestock, particularly young cattle. The occurrence of secondary spread within households or play-groups following zoonotic exposure has also been reported (Casemore *et al.*, 1997). Although farm workers and visitors to farms are considered to have contracted cryptosporidiosis by direct contact, but indirect zoonotic transmission of *Cryptosporidium* of livestock origin via water has been considered to be the most important zoonotic source of human infection.

In 1991, restriction fragment length polymorphism (RFLP) analysis revealed differences between *Cryptosporidium* of cattle and human origin (Ortega *et at.*, 1991). Throughout the globe cryptosporidiosis in humans caused by zoonotic species (*C. parvum*) has been documented. Many food-borne and waterborne outbreaks of cryptosporidiosis have been caused by *C. parvum* in North America and Europe. In Australia *C. parvum* has also been attributed for an outbreak of cryptosporidiosis (Harper *et al.*, 2002). Outbreaks of cryptosporidiosis in children and veterinary students because of bovine contact have been reported (Gait *et al.*, 2008).

In recent time number of molecular tools have been developed for the 'tracking' of infection sources and consequently, for the surveillance of cryptosporidiosis. One of the most commonly used tools is the sequencing of a 60 kDa glycoprotein (gp60) gene, which allows the definition of *C. hominis* Ia, Ib, Id-If and C. parvum IIa-IIk (reviewed by Xiao, 2010). Except for IIj and IIk, all of the above mentioned 'subtype families' have been detected in humans, whereas exclusively IIa, IId and IIj have been found in cattle. Many of the common bovine IIa subtypes in North America, Europe and Australia are also dominant *C. parvum* subtypes in humans in these areas (Xiao *et al.*, 2010). For example, the predominant *C. parvum* subtype in calves in Portugal, Slovenia and the Netherlands, IIaA15G2R1, is also the major *C. parvum* subtype in humans in these countries (Alves *et al.*, 2006; Soba and Logar, 2008; Wielinga *et al.*, 2008). This and other IIa subtypes previously found in calves in Michigan and Ontario also frequently infect humans in Wisconsin and Ontario (Feltus *et al.*, 2006; Trotz-Williams *et al.*, 2006). Likewise, humans in the Republic of Ireland and Northern Ireland are infected with most common IIa subtypes found in calves in Northern Ireland, with the IIaA18G3R1 as the dominant subtype (Thompson *et al.*, 2007; Zintl *et al.*, 2009). This subtype was also the most common subtype in calves and humans in Australia. Another less common bovine *C. parvum* subtype family, IId, may potentially also be responsible for some zoonotic infections in Europe. Four IId subtypes were found in HIV+ persons in Portugal, two of which were previously found in calves and lambs in the same area (Alves *et al.*, 2006). All these are further indicators of differences in the role of zoonotic transmission of C. parvum among geographic areas. Recently, Helmy *et al.* (2013) in Egypt using gp60 gene analysis revealed high prevalence and identical genotype of C. parvum in animals and human indicating zoonotic transmission due to contact with animals, where IIdA20G1 was the most frequent subtype. In India, although *C. parvum* has been documented as a cause of diarrhoea in Indian children (Das *et al.*, 2006; Nagmani, *et al.*, 2007), and in HIV infected patients (Ajjampur *et al.*, 2007) but till date no sub typing studies has been carried for understanding the zoonotic significance of *C. parvum*.

Treatment and control

The major problem concerning cryptosporidiosis is the lack of an effective means for prevention and therapy of this disease. Because oocysts are highly resistant to environmental stress and to many disinfectants, hygienic measures on their own are in general not sufficient to reliably eliminate oocysts from animal housing facilities and thus to avoid infection (O'Donoghue, 1995). More than 200 substances have been tested against cryptosporidiosis (Gargala, 2008). Some exhibit promising effects but none of them were able to consistently control clinical signs or completely eliminate the infection (Delafosse *et al.*, 2006). However, use of some drugs can reduce oocyst shedding, which presumably also reduces environmental pathogen load and subsequent exposure and infection of susceptible hosts. Since drug application or hygiene is not sufficient alone to combat this disease, the combination of both measures is necessary for effective control of cryptosporidiosis. Although no specific drug is recommended for the treatment of cryptosporidiosis in animals, but some chemicals as listed in Table 2 have resulted in decreased oocyst output and improved growth of the infected animals.

In immunocompetent patients the infection is usually self-limiting, with possible need only for restoration of fluid and electrolyte levels.

Short-term azithromycin treatment for cryptosporidial diarrhoea in AIDs patients gave good clinical improvement but parasitological benefit was doubtful (Kadappu *et al.*, 2002). Among anti-diarrhoeals for management of childhood diarrhoea, nitazoxanide had been reported to have high efficacy against cryptosporidial diarrhoea only (Alam and Bhatnagar, 2006). Oral azithromycin for 5 days (Karanth *et al.*, 2007) resulted in reduced frequency of stools, and negative results of stool examination in a severe human case of cryptosporidiosis.

Table 2: Drug therapy of *Cryptosporidium* infection in animals

Drugs	Animal and Dosages	References
Azithromycin	Ruminants: 1500 mg/day per calf for 7 days Dog, cat: 10 mg/kg BW, PO, every 24 h until clinical signs resolved Horse: 10 mg/kg BW, PO, every 24 h for 5 days, then every 48 h until resolution of clinical signs	Elitok *et al.* (2005), Robinson *et al.* (2008)
Nitazoxanide	Ruminants: 15 mg/kg BW or per animal 100 mg BIDb for 5 days in animals 24–47 months old; 200 mg BID for 5 days in animals 4–11 years old. Recently, a regimen was approved to treat adults Dog, cat: 25 mg/kg BW, PO, every 12 h for at least 7 days	Scorza and Lappin (2007), Schnyder *et al.* (2009)
Paromomycin	Ruminant: 100 mg/kg BW for 21 days Johnson *et al.* (2000) Dog, cat: 125–165 mg/kg BW, PO, every 12–24 h for at least 5 days Horse: 100 mg/kg BW, PO, every 24 h for 5 days	Johnson *et al.* (2000)
Halofuginone	Ruminant: 0.1 mg/kg BW for 7 consecutive days	Jarvie *et al.* (2005) Randhawa *et al.* (2012)
Tylosin Decoquinate	Dog, cat: 10–15 mg/kg BW, PO, every 8–12 h for 21 days	Scorza and Lappin (2006) Moore *et al.* (2003)

Conclusion and future prospects

The last two decades have been devoted to the development and application of molecular tools to solve about the epidemiology and zoonotic potential of *Cryptosporidium* spp. These findings have been very successful and have helped to elucidate cycles of transmission. The recent finding of *C. hominis* from a calf in Southern India, as well as the reports of clinical form of cryptosporidiosis from various parts of the world due to lessen known *Cryptosporidium* spp. like *C. andersoni* have raised eyebrows.

The broad host range, the cross infectivity among the hosts, the zoonotic potential, high human and livestock population, the strong biotic potential under the tropical climatic conditions of the country and the unsatisfactory hygiene and sanitary conditions are the incriminatory factors for the endemicity of cryptosporidiosis in the country. This disease goes largely unnoticed because of ignorance among the medical and veterinary clinicians. In India, except few studies on epidemiology, no work has been carried on other aspects like host-parasite interactions. Thus, in near future work should focus on molecular based epidemiology for species and subtype identification, immunology, treatment and control measures of cryptosporidiosis in different livestock and human. These studies will result in minimum production losses and better understanding of zoonotic significance, of cryptosporidiosis. The studies on disinfectant and disinfection procedures in farm are also required for prevention of disease transmission among young livestock and too human.

References

Agarwal, A., Ningthouja, S., Sharma, D., Mohen, Y. and Singh, N.B. (1998). *Cryptosporidium* and HIV. *J. Indian Med. Assoc.*, 96: 276-277.

Ajjampur, S.S.R., Asirvatham, J.R., Muthusamy, D., Gladston, B.P., Abraham O.C., Mathai, D., Ward, H., Wanke, C. and Kang, G. (2007). Clinical features and risk factors associated with cryptosporidiosis in HIV infected adults in India. *Indian J. Med. Res.*, 126: 553-557.

Ajjampur, S.S.R., Sankaran, P. and Kang, G. (2008). *Cryptosporidium* species in HIV infected individuals in India: An overview. *Natl. Med. J. India*, 21: 178-184.

Alam, S. and Bhatnagar, S. (2006). Current status of anti-diarrhoeal and anti-secretory drugs in the management of acute childhood diarrhoea. *Indian J. Ped.*, 73: 693–96.

Alles, A.J., Waldron, M., Sierra, L.S. and Maslia, A.R. (1995). Prospective comparison of direct immunofluorescence and conventional staining methods for detection of *Giardia* and *Cryptosporidium* spp. in human fecal specimens. *J. Clin. Microbiol.*, 33: 1632-34.

Alves, M., Xiao, L., Antunes, F. and Matos, O. (2006). Distribution of *Cryptosporidium* subtypes in humans and domestic and wild ruminants in Portugal. *Parasitol. Res.*, 99: 287–292.

Anusz, K.Z., Mason, P.H., Riggs, M.W. and Perryman, L.E. (1990). Detection of *Cryptosporidium parvum* oocysts in bovine faeces by monoclonal antibody caputre enzyme-linked immunosorbent assay. *J. Clin. Microbiol.*, 28: 2770-2774.

Arrowood, M.J. and Donaldsen, K. (1996). Improved purification methods for calf derived *Cryptosporidium parvum* oocysts using discontinuous sucrose and caesium chloride gradients. *J. Eukaryot. Microbiol.*, 43: 895.

Arrowood, M.J. and Sterling, C.R. (1987). Isolation of *Cryptosporidium* oocysts and sporozoites using discontinuous sucrose and isopycnic percoll gradients. *J. Parasitol.*, 78: 314-319.

Balatbat, A.B., Jordan, G.W., Tang, Y.J. and Silva Jr., J. 1996. Detection of *Cryptosporidium parvum* DNA in human feces by nested-PCR. *J. Clin. Microbiol.*, 34: 1769-1772.

Barwick, R.S., Mohammed, H.O., White, A.B. and Bryan, R.T. (2000). Detection of *Cryptosporidium parvum* and *Cryptosporidium muris* in soil samples. *Biol. Fertile Soils,* 31: 385-390.

Becher, K.A., Robertson, I.D., Fraser, D.M., Palmer, D.G. and Thompson, R.C.A. (2004). Molecular epidemiology of *Giardia* and *Cryptosporidium* infections in dairy calves originating from three sources in Western Australia. *Vet. Parasitol.*, 123 : 1-9.

Becker, M.L., Cohen, C.R., Cheang, M., Washington, R.G., Blanchard, J.F. and Moses, S. (2007). Diarrhoeal disease among HIV-infected adults in Karnataka, India: Evaluation of risk factors and etiology. *Amer. J. Trop. Med. Hyg.*, 76: 718–722.

Bhat, S.A., Juyal, P.D., Dingh, N.K., Singla, L.D., Singh, A.P., Sharma, A. and Kaur, P. (2012). Cryptosporidiosis and calf diarrhoea in Ludhiana district of Punjab. In: Proceedings of 23rd National Congress of Veterinary Parasitology, Guwahati, Assam, India, Dec. 12-14, 2012.

Bhattacharya, M.K., Teka, T., Faruque, A.S. and Fuchs, G.J. (1997). *Cryptosporidium* infection in children in urban Bangladesh. *J. Trop. Ped.*, 43: 282-286.

Bonnin, A., Fourmaux, M.N., Dubremetz, J.F., Nelson, R.G., Gobet, P., Harly, G., Buisson, M., Pyugauthier-Toubas, D., Gabriel-Pospisil, F., Naciri, M. and Camerlynch, P. (1996). Genotyping human and bovine isolates of *Cryptosporidium parvum* by polymerase chain reaction-restriction fragment length polymorphism analysis of a repetitive DNA sequence. FEMS Microbiol. Letters, 137: 207-211.

Brook, E.J., Anthony Hart, C., French, N.P. and Christley, R.M. (2008). Prevalence and risk factors for *Cryptosporidium* spp. in young calves. *Vet. Parasitol.,* 152: 46-52.

Buret, A.G., Chin, A.C. and Scott, K.G.E. (2003). Infection of human and bovine epithelial cells with *Cryptosporidium andersoni* induces apoptosis and disrupts tight junction ZO-I: effects of epidermal growth factor. *Int. J. Parasitol.,* 33: 1363-1371.

Carraway, M., Tzipori, S. and Widmer, G. (1996). Identification of genetic heterogeneity in the *Cryptosporidium parvum* ribosomal repeat. *App. Environ. Microbiol.,* 62: 712-716.

Carvalho-Costa, F.A., Gonçalves, A.Q., Lassance, S.L., Albuquerque, C.P., Leite, J.P. and Bóia, M.N. (2007). Detection of *Cryptosporidium* spp. and other intestinal parasites in children with acute diarrhoea and severe dehydration in Rio de Janeiro. Revista da Sociedade Brasileira de Medicina Trop., 40: 346-348.

Casemore, D.P., Wright, S.E. and Coop, R.L. (1997). Cryptosporidiosis-human and animal epidemiology. In: R. Fayer, (ed.), *Cryptosporidium* and Cryptosporidiosis, CRC Press Inc., Boca Raton, pp. 65–92.

Castro-Hermida, J.A., Gonzalez-Losada, Y.A. and Ares-Mazas, E. (2002). Prevalence of and risk factors involved in neonatal bovine cryptosporidiosis in Galicia (NW Spain). *Vet. Parasitol.,* 106: 1-10.

Certad, G., Arenas-Pinto, A., Pocaterra, L., Ferrara, G., Castro, J., Bello, A. and Núñez, L. (2005). Cryptosporidiosis in HIV-infected Venezuelan adults is strongly associated with acute or chronic diarrhea. *Am. J. Trop. Med. Hyg.,* 73: 54-57.

Chalmers, R.M., Sturdee, A.P., Bull, S.A., Miller, A. and Wright, S.E. (1997). The prevalence of *Cryptosporidium parvum* and *C. muris* in Musca domesticus, Apodemus sylvaticus and Clethrionomys glareolus in an agricultural system. *Parasitol. Res.,* 83 (5): 478–82.

Chattopadhyay, U.K., Chowdhury, D., Dasgupta, C.K. and Pramanik, A.K. (2000). Prevalence of cryptosporidiosis in man and animals in and around Calcutta. *J. Vet. Parasitol.,* 14: 167-168.

Cocklin, T., Uehlinger, F.D., Farber, J., Barkmen, H.W., O' Handley, R.M. and Dixon, B. (2006). *Cryptosporidium* spp. in dairy calves from 11 farms in Prince Edward Island, Canada. *Vet. Parasitol.*, 160: 323-326.

Cocklin, T., Farber, J., Parrington, L. and Dixon, B. (2007). Prevalence and molecular characterization of *Giardia duodenalis* and *Cryptosporidium* spp. in dairy cattle in Ontario, Canada. *Vet. Parasitol.*, 150: 297-305.

Corso, P.S., Kramer, M.H., Blair, K.A., Addiss, D.G., Davis, J.P. and Haddix, A.C. (2003). Cost of illness in the 1993 waterborne *Cryptosporidium* outbreak, Milwaukee, Wisconsin. Emerg. *Infect. Dis.*, 9: 426.

Coupe, S., Sarfati, C., Hamane, S. and Derowin, F. (2005). Detection of *Cryptosporidium* and identification to species level by Nested PCR and Restriction fragment length polymorphism. *J. Clin. Microbiol.*, 43: 1017-1023.

Current, W.L. (1990). Techniques and laboratory maintenance of *Cryptosporidium*. In: J.P. Dubey, C.A. Speer and R. Fayer (eds.), Cryptosporidiosis of man and animals, Boca Raton, FL, Press. pp. 31-39.

Current, W.L., Reese, N.C., Ernst, J.V., Bailey, W.S., Heyman, M.B. and Weinstein, W.M. 1983. Human cryptosporidiosis in immunocompetent and immunodeficient persons. Studies on outbreak and experimental transmission. *N. Eng. J. Med.*, 308: 1252-1258.

Current, W.L., Upton, S.J. and Haynes, T.B. (1986). The life cycle of *C. baileyi* spp. (Apicomplexa: Cryptosporidiidae) infecting chickens. *J. Protozool.*, 33: 289-296.

Das, G., Changkija, B., Sarkar, S. and Das, P. (2011). Genotyping of *Cryptosporidium parvum* isolates in bovine population in Kolkata and characterization of new bovine genotypes. *Res. Vet. Sci.*, 91: 246-250.

Das, G., Sarkar, S., Panja, P. and Das, P. (2004). PCR based detection of *Cryptosporidium parvum* in cattle. *J. Vet. Parasitol.*, 18: 43-44.

Das, P., Roy, S.S., Mitra, Dhar, K., Dutta, P., Bhattacharya, M.K., Sen, A., Ganguly, S., Bhattacharya, S.K., Lal, A.A. and Xiao, L. (2006). Molecular characterization of *Cryptosporidium* spp. in children in Kolkata, *India. J. Clin. Microbiol.*, 44 : 4246–4249.

Delafosse, A., Castro-Hermida, J. A., Baudry, C., Ares-Mazas, E. and Chartier, C. (2006). Herd-level risk factors for *Cryptosporidium* infection in dairy goat kids in western France. Prev. *Vet. Med.*, 77: 109–121.

Dela Fuente, R., Luon, M., Ruiz-Santa-Quiteria, J.A., Garcia, A., Cid, D., Orden, J.A., Garcia, S., Sanz, R. and Gomez-Bautista, M. (1999). *Cryptosporidium* and concurrent infections with other major enteropathogens in 1-30 days old diarrhoeic dairy calves in central Spain. *Vet. Parasitol.*, 8: 119-185.

Del Coco, V.F., Cordoba, M.A. and Basualdo, J.A. (2008). *Cryptosporidium* infection in calves from a rural area of Buenos Aires, Argentina. *Vet. Parasitol.*, 158: 31-35.

Dubey, J.P., Fayer, R. and Rao, J.R. (1992). Cryptosporidial oocysts in faeces of water buffalo and zebu calves in India. *J. Vet. Parasitol.*, 6: 55-56.

Elitok, B., Ozgul, M.E. and Huseyin, P. (2005). Efficacy of azithromycin dehydrate in treatment of cryptosporidiosis in naturally infected dairy calves. *J. Vet. Int. Med.*, 19: 590–593.

El-Khodery S.A. and Osman, S.A. (2008). Cryptosporidiosis in buffalo calves (Bubalus bubalis): Prevalence and potential risk factors. *Trop. Anim. Hlth. Prod.*, 40: 419-426.

El-Rahim, R. (1997). Bovine cryptosporidiosis in new born buffalo calves. In: Proceedings 5th world buffalo congress, Caserta, Italy, p. 37.

Ernest, J.A., Blagburn, B.L., Lindsay, D.S. and Current, W.L. (1986). Infection dynamics of *Cryptosporidium parvum* (Apicomplexa: Cryptosporiidae) in neonatal mice (Mus musculus). *J. Parasitol.*, 72: 796.

Farthing, M.J.G. (2000). Clinical aspects of human cryptosporidiosis. In: Percy, F. (ed.) Cryptosporidiosis and microsporidiosis. Contrib Microbiol Basel, Karger, 6: 50-74.

Fayer, R. (2004). *Cryptosporidium*: a water-borne zoonotic parasite. *Vet. Parasitol.*, 126: 37-56.

Fayer, R. and Ungar, B.L.P. (1986). *Cryptosporidium* spp. and cryptosporidiosis. Microbiol. Reviews, 50: 458.

Fayer, R., Gasbarre, L., Pasquali, P., Canals, A., Almeria, S. and Zarlenga, D. (1998). *Cryptosporidium parvum* infection in bovine neonates: dynamic, clinical, parasitic and immunologic patterns. *Int. J. Parasitol.*, 28: 49-56.

Fayer, R., Santin, M., Trout, J.M. and Greiner, E. (2006). Prevalence of species and genotypes of *Cryptosporidium* found in 1-2 year old dairy cattle in the eastern United States. *Vet. Parasitol.*, 135: 105-112.

Fayer, R., Santin, M. and Trout, J.M. (2007). Prevalence of *Cryptosporidium* spp. and genotypes in mature dairy cattle on farms in Eastern United States compared with younger cattle from the same locations. *Vet. Parasitol.*, 145: 260-266.

Fayer, R., Santin, M. and Xiao, L. (2005). *Cryptosporidium bovis* n. sp. (Apicomplexa: Cryptosporiidae) in cattle (Bos taurus). *J. Parasitol.*, 91: 624-629.

Fayer, R., Speer, C.A. and Dubey, J.P. (1997). The general biology of *Cryptosporidium*. In: Fayer, R., (ed.) *Cryptosporidium* and Cryptosporidiosis. Boca Raton, CRC Press, pp. 1-42.

Fayer, R., Trout, J.M., Graczyk T.D. and Lewis, E.J. (2000). Prevalence of *Cryptosporidium, Giardia* and *Eimeria* infections in post-weaned and adult cattle on three Maryland farms. *Vet. Parasitol.,* 93: 103-112.

Feltus, D.C., Giddings, C.W., Schneck, B.L., Monson, T., Warshauer, D. and McEvoy, J.M. (2006). Evidence supporting zoonotic transmission of *Cryptosporidium* in Wisconsin. *J. Clin. Microbiol.,* 44: 4303–4308.

Feng, Y., Ortega, Y., He, G., Das, P., Xu, M., Zhang, X., Fayer, R., Gatei, W., Cama, V. and Xiao, L. (2007). Wide geographic distribution of *Cryptosporidium parvum* and deer like genotype in bovines. *Vet. Parasitol.,* 144: 1-9.

Fukushima, K. and Helman, R.G. (1984). Cryptosporidiosis in a pup with distemper. *Vet. Pathol.,* 21: 247–48.

Gait, R., Soutar, R.H., Hanson, M., Fraser, C. and Chalmers, R. (2008). Outbreak of cryptosporidiosis amongst veterinary students. *Vet. Rec.,* 162: 843-845.

Garcia, L.S., Shimizu, R.Y., Novak, S., Carroll, M. and Chan, F. (2003). Commercial assay for detection of *Giardia lamblia* and *Cryptosporidium parvum* antigens in human fecal specimens by rapid solid-phase qualitative immunochromatography. *J. Clin. Microbiol.,* 41: 209 - 212.

Gargala, G. (2008). Drug treatment and novel drug target against *Cryptosporidium. Parasite,* 15: 275–281.

Gatei, W., Barrett, D., Lindo, J.F., Eldemire-Shearer, D., Cama, V. and Xiao, L. (2008). Unique *Cryptosporidium* population in HIV-infected persons, *Jamaica. Emer. Infect. Dis.,* 14: 841–843.

Gatei, W., Greensill, J., Ashford, R.W., Cuevas, L.E., Parry, C.M., Cunliffe, N.A., Beeching, N. J. and Hart, C.A. (2003). Molecular analysis of the 18 SrRNA gene of *Cryptosporidium* parasites from patients with or without human immunode?ciency virus living in Kenya, Malawi, Brazil, the United Kingdom and Vietnam. *J. Clin. Microbiol.,* 41: 1458–1462.

Gatei, W., Wamae, C.N., Mbae, C., Waruru, A., Mulinge, E., Waithera, T., Gatika, S.M., Kamwati, S.K., Revathi, G. and Hart, C.A. 2006. Cryptosporidiosis: prevalence, genotype analysis, and symptoms associated with infections in children in Kenya. *Am. J. Trop. Med. Hyg.,* 75: 78-82.

Geurden, T., Berkvens, D., Martens, C., Casaert, S., Vercruysse, J. and Claerebout, E. (2007). Molecular epidemiology with subtype analysis of *Cryptosporidium* in calves in Belgium. *Parasitol.,* 134:1981–1987.

Geurden, T., Gomab, F.Y., Siwilab, J., Phirib, I.G.K., Mwanzab, A.M., Gabriela, S. Claerebouta, E. and Vercruyssea, J. (2006). Prevalence and genotyping of *Cryptosporidium* in three cattle husbandry systems in Zambia. *Vet. Parasitol.,* 138: 217-222.

Ghimire, P., Sapkota, D., Prasad, S. and Manandhar, J. (2004). Cryptosporidiosis: Opportunistic Infection in HIV/AIDS Patients in Nepal. Trop. *Med. Parasitol.*, 27:7-10.

Ghorpade, M.V., Kulkarni, S.A. and Kulkarni, A.G. (1996). *Cryptosporidium, Isospora* and *Strongyloides* in AIDS. *Natl. Med. J. Ind.*, 9: 201.

Gibbons, C.L., Gazzard, B.G., Ibrahim, M., Morris-Jones, S., Ong, C.S.L. and Awad-E-Kareim, F.M. (1998). Correlation between markers of strain variation in *Cryptosporidium parvum*: evidence of clonality. *Parasitol. Int.*, 47: 139-147.

Godiwala, N.T., Vandewalle, A., Ward, H.D. and Leav, B.A. (2006). Quantification of in vitro and in vivo *Cryptosporidium parvum* by using Real-time PCR. App. Environ. *Microbiol.*, 72: 4484-4488.

Guarino, A., Canani, R.B., Casola, A., Pozio, E., Russo, R., Bruzzese, E., Fontana, M. and Rubino, A. (1995). Human intestinal cryptosporidiosis: secretory diarrhoea and enterotoxic activity in CaCo-2 cells. *J. Infect. Dis.*, 171: 976-983.

Hallier-Soulier, S. and Guillot, E. (2003). An immunomagnetic separation-reverse transcription polymerase chain reaction (IMS-RT-PCR) test for sensitive and rapid detection of viable waterborne *Cryptosporidium parvum*. App. Environ. *Microbiol.*, 5: 592-598.

Hamnes, I.S., Gjerde, B. and Robertson, L. (2006). Prevalence of *Giardia* and *Cryptosporidium* in dairy calves in three areas of Norway. *Vet. Parasitol.*, 140: 204-216.

Harper, C.M., Cowell, N.A., Adams, B.C., Langley, A.J. and Wohlson, T.D. (2002). Outbreak of *Cryptosporidium* linked to drinking unpasteurized milk. *Comm. Dis. Int.*, 26: 449-450.

Helmy, Y.A., Krucken, J., Nockler, K., Samson-Himmelstjerna, G. and Zessin, K.H. (2013). Molecular epidemiology of *Cryptosporidium* in livestock animals and human in the Ismailia province of Egypt. *Vet. Parasitol.*, 193: 15-24.

Henricksen, S.A. and Pohlenz, J.F.L. (1981). Staining of cryptosporidia by a modified Ziehl-Neelsen technique. *Acta Vet. Scand.*, 22: 594.

Hunter, P.R. and Nichols, G. (2002). Epidemiology and clinical features of *Cryptosporidium* infection in immunocompromised patients. *Clin. Microbiol. Rev.*, 15: 145–154.

International Commission on Zoological Nomenclature (1999). International Code of Zoological Nomenclature. International Trust for Zoological Nomenclature.

Jayalakshmi, J., Appalaraju, B. and Mahadevan, K. (2008). Evaluation of an enzyme-linked immunoassay for the detection of *Cryptosporidium* antigen in fecal specimens of HIV/AIDS patients. *Indian J. Path. Microbiol.,* 51: 137-138.

Jarvie, B.D., Trotz-Williams, L.A., McKnight, D.R., Leslie, K.E., Wallace, M.M., Todd, C.G., Scharpe, P.H. and Peregrine, A.S. (2005). Effect of halofuginone lactate on the occurrence of *Cryptosporidium parvum* and growth of neonatal dairy calves. *J. Dairy Sci.,* 88: 1801–1806.

Johnson, E.H., Windsor, J.J., Muirhead, D.E., King, G.J. and Al-Busaidy, R. (2000). Confirmation of the prophylactic value of paromomycin in a natural outbreak of caprine cryptosporidiosis. *Vet. Res. Comm.,* 24: 63–67.

Jeyabal, L. and Ray, D.D. (2005). Cryptosporidial infection in cattle and buffaloes. *J. Vet. Parasitol.,* 19: 165-166.

Kadappu, K.K., Nagaraja, M.V., Rao, P.V. and Shastry, B.A. (2002). Azithromycin as treatment for cryptosporidiosis in human immunodeficiency virus disease. *J. Postgrad. Med.,* 48: 179–181.

Karanth, N.V., Karanth, P.N., Gupta, S., Nair, R. and Parikh, P.M. (2007). Cryptosporidiosis in a relapsed case of Hodgkin's disease. *Indian J. Med. Sci.,* 61: 419–21.

Kaur, R., Rawat, D., Kakkar, M., Uppal, B. and Sharma, V.K. (2002). Intestinal parasites in children with diarrhea in Delhi, India. *Southeast Asian J. Trop. Med. Pub. Hlth.,* 33: 725–729.

Kaushik, K., Khurana, S., Wanchu, A. and Malla, N. (2008). Evaluation of staining techniques, antigen detection and nested-PCR for the diagnosis of cryptosporidiosis in HIV seropositive and seronegative patients. *Acta Trop.,* 107: 1–7.

Kehl, K.S.C., Cicirello, H. and Havens, P.L. (1995). Comparison of four different methods for detection of *Cryptosporidium* species. *J. Clin. Microbiol.,* 33: 416-418.

Keshavarz, A., Haghighi, A., Athari, A., Kazemi, B., Abadi, A. and Mojarad, E.N. (2009). Prevalence and molecular characterization of bovine *Cryptosporidium* in Qazvin province, Iran. *Vet. Parasitol.,* 160: 4316-4318.

Khan, S.M., Debnath, C., Pramanik, A.K., Xiaoc, L., Nozakid, T. and Gangulya, S. (2010). Molecular characterization and assessment of zoonotic transmission of *Cryptosporidium* from dairy cattle in West Bengal, India, *Vet. Parasitol.,* 171: 41-47.

Kilani, R.T. and Sekla, L. (1987). Purification of *Cryptosporidium* oocysts and sporozoites by caesium chloride and percoll gradients. *Am. J. Trop. Med. Hyg.,* 36: 505.

Kumar, D., Sreekrishnan, R. and Das, S.S. (2004). Cryptosporidiosis in man and animals in Pondicherry. *Indian J. Anim. Sci.,* 74: 261-263.

Kumarasamy, N., Solomon, S., Jayaker, Paul, S.A., Venilla, R. and Amalraj, R.E. (1995). Spectrum of opportunistic infections among AIDS patients in Tamil Nadu, *India. Int. J. STD AIDS,* 6: 447–449.

Kváè, M., Kouba, M. and Vítovec, J. (2006). Age-related and housing-dependence of *Cryptosporidium* infection of calves from dairy and beef herds in South Bohemia, Czech Republic. *Vet. Parasitol.,* 137: 202-209.

Leoni, F., Mallon, M.E., Smith, H.V., Tait, A. and McLauchlin, J. (2007). Multilocus analysis of *Cryptosporidium hominis* and *Cryptosporidium parvum* from sporadic and outbreak-related human cases and C. parvum from sporadic cases in livestock in the UK. *J. Clin. Microbiol.,* 45: 3286–3294.

Levine, N.D. (1985). Phylum II. Apicomplexa In: illustrated Guide to the Protozoa, Lee, J.J., Hutner, S.H. and Bovee, E.C. (eds.), Society of Protozoologists, Lawrence, pp. 322.

Lindergard, G., Nydam, D.V., Wade, S.E., Schaaf, S.L. and Mohammed, H.O. (2003). A novel multiplex polymerase chain reaction approach for detection of four human infective *Cryptosporidium* isolates: *Cryptosporidium parvum,* types H and C, *Cryptosporidium canis* and *Cryptosporidium felis* in fecal and soil samples. *J. Vet. Diag. Invest.,* 15: 262-267.

Llorente, M.T., Clavel, A., Varea, M., Olivera, S., Castillo, F.J., Sahagun, J., Rubio, M.C. and Gomez-Lus, R. (2002). Evaluation of an Immuno-chromatographic dip-strip test for the detection of *Cryptosporidium* oocysts in stool specimens. Eur. *J. Clin. Microbiol. Infec. Dis.,* 21: 624–625.

Maddox-Hyttel, C., Langkjaer, R.B, Enemark, H.L. and Vigre, H. (2006). *Cryptosporidium* and *Giardia* in different age group of Danish cattle and pigs- occurrence and management associated risk factors. *Vet. Parasitol.,* 141: 48-59.

Malla, N., Sehgal, R., Ganguly, N.K. and Mahajan, R.C. (1987). Cryptosporidiosis in children in Chandigarh. *Indian J. Med. Res.,* 86: 722–725.

Mallinath, R.H.K., Chikkachowdappa, P.G., Gowda, A.K.J. and D'Souza, P.E. (2009). Studies on the prevalence of cryptosporidiosis in bovines in organized dairy farms in and around Bangalore, south India. *Vet. Arhiv,* 79: 461-470.

Manabe, Y.C., Clark, D.P., Moore, R.D., Lumadue, J.A., Dahlman, H.R., Belitsos, P.C., Chaisson, R.E. and Sears. C.L. (1998). Cryptosporidiosis in patients with AIDS: correlates of disease and survival. Clin. *Infect. Dis.,* 27: 536-542.

Maurya, P.S., Rakesh, R.L., Mandal, M., Kumar, S., Kundu, K., Ram, H., Garg, R. and Banerjee, P.S. (2012). *Cryptosporidium* oocysts shedding pattern in new born dairy calves. In: proceedings of 23rd National Congress of Veterinary Parasitology. Guwahati, Assam, India, Dec. 12-14, 2012.

Maurya, P.S. (2011). Molecular characterization of *Cryptosporidium* spp. isolates from domestic animals. M.V.Sc. thesis submitted to Deemed University, Indian Veterinary Research Institute, Izatnagar, UP, India.

Mawdsley, J.L., Brooks, A.E. and Merry, R.J. (1996). Movement of the protozoan pathogen *Cryptosporidium parvum* through three contrasting soil types. *Biol. Fert. Soils*, 21: 30–36.

McAllister, T.A., Olson, M.E., Fletch, A., Wetzstein, M. and Entz, T. (2005). Prevalence of *Giardia* and *Cryptosporidium* in beef cows in southern Ontario and in beef calves in southern British Columbia. *Can. Vet. J.*, 46: 47–55.

McKenzie, W.R., Hoxie, N.J., Proctor, M.E., Gradus, S., Blair, K.A., Peterson, D.E. and Lazmlerczak, J.J. (1994). A massive outbreak in Milwaukee of *Cryptosporidium* infection transmitted through the public water supply. *N. Eng. J. Med.*, 331: 161-167.

McLauchlin, J., Amar, C., Pedraza-Diaz, S. and Nichols, G.L. (2000). Molecular epidemiological analysis of Cryptosporidium spp. in the United Kingdom: results of genotyping *Cryptosporidium* spp. in 1,705 fecal samples from humans and 105 fecal samples from livestock animals. *J. Clin. Microbiol.*, 38: 3984–3990.

Meloni, B.P. and Thompson, R.C.A. (1996). Simplified method for obtaining purified oocysts from mice and growing *Cryptosporidium parvum* in vitro. *J. Parasitol.*, 82: 757-762.

Mohammed, H.O., Wade, S.E. and Schaaf, S. (1999). Risk factors associated with *Cryptosporidium parvum* infection in dairy cattle in southeastern New York State. *Vet. Parasitol.*, 106: 1-10.

Molbak, K., Andersen, M., Aaby, P., Hojlyng, N., Jakobsen, M., Sodemann, M. and da Silva. A.P. (1997). *Cryptosporidium* infection in infancy as a cause of malnutrition: a community study from Guinea-Bissau, West Africa. *Am. J. Clin. Nut.*, 65: 149–152.

Molloy, S.F., Smith, H.V., Kirwan, P., Nichols, R.A.B., Asaolu, S.O., Connelly, L. and Holland, C.V. (2010). Identification of a high diversity of *Cryptosporidium* species genotypes and subtypes in a pediatric population in Nigeria. *Am. J. Trop. Med. Hyg.*, 82: 608-613.

Moore, D.A., Atwill, E.R., Kirk, J.H., Brahmbhatt, D., Herrera Alonso, L., Hou, L., Singer, M. D. and Miller, T.D. (2003). Prophylactic use of decoquinate for infections with *Cryptosporidium parvum* in experimentally challenged neonatal calves. *J. Am. Vet. Med. Assoc.*, 223: 839–845.

Mukhopadhya, A., Ramakrishna, B.S., Kang, G., Pulimood, A.B., Mathan, M.M., Zachariah, A. and Mathai, D.C. (1999). Enteric pathogens in southern Indian HIV-infected patients with and without diarrhoea. *Indian J. Med. Res.*, 109: 85-89.

Muthusamy, D., Rao, S.S., Ramani, S., Monica, B., Banerjee, I., Abraham, O.C., Mathai, D.C., Beryl, P., Muliyil, J., Wanke, C.A., Ward, H.D. and Kang, G. (2006). Multilocus Genotyping of *Cryptosporidium* spp. isolates from human immuno-deficiency virus-infected individuals in South India. J. Clin. *Microbiol.*, 44: 632–634.

Naciri, M., Lefay, M.P., Mancassola, R., Poirier, P. and Chermette, R. (1999). Role of *Cryptosporidium parvum* as a pathogen in neonatal diarrhoea complex in suckling and dairy calves in France. *Vet. Parasitol.*, 85: 245–257.

Nagamani, K., Rajkumari, A. and Gyaneshwari. (2001). Cryptosporidiosis in a tertiary care hospital in Andhra Pradesh. *Indian J. Med. Microbiol.*, 19: 215-216.

Nagamani, K., Pavuluri, P.R.R., Gyaneshwari, M., Prasanthi, K., Rao, M.I.S. and Saxena, N.K. (2007). Molecular characterization of *Cryptosporidium*: An emerging parasite. *Indian J. Med. Microbiol.*, 25: 133-136.

Navin, T.R. and Juranek, D.D. (1984). Cryptosporidiosis: Clinical, epidemiologic and parasitologic review. *Rev. Infect. Dis.*, 6: 313.

Nchito, M., Kelly, P., Sianongo, S., Luo, N.P., Feldman, R., Farthing, M. and Baboo, K.S. (1998). Cryptosporidiosis in urban Zambian children: an analysis of risk factors. *Am. J. Trop. Med. Hyg.*, 59: 435–437.

Newman, R.D., Jaeger, K.L., Wuhib, T., Lima, A.A., Guerrant, R.L. and Sears, C.L. (1993). Evaluation of an antigen capture enzyme-linked immunosorbent assay for detection of *Cryptosporidium* oocysts. *J. Clin. Microbiol.*, 31: 2080–2084.

Nooruddin, M. and Sarma, D.K. (1987). Role of *Cryptosporidium* in calf diarrhoea: In annual report Livestock Advisor, 12: 49.

O'Connor, R.M., Wanyiri, J.W., Cevallos, A.M., Priest, J.W. and Ward, H.D. (2007). *Cryptosporidium parvum* glycoprotein gp40 localizes to the sporozoite surface by association with gp15. *Mol. Biochem. Parasitol.*, 156: 80–83.

O'Donoghue, P.J. (1995). *Cryptosporidium* and cryptosporidiosis in man and animals. *Int. J. Parasitol.*, 25 (2): 139–95.

OIE (2008). Cryptosporidiosis. Chapter 2.9.4. In: OIE Terrestrial Manual, pp. 1192-1215.

Ortega, Y.R., Sheehy, R.R., Cama, V.A., Oishi, K.K. and Sterling. C.R. (1991). Restriction fragment length polymorphism analysis of *Cryptosporidium parvum* isolates of bovine and human origin. *J. Protozool.*, 38: 40S–41S.

Panciera, R. J., Thomassen, R.W. and Garner, F. M. (1971). Cryptosporidial infection in a calf. *Vet. Pathol.*, 35: 249-252.

Pradeep, B. (2008). Cloning and characterization of a surface glycoprotein gene of *Cryptosporidium* spp. of bovine origin. M.V.Sc. thesis submitted to Deemed University, Indian Veterinary Research Institute, Izatnagar, UP, India.

Parker, J.F.W. and Smith, H.V. (1994). The recovery of *Cryptosporidium* spp. oocysts from water samples by immunomagnetic separation. *Trans. R. Soc. Trop. Med. Hyg.*, 88: 25-28.

Paul, S., Chandra, D., Ray, D.D., Tewari, A.K., Rao, J.R., Banerjee, P.S., Baidya, S. and Raina, O.K. (2008). Prevalence and molecular characterization of bovine *Cryptosporidium* isolates in India. *Vet. Parasitol.*, 153: 143-146.

Paul, S., Chandra, D., Tewari, A.K., Banerjee, P.S., Ray, D.D., Raina, O.K. and Rao, J.R. (2009a). Prevalence of *Cryptosporidium andersoni*: A molecular epidemiological survey among cattle in India. *Vet. Parasitol.*, 161: 31-35.

Paul, S., Chandra, D., Tewari, A.K., Banerjee, P.S., Ray, D.D., Boral, R. and Rao, J.R. (2009b). Comparative evaluation and economic assessment of coprological diagnostic methods and PCR for detection of *Cryptosporidium* spp. in bovines. *Vet. Parasitol.*, 164: 291-295.

Pedersen, C., Danner, S., Lazzarin, A., Glauser, M.P., Weber, R., Katlama, C., Barton, S.E. and Lundgren, J.D. (1996). Epidemiology of cryptosporidiosis among European AIDS patients. *Genitourin Med.*, 72: 128-131.

Pohjola, S., Jokipii, L. and Jokipii, A.M.M. (1984). Dimethylsulphoxide-Ziehl-Neelsen staining technique for the detection of cryptosporidial oocysts. *Vet. Rec.*, 115: 442-443.

Prakash, S., Prabu, K. and Palanivel, K. 2009. Prevalence of cryptosporidiosis in dairy calves in Chennai. Tamilnadu. *J. Vet. Anim. Sci.*, 5: 41-46.

Ralston, B.J., Cockwill, E.L., Guselle, N.J., Van Herk, F.H., McAllister, T.A. and Olson, M.E. (2003). Prevalence of *Giardia* and *Cryptosporidium* andersoni and their effects on performance in feedlot beef calves. *Can. J. Ani. Sci.*, 83: 153-159.

Randhawa, S.S., Zahid, U.N., Randhawa, S.S., Juyal, P.D., Singla, L.D. and Uppal, S.K. (2012). Therapeutic management of cryptosporidiosis in cross bred dairy calves. *Ind. Vet. J.*, 82: 17-19.

Ramirez, N.E. and Sreevatsan, S. (2006). Development of a sensitive detection system for *Cryptosporidium* in environmental samples. *Vet. Parasitol.*, 136: 201-213.

Rinaldi, L., Musella, V., Condoleo, R., Saralli, G., Veneziano, V., Bruni, G., Condoleo, R.U. and Cringoli, G. (2007). *Giardia* and *Cryptosporidium* in water buffaloes (Bubalus bubalis). *Parasitol. Res.,* 100: 1113-1118.

Robinson, G., Elwin, K. and Chalmers, R.M. (2008). Unusual Cryptosporidium genotypes in human cases of diarrhoea. Emerg. *Infect. Dis.,* 14: 1800–1802.

Rosenblatt, J.E. and Sloan, L.M. (1993). Evaluation of an enzyme linked immunosorbent assay for detection of *Cryptosporidium* spp. in stool specimens. *J. Clin. Microbiol.,* 31: 1468-1471.

Roy, S.S., Sarkar, S., Batabyal, S., Pramanik, A.K. and Das, P. (2006). Observation on the epidemiology of bovine cryptosporidiosis in India. *Vet. Parasitol.,* 141: 330-333.

Sahu, B.D., Maiti, S.K., Sanyal, P.K. and Pal, S. (2010). Morphologic study of *Cryptosporidium* oocysts in diarrhoeic calves. *J. Vet. Parasitol.,* 24:105-106.

Santin, M., Trout, J.M. and Fayer, R. (2008). A longitudinal study of Cryptosporidiosis in dairy cattle from birth to 2 years of age. *Vet. Parasitol.,* 155: 15-23.

Santin, M., Trout, J.M., Xiao, L., Zhou, L., Greiner, E. and Fayer, R. (2004). Prevalence and age related variation of *Cryptosporidium* species and genotypes in dairy calves. *Vet. Parasitol.,* 122: 103–117.

Spano, F., Putignani, L., McLauchlin, J., Casemore, D.P. and Crisanti, A. (1997). PCR-RFLP analysis of the *Cryptosporidium* oocyst wall protein (COWP) gene discriminates between *C. wrairi* and *C. parvum*, and between C. parvum isolates of human and animal origin. FEMS Microbiol. Letters, 150: 209-217.

Saraswathi, K., Pandit, D.V., Deodhar, L.P. and Bichiles, L.S. (1988). Prevalence of Cryptosporidia in patients with diarrhoea in Bombay. *Ind. J. Med. Res.,* 87: 221-224.

Schnyder, M., Kohler, L., Hemphill, A. and Deplazes, P. (2009). Prophylactic and therapeutic efficacy of nitazoxanide against *Cryptosporidium parvum* in experimentally challenged neonatal calves. *Vet. Parasitol.,* 160: 149–154.

Scorza, A.V. and Lappin, M.R. (2006). An update in three important protozoan parasitic infections in cats: cryptosporidiosis, giardiasis, and tritrichomoniasis. *Vet. Med.,* 18-32 (Suppl.).

Scorza, A.V. and Lappin, M.R. (2007). Co-infection of *Cryptosporidium* and *Giardia* in naturally infected cats. In: Diagnosis and Treatment of cryptosporidiosis and giardiasis in cats and dogs in the United States. Clinical Sciences, Colorado State University, Fort Collins, CO.

Shobhamani, B., Singari, N.A. and Syamasundar, N. (2006). A study on clinical manifestations of cryptosporidiosis in calves. *Ind. Vet. J.,* 83: 677-678.

Silverlas, C., Naslund, K., Bjorkman, C. and Mattsson, J.G. (2010). Molecular characterization of *Cryptosporidium* isolates from Swedish dairy cattle in relation to age, diarrhoea and region. *Vet. Parasitol.,* 169: 289–295.

Singh, B.B., Sharma, R., Kumar, H., Banga, H.S., Aulakh, R.S., Gill, J.P.S. and Sharma, J.K. (2006). Prevalence of *Cryptosporidium parvum* infection in Punjab and its association with diarrhoea in neonatal dairy calves. *Vet. Parasitol.,* 140: 162-165.

Smith, H.V. (1998). Detection of parasites in the environment. Parasitol., 117: S113–S141.

Smith, H.V., McDiarmid, A., Smith, A.L., Hinson, A.R. and Gilmour, R.A. (1989). An analysis of staining methods for the detection of *Cryptosporidium* spp. oocysts in water-related samples. *Parasitol.,* 99: 323-327.

Soave, M.P.R. (1983). Three-step stool examination for cryptosporidiosis in 10 homosexual men with protracted watery diarrhoea. *J. Infect. Dis.,* 147: 824-828.

Soba, B. and Logar, J. (2008). Genetic classification of *Cryptosporidium* isolates from humans and calves in Slovenia. *Parasitol.,* 135: 1263-1270.

Sorvillo, F., Beall, G., Turner, P.A., Beer, V.L., Kovacs, A., Kraus, P., Masters, D. and Kerndt, P.R. (1998). Seasonality and factors associated with cryptosporidiosis among individuals with HIV infection. Epidimiol. *Infect.,* 121: 197-204.

Spano, F. and Crisanti, A. (2000). *Cryptosporidium parvum*: the many secrets of a small genome. *Int. J. Parasitol.,* 30 (4): 553–65.

Striepen, B., White, M.W., Li, C., Guerini, M.N., Malik, S.B., Logsdon, J.M., Lin, C. and Abrahamsen, M.S. (2002). Genetic complementation in apicomplexan parasites. *Proceed. Natl. Acad. Sci.,* 99: 6304-6309.

Sturbaum, G.D., Reed, C., Hoover, P.J., Jost, B.H., Marshall, M.M. and Sterling, C.R. (2001). Species-specific Nested PCR-Restriction Fragment Length Polymorphism detection of single *Cryptosporidium parvum* Oocysts. App. Environ. *Microbiol.,* 67: 2665 - 2668.

Subramanyam, V.R., Broadhead, R.L., Pal, B.B., Pati, J.B. and Mohanty, G. (1989). Cryptosporidiosis in children of eastern India. *Ani. Trop. Paed.,* 9: 122-125.

Sulaiman, I.M., Xiao, L., Yang, C., Escalante, L., Moore, A., Beard, C.B., Arrowood, M.J. and Lal, A.A. (1998). Differentiating human from animal isolates of *Cryptosporidium parvum*. *Emerg. Infect. Dis.,* 4: 681-685.

Sulaiman, I.M., Morgan, U.M., Thompson, R.C., Lal, A.A. and Xiao, L. (2000). Phylogenetic relationships of *Cryptosporidium* parasites based on the 70-kilodalton heat shock protein (HSP 70) gene. *Appl. Environ. Microbiol.,* 66: 2385-2391.

Sulaiman, I.M., Hira, P.R., Zhou, L., Al-Ali, F.M., Al-Shelahi, F.A., Shweiki, H.M., Iqbal, J., Khalid, N. and Xiao, L. (2005). Unique endemicity of cryptosporidiosis in children in Kuwait. *J. Clin. Microbiol.,* 43: 2805-2809.

Thompson, R.C.A., Olson, M.E., Zhu, G., Enomoto, S., Abrahamsen, M.S. and Hijjawl, N.S. (2005). *Cryptosporidium* and Cryptosporidiosis. *Adv. Parasitol.,* 59: 77-158.

Thompson, H.P., Dooley, J.S., Kenny, J., McCoy, M., Lowery, C.J., Moore, J.E. and Xiao, L. (2007). Genotypes and subtypes of *Cryptosporidium* spp. in neonatal calves in Northern Ireland. *Parasitol. Res.,* 100: 619–624.

Trotz-Williams, L.A., Martin, D.S., Gatei, W., Cama, V., Peregrine, A.S., Martin, S.W., Nydam, D.V., Jamieson, F. and Xiao, L. (2006). Genotype and subtype analyses of *Cryptosporidium* isolates from dairy calves and humans in Ontario. *Parasitol. Res.,* 99: 346–352.

Tyzzer, E. (1907). A sporozoon found in the peptic glands of the common mouse. Proceed. Soc. Exp. Biol. Med., 5: 12-13.

Tyzzer, E. (1910). An extracelluar coccidium, *Cryptosporidium muris* (gen. and sp. nov.), of the gastric glands of the common mouse. *J. Med. Res.,* 18: 487-509.

Tyzzer, E. (1912). *Cryptosporidium parvum* (sp. nov.), a coccidium found in the small intestine of the common mouse. *Arch Protisenkd.,* 26: 394-412.

Tzipori, S. and Ward, H. (2002). Cryptosporidiosis: biology, pathogenesis and disease. *Microbes and Infection,* 4: 1047-58.

Tzipori, S. and Widmer, G. (2008). A hundred year retrospective on cryptosporidiosis. *Trends Parasitol.,* 24: 184-189.

Tzipori, S., Angus, K.W., Campbell, I. and Gray, E.W. (1980). *Cryptosporidium*: evidence for a single-species genus. *Infect. Immun.,* 30: 884–886.

Tzipori, S., Smith, M., Halpin, C., Angus, K.W., Sherwood, D. and Campbell, I. (1983). Experimental cryptosporidiosis in calves: clinical manifestations and pathological findings. *Vet. Rec.,* 112: 116-118.

Uga, S., Matsuo, J., Kono, E., Kimura, K., Inoue, M., Rai, S.K. and Ono, K. (2000). Prevalence of *Cryptosporidium parvum* infection and pattern of oocysts shedding in calves in Japan *Vet. Parasitol.,* 94: 27-32.

Ungar, B. (1990). Cryptosporidiosis in humans. In JP Dubey, CA Speer, R Fayer (eds), Cryptosporidiosis of Man and Animals, CRC Press, Boca Raton, USA, pp. 59-82.

Upton, S.J. and Current, W.L. (1985). The species of *Cryptosporidium* (Apicomplexa: Cryptosporidiidae) infecting mammals. *J. Parasitol.,* 71: 625-629.

Vakil, N.B., Schwartz, S.M., Buggy, B.P., Brummitt, C.F., Kherellah, M., Letzer, D.M., Gilson, I.H. and Jones, P.G. (1996). Biliary cryptosporidiosis in HIV-infected people after the waterborne outbreak of cryptosporidiosis in Milwaukee. *N. Eng. J. Med.*, 334: 19-23.

Venu, R., Latha, B.R., Basith, S.A., Sreekumar, C., Dhinakarraj, G. and Raman, M. (2011). Molecular detection and typing of *Cryptosporidium* in dairy calves. In proceedings of 22nd National congress of Veterinary Parasitology, Mumbai, *India, Jan.* 5-7, 2011.

Venu, R., Latha, B.R., Basith, A.S., Raj, D.G., Sreekumar, C. and Raman, M. (2012). Molecular prevalence of *Cryptosporidium* spp. in dairy calves in southern states of India. *Vet. Parasitol.*, 188: 19-24.

Weber, R., Bryan, R.T., Bishop, H.S., Wahlquist, S.P., Sullivan, J.J. and Juranek, D.D. (1991). Threshold of detection of *Cryptosporidium* oocysts in human stool specimens: evidence of low sensitivity in current diagnostic methods. *J. Clin. Microbiol.*, 29: 1323-1327.

Webster, K.A., Smith, H.V., Giles, M., Dawson, L. and Robertson, L.J. (1996). Detection of *Cryptosporidium parvum* oocysts in faeces: Comparison of conventional coproscopical methods and the polymerase chain reaction. *Vet. Parasitol.*, 61: 5-13.

Wielinga, P.R., de Vries, A., Vander Goot, T.H., Mank, T., Mars, M.H., Kortbeek, L.M. and Vander Giessen, J.W. (2008). Molecular epidemiology of *Cryptosporidium* in humans and cattle in the Netherlands. *Int. J. Parasitol.*, 38: 809–817.

Xiao, L., Bern, C., Limor, J., Sulaiman, I., Roberts, J., Checkley, W., Cabrera, L., Gilman, R.H. and Lal, A.A. (2001a). Identification of 5 types of *Cryptosporidium* parasites in children in Lima, Peru. *J. Infect. Dis.*, 183: 492-497.

Xiao, L., Escalante, L., Yang, C., Sulaiman, I., Escalante, A.A., Monsali, R.J., Fayer, R. and Lal, A.A. (1999). Phylogenetic analysis of *Cryptosporidium* parasites based on the ssu rRNA gene locus. *Appl. Environ. Microbiol.*, 65: 1578-1583.

Xiao, L., Fayer, R., Ryan, U. and Upton, S.J. (2004). *Cryptosporidium* taxonomy: recent advances and implications for public health. *Clin. Microbiol. Rev.*, 17: 72–97.

Xiao, L. (2010). Molecular epidemiology of cryptosporidiosis: an update. Exp. *Parasitol.*, 124: 80-89.

Yadav, A., Katoch, R., Katoch, M., Agrawal, R., Khajuria, J.K., Borkataki, S. and Kumar, S. (2010). Prevalence of bovine cryptosporidiosis in Jammu region. XX National Congress of Veterinary Parasitology, Hisar, Feb. 18-20, 2010.

Yadav, A., Katoch, R., Katoch, M., Agrawal, R., Khajuria, J.K. Godara, R. and

Kalha, R. (2012). Cross-sectional study and analysis of potential risk factors for *Cryptosporidium* spp. infection in buffalo calves in Jammu. *Vet. Pract.*, 13(2): 278-281.

Zintl, A., Proctor, A.F., Read, C., Dewaal, T., Shanaghy, N., Fanning, S. and Mulcahy, G. (2009). The prevalence of *Cryptosporidium* species and subtypes in human faecal samples in Ireland. *Epid. Infect.*, 137: 270–277.

□□□

Chapter 5

Epidemiology and Management of Gastrointestinal Nematodes in Ruminants

S.S. Chaudhri and V. Bhanot
Lala Lajpat Rai University of Veterinary and Animal Sciences, Veterinary Unit Substation, Teaching Veterinary Clinical Complex, Uchani, Karnal, India

Introduction

Livestock population including cattle-185.2, buffaloes- 97.9, sheep- 61.5, goats-124.4 and camels- 0.6 million in India ranks first in respect of buffalo, second in cattle and goat, third in sheep and sixth in camel population in the world (Anon, 2003).The country's milk production in the year 2008-09 stood at about 108.5 million tones, which is highest in the world but in spite of a higher growth rate, per capita availability of milk in India is only 252 grams per day in comparison to world average 265 grams per day. This sector has also contributed other food products including wool and meat to the global market. Thus, livestock sector plays an important role in the rural economy by supplementing family income and generating gainful employment in the rural sector.

Since productivity is a key to growth, livestock productivity will have to be raised through scientific breeding, feeding and management of diseases and metabolic disorders. The diseases in animals are caused by infectious and non-infectious agents and among them gastrointestinal (GI) nematodes leading to parasitic gastroenteritis (PGE) are major constraints for livestock production by lowering their working capacity, growth, body weight, milk yield, etc. (Mehlhorn, 1988). Though information on incidence of GI nematodes involved in PGE and several epidemiological factors influencing their spread and intensity in some agro-climatic zones of India is available (Gupta *et al.*, 1987; Sanyal and Singh, 1995; Singh *et al.*, 1997; Yadav *et al.*, 2006; Bhat *et al.*, 2007) but continuous monitoring and surveillance is required for effective control. Integrated control of these infections will also require highly specific and sensitive methods to detect tissue stages of these infections and also to monitor anthelmintic resistance in different nematode species, but studies conducted on these aspects are limited (Ghosh and Banerjee, 1998; Jas *et al.*, 2010; Jyoti *et al.*, 2011a,b). The available literature on GI nematodes infecting small and large ruminants with particular reference to epidemiology, animal husbandry practices, effective diagnostic methods and anthelmintics in different agro-climatic zones has been reviewed to devise integrated control measures.

Epidemiology

Planning Commission has demarcated the geographical area of India based on agro-climatic features, particularly soil type, climate including temperature, rainfall and water resources availability into 15 agro-climatic regions. Pasture contamination with more free living stages of *Haemonchus contortus*, the dominant GI nematode responsible for causing PGE in ruminants, during rainy and post rainy seasons is due to favourable climatic conditions influencing rate of larval migration (Ogbourne, 1972; Croll, 1973). Higher rate of infection in animals during rainy months may be attributed to suitable molarity of salt present in soil which is an important factor for ecdysis of larvae (Ahmad and Ansari, 1987; Katoch *et al.*, 2000; Gagan *et al.*, 2003). The agro-climatic conditions, animal husbandry practices and pasture management largely determine the incidence and the severity of parasitic diseases affecting grazing animals (Jithendran and Bhat, 1999). While evaluating preponderance of infective L_3 of GI nematodes in grazing areas of North-eastern zone in Tamil Nadu in relation to various meteorological parameters, rainfall was observed to have positive influence on GI nematode egg load during Northwest and Southwest monsoon seasons (Basith *et al.*, 2010). Thus epizootiological determinants including agro-climate, prolonged winter, rainfall etc. have been observed to affect the survival and development of free living stages of GI nematodes. The data has been reviewed on the prevalence, epidemiological pattern and management of GI nematodosis in ruminants in some major agro-climatic zones.

Western Himalayan region

This is the mountainous region having temperate climate and it is comprised of Jammu and Kashmir,Himachal Pradesh and Uttrakhand. Mainly sheep and goats are reared in this region and population of cows and buffalos is very less.In Kashmir valley,there is precipitation of snow and rain during winter (December to February). Sheep flocks are reared on lush green pastures during summer. Increasing trend in nematode infections of ruminants in Kashmir has been observed from March to May (spring) and from June to November (Makhdoomi *et al.*, 1995; Tariq *et al.*, 2008). Seasonal incidence of GI nematodes including *Haemonchus* spp., *Nematodirus* spp. and *Marshallagia* spp. was highest in summer (67.1%), followed by autumn (64.9%) (Nasreen *et al.*, 2005).High egg per gram (EPG) values have also been reported in goats during rainy season (July to September) from Jammu region (Yadav *et al.*, 2006) and such high counts may be due to suitable temperature and humidity required for the development and survival of preparasitic stages (Soulsby, 1982).

High mortality was recorded due to *H.contortus* in lambs and ewes of Corriedale breed following their migration from highland pastures to sheep breeding farm, Shuhama of Kashmir valley (Darzi *et al.*, 2004). Later, sheep in this farm and highland pastures were recorded with much higher incidence of strongyles (85-94.1%) and high susceptibility in hoggets than weaners (Bhat *et al.*, 2007). The exotic breeds of organized farm and high land pasture had higher incidence of strongyles (64-73.2%) than native breeds (26.8-35.3 %), and among GI nematodes, *Nematodirus* spp. were most common in farm, whereas *Haemonchus,* followed by *Marshallagia* was most abundant at grassland pasture. The epidemiological studies on GI nematodes in sheep managed under traditional husbandry in Kashmir valley revealed its overall prevalence from 58.4 to 64.8% and parasites encountered in decreasing order were *H. contortus, O. circumcincta, B. trigonocephalum, Chabertia ovina, Trichostrongylus* spp., *N. spathiger, O. columbianum, T. ovis* and *M. marshalli* (Tariq *et al.*, 2008). Lower age group of animals had more infection than the others.*H. contortus, Trichostrongylus, Oesophagostomum, Strongyloides, Ostertagia, Chabertia* and *Trichuris* were recovered during an outbreak of PGE in sheep from plains of Jammu division(Khajuria *et al.*, 2009). The affected animals were weak, anorectic and diarrhoeic with 80% morbidity and 8% mortality.

GI nematodes in animals of Jammu and Kashmir included *T. axei, T. colubriformis, H. contortus, B. trigonocephalum, C. ovina. C. himalayana,*

N.spathiger, Skrjabinema ovis, O. ovis, T. globulosa, Cooperia spp., *S.papillosus* and *Marshallagia* in sheep; *N. spathiger, S. ovis, O. ovis, T. globulosa* and *Ostertagia* in goats; *Ostertagia* and *Cooperia* in yaks and *T. vitulorum* in cow calves (Sharma and Godara, 2010). Species-wise incidence of *Trichostrongylus* spp. and *Marshallagia* spp. was highest in winter and that of *Haemonchus* and *Nematodirus* was highest in summer. The incidence of *C. ovina* in sheep was recorded with peak levels during autumn and winter months.

High mortality was seen in sheep on a high altitude farm in Himachal Pradesh (HP) due to *Haemonchus* spp., *Strongyloides* spp., *Trichostrongylus* spp. and*Nematodirus* spp. (Katoch *et al.*, 1998). The migrating flocks of sheep in Himachal Pradesh were observed with high intensity of GI nematodes from July to September (Jithenderan, 1998). The prevalence of GI nematodes viz., *Strongyloides, Trichostrongylus, Haemonchus, Oesophagostomum, Bunostomum* and *Mecistocirrus* was recorded with overall monthly mean faecal egg counts ranging from 85 to 1720 in cattle and 90 to 1625 in buffaloes, with peak during the months of July to September(Jithenderan and Bhat, 1999). Review of literature about the prevalence of GI nematodes in ruminants of Himachal Pradesh could revealed the presence of *T. axei, T. colubriformis, H. contortus, Strongyloides spp., B. trigonocephalum, Chabertia* spp., *Ostertagia* spp.and *Oesophagostomum* in sheep and goats, and *T. axei, T. colubriformis, H. contortus, Strongyloides* spp., *Trichuris, Capillaria* spp., *Oesophagostomum, Paracooperia* spp. and *T. vitulorum* in bovines (Sharma and Godara, 2010).

Sheep and goats of tarai region in Uttrakhand were seen to have higher prevalence (66.6-67.0%) of GI nematodesthan that of hill region (33.3-45.0%) and risk-wise animals of tarai region suffered from GI nematodosis in September and October, whereas those of hill region suffered during May to July (Yadav *et al.*, 2008a; 2009). *H. contortus* was the predominant parasite, followed by *T.colubriformis* and *O. columbianum*. Cattle (17.8%) and buffaloes (9.8%) in hills and tarai regions of Uttrakhand were observed to be infected with *H.contortus* as predominant parasite, followed by *Trichostrongylus* spp., *Oesophagostomum* spp., *Bunostomum* spp., *Ostertagia* spp. and *Cooperia* spp. in cattle and *Paracooperia* spp. in buffaloes with more or less similar infection incattle of hills and tarai region and lowerinfection in hill buffaloes (2.9%) than thatof tarairegion (16.8%) (Yadav *et al.*, 2008b).

Eastern Himalayan region

Sheep, goats, yak and buffaloes in this region are used for transport, food, fiber and their dung is used as a source of fuel. Cattle and mithun (*Bos frontalis*) play amajor role in improving socio-economic conditions of people in North-eastern Himalayan region comprised of Assam, Meghalaya, Arunachal Pradesh, Nagaland, Mizoram, Manipur, Tripura and Sikkim. Mithun is a crossbred between Gaur (*Bos gaurus*) and domestic cattle (*Bos indicus*) and under similar environmental conditions, there is every possibility that they suffer from parasitic diseasessimilar to cattle. The calves of mithun, 1-3 months of age from Arunachal Pradesh, Manipur, Mizoram and Nagaland had higher infection of *T. vitulorum* and *Strongyloides* and number of animals infected with these GINs decreased with the age, whereas reverse was seen with strongyle infection (Rajkhowa*et al.*, 2003, 2005). These observations were similar to those made in buffalo and cow-calves from other parts of India (Gupta *et al.*, 1985;Pradhan *et al.*, 1991). Mithun calves, one year old, from Jharna Panifarm of Assam were observed to be infected with *Toxocara, Strongyloides* and *Trichuris* spp. (Chamuah *et al.*, 2009). The prevalence of *Toxocara* was more in monsoon season, whereas *Strongyloides* had no seasonal effect. The most common strongyle worms in these calves were *Haemonchus* and *Trichostrongylus* spp. and less common were *Cooperia* spp. and *Bunostomum* spp.

The goats from some villages and from organized farms in temperate and humid zones of Sikkim had *H. contortus* in abomasii, *B. trigonocephalum, T. colubriformis* and *N. fillicolis* in small intestine, and *O. columbianum, T. globulosa* and *T. ovis* in large intestine (Pal and Bandyopadhyay, 2004). *Haemonchus* spp. was most prevalent GIN throughout the year, whereas other parasites were recorded during two seasons, the first in the months of March-April and the later in September-November.Season-wise prevalence of GINs in goats from Meghalaya was more in summer, followed by monsoon and winter (Laha *et al.*, 2010). Yaks, multi-utility animals in northern and eastern districts of Sikkim, had GINs including strongyles (16.9%), *Strongyloides* (4.9%), *Toxocara* (4.4%) and*Trichuris* (3.4%),with faecal egg counts ranging between 100-2900 and high worm loads during rainy and post rainy seasons (Bandyopadhyay *et al.*, 2007). It was further reported that calves of Yak, 1-5 months-old, had *Haemonchus* and *Toxocara* spp. Cattle in Kamrup district of Assam were found to have 21.7% strongyles, 1.66% *Strongyloides* and 5.0% *T. vitulorum,* whereas goats had 45.9% strongyles, 2.6% *Strongyloides* and 1.7% *Trichuris* (Barua *et al.*, 2009).

The review of reports on the prevalence of GINs in animals of this region showed that goats had *T. colubriformis, H. contortus, B. trigonocephalum, O. columbianum,O. aspersum, C. ovina, T. globulosa, T. ovis, Strongyloides* spp. and *Nematodirus,* whereas cattle had *Trichostrongylus* spp. (Sharma and Godara, 2010). The highest intensity of strongyle infection in dairy animals from Assam during monsoon and post monsoon seasons can be attributed to the availability of infective 3rd stage larvae in the months of June to August (Borthakur and Das, 1998).

Gangetic plain region

This region includes Chandigarh, Delhi, Haryana, Punjab, Uttar Pradesh, Bihar and West Bengal. Cattle, buffaloes, sheep, goats and pigs are common in this region. Cattle and buffaloes are kept for milk purpose, whereas sheep, goats and pigs are reared for meat purpose.

The incidence of *T.vitulorum* and strongyles was negatively and positively correlated with the age of the host, respectively (Gupta *et al.*, 1985; Kumar and Verma, 2006). Thus, the calves of two month-old age had more infection of *T.vitulorum* than strongyles. Incidence of *T.vitulorum* in buffalo calves in the age group of 1-2 months from Mathura (UP) was higher than that of cow calves and the earliest age of detection in the former was 13 days in comparison to 18 days in the later (Shankar, 1999). The buffalo-calves from Patna (Bihar) have also been reported to be infected with GI nematodes viz. *T.vitulorum* (38.8%), *Trichuris* (11.2%) *Strongyloides* (9.6%) and strongyles (8.8%) (Kumar and Verma, 2006).*T. vitulorum* was also recordedin 78.6% cow and buffalo calves from Patiala, Punjab (Kaur and Kaur, 2008). Prevalence of *T. vitulorum* and *Strongyloides* has also been recorded in calves up to 4 month-old from organized farms of Ludhiana, Punjab (Jyoti *et al.*, 2011a). The calves get infection of *T. vitulorum* through colostrum of the infected mothers and approximately 90% larvae are excreted in the milk of infected mother till day 9 post calving and almost 100% larvae are released in the milk by day 25 post calving (Roberts *et al.*, 1990). *Strongyloides* spp. in calves occurs through percutaneous route under wet conditions (Copeman, 1982).

H. contortus is considered to be most pathogenic parasite, followed by *T. colubriformis,* while *Bunostomum, Oesophagostomum, Cooperia* and

Strongyloides spp. are less economically important parasitesin northern states, including Haryana (Gupta *et al.*, 1987, 1988) and Punjab (Singh *et al.*, 2005). In the northern plains, surveys indicated higher prevalence rate of GI nematodes during June to October (Gupta *et al.*,1987). *H. contortus* and *Trichostrongylus* spp. persisted in the host throughout the year,while prevalence of *Oesophagostomum* spp. was restricted mainly from August to November and *Ostertagia* spp. was recorded in the month of May (Anon, 2008).However, the survey work of Kumar *et al.* (2008a) from some northern states revealed the prevalence of *O. columbianum* throughout the year, whereas *S. papillosus* and *B. trigonocephalum* were seen during some months only. GI nematode, *C. ovina*, which is normally encountered from Jammu and Kashmir, has also been reported from one of the sheep from Karnal. It may be due to recovery of GI nematodes from the migratory sheep. Outbreaks of PGE resulting from *Ostertagia, Haemonchus* and *Trichostrongylus* spp. have also been reported from sheep and goats of Punjab, with clinical signs including diarrhoea, emaciation, dehydration and death within 1-2 days and 6460±1034.6 faecal egg counts (Bal *et al.*, 2007). Prevalence of GI nematodes consisted of predominantly *H. contortus,* followed by *T. colubriformis, T. ovis* and *S. papillosus* in sheep and goats has also been made from Patna, Bihar (Kumari *et al.*, 2010).

Teladorsagia circumcincta was identified in goats from Bareilly (UP) based on morphological and molecular assay by using PCR–RFLP. It is one of the most common and economically important parasites of sheep and goats in temperate zone throughout world and this was the first report of specific identification based on PCR-RFLP of B-tubulin gene from India (Shankar *et al.*, 2007). Species-wise sheep had higher infection than goats (Kumar *et al.*, 2008a).

The worm burden in one of the outbreaks of GI nematodosis in calves from Haryana was constituted mostly by *H.placei* (98%), followed by *Oesophagostomum* spp., *Bunostomum* spp., and *Trichuris* spp. (Yadav and Sardana, 1999). There is increasing evidence that *H. contortus* and *H. placei* is a single species with only strain adaptation forsheep and cattle, respectively (Taylor *et al.*, 2007). Later, Kaur and Kaur (2008) from Patiala, Punjab also reported *Haemonchus* spp. to be predominant, followed by *Oesophagostomum* spp. and *Trichuris* spp. in cattle/buffaloes. Based on faecal examination of animals from eastern districts of Haryana from 2003-2009, strongyles were found in 32.2% cattle, 6.7% buffaloes and 74.6% sheep with high incidence during rainy season (Chaudhri *et al.*,2010). A study on incidence of GI nematode infection in sheep, goats, cattle and buffaloes from Mathura, UP also showed *H. contortus* as dominant parasite,followed by *Strongyloides* and *Trichostrongylus,*with high incidence during monsoon season (Shankar *et al.*, 2010).

The camels from western Haryana have been reported to be infected with *H. longistipes* (58-64%), *T. colubriformis* (31-35%) and *S. papillosus* (5-8%) (Yadav and Kumar, 1990).Two main nematode parasites, *H. longistipes* and *T. colubriformis*, have been reported to cause morbidity and mortality in camels. Although goats are usually reared with camels in the combined animal husbandry system prevailing in northern India, these parasites have not been reported in goats. An experimental cross-transmission study in camels and goats revealed that camel isolates, *H. longistipes* and *T. colubriformis*, can result in GI nematodosis in goats (Singh *et al.*, 1993).

Western semi-arid and dry region

It includes Rajasthan, which has extremely hot weather conditions and famous for cattle (Rathi,Tharparker. Marwari, Jaisalmeri) and sheep (Nali) breeds. Sheep produce wool, whereas cattle breeds are kept for dairy purpose. High incidence of *Haemonchus* spp., *Bunostomum* spp., *Gaigeria* spp., *Oesophagostomum* spp., *Trichostrongylus* spp., *Chabertia* spp. and low incidence of *Trichuris* spp. and *S. papillosus* have been reported in adult sheep, followed by hoggets and weaners from Avikanagar, Rajasthan (Swarnkar *et al.*,1996). Crossbred sheep had higher level of infection than native breeds. Monthly rainfall of ≥50mm and monthly maximum temperature≥18.3°C provide optimal conditions for development and survival of preparasitic stages of *H.contortus* (Gordon, 1953). Weather data revealed that required temperature in semi-arid region of Rajasthan persisted throughout the year but monthly rainfall 50 mm was generally seen from July to October. It was observed that moderate temperature≥25°C and adequate rainfall (50 mm per month) were conducive for an increase in larval population and these conditions persisted from July to September (Swarnkar *et al.*, 1997). Incidence of GINs was high during monsoon in all climatic regions of Rajasthan and it was higher in organized farms as compared to farmers flocks.

H. contortus was predominant parasite in sheep and faecal egg counts due to GINs were at peak from July to early September in adult sheep and from August to early November in young sheep (Singh *et al.*, 1997; Khan *et al.*, 1999). Season-wise, *H. contortus* and *S. papillosus* were present throughout the year, whereas *Trichostrongylus* and *O. columbianum* were present during premonsoon, summer and monsoon, respectively (Singh *et al.*, 1997). Prevalence of GINs including strongyles (22.1 and 35.7%), ascarids (8.6 and 0.0%), *Strongyloides* spp. (3.9 and 5.0%) and *Trichuris* spp. (2.8 and 3.6%) in cattle/buffaloes and sheep/ goats, respectively has been reported on the basis of faecal examination from Jaipur, Rajasthan(Godara and Sharma, 2010).

Haemonchus spp. has been reported predominant infection in camels also. *Nematodirella dromedarii* has been reported for the first time from Indian camels in the arid zones of Rajasthan (Lodha and Raisinghani, 1979). The camels from Bikaner, the arid region of western Rajasthan, were found to have higher strongyle infection, followed by *Nematodirella, Strongyloides* and *Trichuris,* with high infection in field than farm camels (Partani *et al.*, 1996). Among strongyle infection, *H. longistipes* (86.4%) was the main contributor, followed by *Trichostrongylus* (13.6%) and the highest prevalence was seen during rainy season. The camels of more than 3 years of age from Bikaner, Jaisalmer, Udaipur and Hanumangarh of Rajasthan were more susceptible to GI nematodes, predominantly *Haemonchus,* followed by *Nematodirus,Strongyloides* and *Trichuris* during all the three seasons (Kumar *et al.*, 2010). It was further observed that infection rate was more in Jaisalmer (38.5%) and Hanumangarh (29.3%) districts followed by Udaipur (18.7%) and Bikaner (15.3%).

Gujarat plains and hills region

This region includes the states of Gujarat, Dadra and Nagar Haveli, Daman and Diu. Arabian goats are reared here and are good milkers. Camels were infected with *Strongyloides, Nematodirus, Nematodirella* spp. with higher prevalence in 1-3 year-old males than females and in Kachchhi breed than others (Sena *et al.*, 2000). The common GI nematodes reported in camels of Gujarat include *Haemonchus, Nematodirella, Nematodirus, Trichostrongylus, Strongyloides, Ostertagia, Cooperia, Trichuris, Marshallgia* and *Camelostrongylus* (Parsani *et al.*, 2008). The prevalence and intensity of these infections were maximum in rainy season and minimum in summer season and age of the animal also played a significant role in acquiring these infections. Among GI nematodes, *Nematodirella* showed highest incidence throughout the year on organized farms, whereas in field, *Haemonchus* spp. was most common and main causative agent of GI nematodosis.

Eastern, Central and Western Plateau and hill regions

This includes Chhattisgarh, Jharkhand, Madhya Pradesh, Maharashtra and Orissa.The buffalo and cowcalves up to 3 months of age from Marathwada area were found to be infected with *T.vitulorum* (34.9 and 7.8%), *S.papillosus* (24.7 and 16.3%) and strongyles (6.6 and 9.2%) (Bharkad *et al.*, 1999). Peak incidence of *T. vitulorum* and *S. papillosus* was observed in buffalo calves of 31-45 days of age, whereas highest incidence of strongyles was observed in buffalo calves of 75-90 days of age. The observations of higher rate of infection in buffalo calves (34.97%) than cow calves (7.8%) indicate more susceptibility of the former than the later as observed from Orissa (Das and Singh, 1955) and Haryana (Gupta and Pruthi, 1982).Higher incidence of *T. vitulorum* has also been reported from buffalo calves of age group of 2-3 months from Orissa (Shahoo *et al.*, 1991).

Goats from Chhattisgarh plains have been reported to have high risk of GINs from June to August (Dey *et al.*, 2008). *H. contortus* was the dominant species throughout the year,whereas *Cooperia, Bunostomum* and *Trichostrongylus* had occasional presence during rainy season.

Sub-temperate southern humid region

The buffalo calves around Hyderabad were also observed to have 30% infection of *T. vitulorum* with highest infection in age group of 30 days (42.5%) and lowest in age group of ≥90 days (4.1%) (Rao *et al.*, 2000).The buffalo-calves, 1-2 month-old, around Bidar, Karnataka, have been observed with high prevalence of *T. vitulorum* during South-west monsoon and post monsoon season, June to December (Halmandge *et al.*, 2005). The variation in incidence rate in different regions might be due to differences in climatic conditions and managemental practices.

Peak parasitism in sheep was observed from November to January in Tamil Nadu and it was associated with the rainfall pattern of this region, which receives northeast monsoon during October and November (Gupta and Mathur, 1969). Prevalence of *H. contortus* was higher, followed by *T. colubriformis, O. venulosum* and *Strongyloides* (Sanyal and Gour, 1984). The studies conducted at an organized farm in Kodai hills of Tamil Nadu could reveal June to November months more suitable for survival and migration of exogenous larval stages of GINs (Sanyal, 1989). Migration of infective larvae was more in autumn, whereas pre-parasitic activities were low in winter due to scanty rainfall. The contamination of pastures with infective larvae of GINs was low during December due to low temperature and scanty rains, whereas survivability of infective larvae was 11 weeks in rainy season and larvae were found to migrate vertically up to 15 cm and laterally up to 50 cm (Sanyal, 1989). Higher incidence of GINs has been recorded during Southwest and Northeast monsoon season (Anon, 2004).

The cattle and buffaloes from villages around Madras were observed to be infected with *Haemonchus, Mecistocirrus, Trichostrongylus, Bunostomum, Cooperia, Oesophagostomum* and *Strongyloides* (Raman *et al.,* 1999). Later, a forecasting model was developed for helminthic infections in small ruminants of high rainfall zone of Tamil Nadu (Raman *et al.,* 2009). It was observed that one mm raise in rainfall might be responsible for 19.2 times rise in egg counts. While evaluating preponderance of infective L3 of GINs in grazing areas of North eastern zone in Tamil Nadu in relation to various meteorological parameters from 2001-2007, rainfall was observed to have positive influence on GIN egg load during Northwest and Southwest monsoon seasons (Basith *et al.,* 2010).

Camels from Thrissur, Kerala have been reported to be infected with strongyles, *Strongyloides* and *Trichuris* (Vardharajan, 2002). The migratory camels from Uttar Pradesh, Madhya Pradesh and Rajasthan were found to be infected with *Trichuris* spp. (50%), *Strongyloides* spp. (32%), *Trichostrongylus* spp. (10.7%), *Nematodirus* spp. (10.3%) and *Haemonchus* spp. (14.2%) in Nagpur, Maharashtra (Rewatkar *et al.,* 2009).

Based on survey of parasite epidemiology in dairy animals in seven agro-climatic zones of India, Sanyal and Singh (1995) indicated an increased parasitic burden in the host and on the pasture during rainy season.Though the animals suffer from mixed infections of GI nematodes but predominance of *Haemonchus* spp., has been reported from most of the states including Haryana (Gupta *et al.,* 1987, 1988), Punjab (Singh *et al.,* 2005), Assam (Borthakur and Das, 1998), Tamil Nadu (Sanyal and Gour, 1984; Raman *et al.,* 1999), Uttrakhand (Yadav *et al.,* 2008a, b), Rajasthan (Singh *et al.,* 1997; Khan *et al.,* 1999) and

Chattisgarh (Dey *et al.*, 2008). Females of *Haemonchus* are prolific egg layers (Urquhart, 1996), and the infective stages of this parasite survive for a longer period on pastures (Soulsby, 1982), therefore these can be picked up constantly by susceptible animals resulting in clinical haemonchosis. *H. contortus* infective larvae did not show geotaxis behavior (Sciacca *et al.*, 2002), whereas moisture was observed to be attractive for the migration of infective larvae of GINs. Three main factors responsible for vertical migration of *H.contortus* infective larvae are moderate temperature, high humidity (continuous precipitation) and low light intensity resulting into migration of greater number of larvae on grass blades in the early morning and in the evening hours than mid-day and night (Gwendolen, 1950).Haemonchosis has been shown to induce stress in lambs (Fleming, 1997) which may get aggravated due to transportation. Deaths in females during postpartum period could be due to increased worm load causing temporary impairment of acquired immune responsiveness along with increased cortisol levels inducing stress in animals (Jacob and Vadodaria, 2000).

The epidemiology of GINs is also influenced by the following factors, which needs to be considered in devising control programmes.

(i) *Host genetic resistance* : Genetic resistance to parasitism is increasingly under investigation. Resistance to GIN parasitic infections has been documented both between and within sheep breeds (Woolastan and Windon, 2001; Yadav, 2004), can be exploited for the control of parasites. Breeding of stocks genetically resistant to parasites may provide a promising strategy at the outset of emerging anthelmintic resistance. Following *H. contortus* infection, the native breeds had significantly less changes in haematological values, body weight gains, abomasal pH and lower establishment of worms in comparison to those of pure bred and their crosses (Yadav *et al.*, 1993). Routine parasitological techniques were demonstrated for identification of the female lambs resistant to *H. contortus* (Hooda *et al.*, 1999). Such resistant females can be selectively used in breeding programmes for increased resistance to *H. contortus.* Genetic variation among Avikalin breed has been reported in terms of GI nematode resistance (Singh *et al.*, 2009), which is moderately inheritable and selection for this resistance is possible without affecting production parameters in semi-arid environment. Pure Parolerams have also been demonstrated with higher resistance for GI nematodes as compared to crosses of Deccani and Awashi breeds (Ghalsasi *et al.*, 2009). The studies on breed susceptibility of goats to natural infection of *H. contortus* revealed that Jamunapari breed was more susceptible than Sirohi (Agrawal *et al.*, 2010).

(ii) *Anthelmintic resistance* : Anthelmintic resistance has been reported for the first time against phenothiazine and thiabendazole in *H. contortus* of sheep from Rishikesh, UP. From 1990 onwards, reports of emerging resistance to benzimidazoles (BZ), probenzimidazoles, imidothiazoles, pyrimidines, rafoxanide, closantel in *H. contortus* of sheep were made from organized (mostly) and unorganized farms of Haryana (Yadav *et al.* 1993, 1995; Kumar and Yadav, 1994;Yadav and Garg, 2004; Das and Singh, 2005; Singh and Yadav, 1997), Rajasthan (Swarnkar *et al.*, 1999; Singh *et al.*, 2002). The level and type of anthelmintic resistance on different farms appeared to be associated with type and frequency of anthelmintic used and with the management practices on the farm concerned (Singh and Yadav, 1997). Anthelmintic resistance in nematodes has great epidemiological significance as the resistant parasites may be more fecund (Kumar *et al.*, 2008b) and pathogenic in the hosts and there is increased survivability of free living stages. Though majority of anthelmintics are still efficacious in ruminants and need to be used for a longer period by adopting suitable modifications proved effective from time to time. Benzimidazoles in ruminants can be used optimally by administering the oral dose correctly to obviate ruminal-bypass by withdrawal of feed for 24 hours before administering oral anthelmintic and offering dry fodder to animals at least 48 hours before treatment and ensuring that animal gets full dose (Sanyal *et al.*, 2003).

(iii) *Hypobiosis:* It is defined astemporary arrested larval development representing one of the most useful adaptations of life cycle to ensure parasitessurvival and it is most widespread among parasitic nematodes. It can thus be of major importance in ensuring survival of the parasite during periods of environmental adversity when conditions for transmission are poor and survival of free-living forms may be minimal. It also enables the parasite to be available in large numbers of infective forms at points in the host reproductive cycle which coincide with the production of the susceptible neonates, thereby greatly facilitating transmission. Hypobiosis phenomenon has been reported in sheep from Kodai Hills (Tamil Nadu), where sudden increase in faecal egg counts, pasture larval burden and worm counts of *H. contortus* was seen in March following extreme winter months (Sanyal, 1988). However, this phenomenon could not be seen in sheep from eastern Haryana where adult parasites persisted in the host throughout the year (Gupta *et al.*, 1986).

(iv) *Peri-parturient rise phenomenon* : It is the phenomenon in which faecal egg counts rise before and after parturitiondue to infection with many species of GI nematodes. Hormonal changes associated with peri-parturition and early lactation suppress immunity and thus allow maturation of developing larvae, increase fecundity of adult female worms and decrease the ability of the hosts to expel adult worms. As it appears to be the major source leading to increase in faecal egg counts, therefore, it is the prime source of infection for the susceptible animals grazing in the contaminated pastures. The climatic conditions favourable for trichostrongyle larvae on pasture from February to April lead to occurrence of peri-parturient rise in faecal egg counts (Gupta *et al.*, 1986). It was interesting to note that different breeds of sheep including Malpura breed of semi-arid western region did not show any peri-parturient rise (Singh *et al.*, 1997, 2008b).

(v) *Spring rise phenomenon*: It is defined as rise in faecal egg counts following maturation of hypobiotic larvae of certain GI nematode species. The studies of Gupta *et al.* (1986) suggest that spring rise may occur due to fresh acquisition of larvae and may be independent of parturition or *en mass* maturation of arrested larvae.

(iv) *Influence of reproductive stages on the intensity of GI nematode infections* : Higher faecal egg counts of GI nematodes were observed in lactating animals of different breeds of goats (Chauhan *et al.*, 2003) and sheep (Yadav *et al.*, 2008C) in comparison to dry and pregnant animals. It may be due to poor nutrition, stress, lack of antigenic stimulation and hormonal suppression of immunity.

Pathogenesis and clinical signs

Damage to GI mucosa is one of the major effects of GI nematodes leading to decreased absorption of minerals. Main clinical signs in

Toxocara infected calves are disinclination to feed on milk, constipation, abdominal pain, pica, dullness, depression, etc. The severely infected and non-treated calves may die of toxaemia. The mixed infection of *S. papillosus, H. contortus* and *T. colubriformis* augment the pathogenicity of *T. vitulorum* and cause PGE in calves (Gupta and Paul, 1990; Gupta *et al.*, 1985).

The commonly observed clinical signs due to *H. contortus* and *Trichostrongylus* in sheep and goats are progressive weakness, decrease in production, bottle jaw condition, anaemia, black coloured faeces, progressive emaciation, pica and decrease in wool yield.

Anaemia resulting from experimental oesophagostomosis causes stimulation of erythropoietic activity in infected animals increasing the demand of iron (Jas *et al.*, 2007), which might be ascribed to the fall in serum iron levels. Hypoproteinaemia with decreased levels of serum albumins is an important consequence of GI nematodosis (Jas *et al.*, 2008a). Further it is aggravated by increased catabolism of albumin and protein malabsorption through the damaged intestinal mucosa (Jas *et al.*, 2008b). *O. columbianum*, the cause of oesophagostomosis, was observed to have a prepatent period of 40-41 days and lead to decreased values of haemoglobin (Hb), packed cell volume (PCV), total erythrocytic counts (TEC), total leukocyte counts (TLC), serum proteins, iron and increased values of globulins (Jas *et al.*, 2010).

The experimental studies on quantitative infection with *C. ovina* in lambs indicate that a primary dose of 1000 infective larvae to lamb of 4-6 month old is highly pathogenic and cause acute disease. The parasite has a prepatent period of 40-48 days and patent disease may result into severe blood loss, diarrhoea due to attachment of mature adults to intestinal mucosa of caecum and colon (Sharma and Godara, 2010).

Biochemical parameters observed in GI nematodosis in camels include decrease in Hb, lymphocytes, total serum proteins, albumin, albumin and globulin ratio and increase in TLC, neutrophils, eosinophils, monocytes, serum glucose and globulins levels (Sena *et al.*, 2000). GI nematodes infected camels were observed to have rough coat, dull and listless eyes, pale conjunctiva, weakness, emaciation, pica, drastic reduction in appetite, loss of body weight and body condition,anaemia and oedematous swellings of lower body parts (Chandel *et al.*, 1992; Partani *et al.*, 1998; Tanwar *et al.*, 2005). The camels infected with *H. longistipes, Trichostrongylus* spp., *S. papillosus, Nematodirella* spp. and *Trichuris* spp. with faecal egg counts from 1,400 to 28,000 were observed to have low Hb, PCV and TEC indicating normochromic normocytic anaemia (Partani *et al.*, 1995a). Lowered values of serum proteins were also observed. There was a direct correlation between faecal egg counts and severity of clinical signs (Partani *et al.* 1998). The most severely affected camels had EPG of 7,500-28,000 mainly due to *H. longistipes* infection.

Diagnosis

GI nematodosis in animals can be diagnosed by faecal examination of animals by saturated salt floatation method and clinical signs shown by infected animals. Species of particular nematode can be identified by coproculture and also by postmortem examination.Yadav and Sardana (1999) from Hisar reported postmortem lesions including edema, hyperaemia, and scattered foci of hemorrhages and bleeding ulcers with abdominal contents and reddish brown fluid in 5 of 13 dairy cattle aged 10-30 months died of *H. placei* worms with a mean worm burden of 5670.

An indirect enzyme linked immunosorbent assay (ELISA) was standardized and evaluated to improve diagnosis of prepatent stage of *O. columbianum* in goats (Jas *et al.*, 2010). Indirect ELISA was standardized using the crude somatic antigen (CSAg) for coating the wells, infected goat sera as binding antibody, anti-goat IgG-HRP conjugate and ortho-phenylenediamine (OPD) with peroxide as substrate and antibodies were detected in sera of infected goats on day 18–27 post-infection with 96.00, 73.91 and 85.42% sensitivity, specificity and accuracy, respectively.

Detection of eggs in faeces using routine techniques may not be helpful in detecting the infection of *C. ovina* infection due to long prepatent period and for those immunological tests for detection of antibodies/antigens needs to be developed.

Detection of eggs in faecal samples is considered gold standard method for the diagnosis of toxocarosis in calves but it is applicable in post patent phase only. Tissue stages of toxocarosis needs to be detected for its control in buffaloes having latent infections. A number of attempts have been made by developing immunological tests including indirect haemagglutination test, counter immunoelectrophoresis tests and ELISA to detect antibodies against *T. vitulorum* tissue stages

(Banerjee *et al.*, 1998; Ghosh and Banerjee, 1998; Singh *et al.*, 2003), but still more research work is required to develop highly specific and sensitive assays. An immunodominant antigen of 66.9KDa was identified in somatic antigens of *T. vitulorum*, which may be used in the development of immunoassays for detection of latent toxocarosis in buffaloes (Jyoti *et al.*, 2011b). This field requires lot of research work to develop highly specific and sensitive assays for their application in management of toxocarosis, which is responsible for high mortality in calves of cattle, buffaloes, mithun and yaks.

Control

Parasitic gastroenteritis, dominated by haemonchosis, is one of the major constraints to profitable ruminant production in India. Prevention of parasitic diseases has considerable production benefits; therefore, approach for management of GI nematodes should be based on the epidemiological knowledge, which is acquired over a number of years. The other factors which need to be taken care of include efficacy of available anthelmintics, application of efficacious drench, reduction in pasture contamination, use of warm hostile climate and nonchemical strategies (Bukhari and Sanyal, 2011). Main aim in control of GI parasites should not be creation of parasite free animals but prevention of clinical disease and production losses (Sanyal, 1998).

(i) Grazing management :The infective larvae of GI nematodes move to the top of herbage when intensity of light is low during morning and evening hours, therefore, grazing of animals should be avoided during this period (Bukhari and Sanyal, 2011). Grazing management with regular monitoring of pasture larval burden (mainly *H. contortus* and *T. colubriformis*) indicated that the combination of anthelmintic treatment and rotational grazing was beneficial (Sanyal, 1991). The studies of Swarnkar *et al.* (2010) on epidemiology and management of GI parasites in sheep flocks of arid Rajasthan revealed that incidence of strongyle worms was >60% during June to September and in December. Based on worm profile, target worm species predominantly *H. contortus*, single strategic drench was given during later half of monsoon as per modified worm management programme (MWMP) in comparison to 3 drenches being given by farmers under conventional programme. It was found that flock performance and net annual income under both programmes was non-significantly different. It was concluded that in lieu of high selection pressure for anthelmintic resistance and limited choice for anthelmintic types, MWMP with

reduced drenching efficiency was effective in managing GI nematodes in sheep without any adverse impact on flock performance and economic return to farmers. This step will also help to increase quantum of refugia which in turn will help in maintenance of anthelmintic efficacy.

(ii) Use of anthelmintics : Anthelmintics including benzimidazole, tetramisole and levamisole, and avermectins can be used for the treatment of GINs in small and large ruminants. A long acting narrow spectrum anthelmintic, closantel has been reported with persistent activity up to 5-8 weeks (Khan *et al.*, 1999; Swarnkar *et al.*, 2000). The repeated use of closantel may change generic profile of strongyle worms with increased proportions of *Oesophagostomum* spp. and *Trichostrongylus* spp. due to their restrictive activity against haematophagous parasites (Swarnkar *et al.*, 2000). Moxidectin, a second generation macrocyclic lactone (milbemycin) having unique chemical structure with dimethyl butenyl side chain instead of disaccharide side chain in avermectin group, is highly effective against resistant ovine strain of *H. contortus* with persistent efficacy up to 45 days (Maharshi *et al.*, 2010).

Treatment of flocks of sheep for GI nematodes in Rajasthan during mid to later part of monsoon will help in removing BZ resistant strains of worms (Maharshi *et al.*, 2010). Helminthes including GI nematodes are controlled mainly by anthelmintics but with the intensification of animal husbandry resulting into widespread use, overuse and misuse of anthelmintics, a new problem called anthelmintic resistance is emerging very fast in different Indian states (Singh and Yadav, 1997; Yadav and Garg, 2004). It warrants regular monitoring of anthelmintic resistance in small ruminants before it becomes a widespread problem.

The increase in bioavailability of BZ anthelmintics given by intraruminal route could be used to optimize the use of anthelmintic for sustained parasite control in small ruminants. The concept of frequent deworming of all sheep in a flock is unsustainable and it has posed a challenge to parasite control programme in the form of emergence of anthelmintic resistance (Singh and Swarnkar, 2010). Targeted selective treatment of sheep has not only decreased the dependency on anthelmintics but also increased the frequency of susceptible alleles in parasite population of *H. contortus*. The breeding of sheep for resistance in Malpura and Avikalin breeds has been observed to reduce the requirement of anthelmintic treatments.

The dairy animals in Himachal Pradesh had highest risk of GI nematodosis and pasture contamination from July to September (Jithendran and Bhat, 1999). The treatment with broad-spectrum anthelmintics in dairy animals at least twice a year, once in March-April and again in July-September, has been observed to reduce the parasitism and to increase the productivity of animals in the region.

Anthelmintic trials in GIN infected camels include albendazole and mebendazole (Yadav and Kumar, 1990), ivermectin (Kumar and Yadav, 1991; Sharma, 1991; Parsani *et al.*, 2008), thiophanate (Yadav and Singh, 1991), levamisole and fenbendazole (Kumar and Yadav, 1991; Partani *et al.*, 1995b), tetramisole hydrochloride and morantel tartrate (Parsani *et al.*, 2008). Benzimidazoles have also been found effective against *Trichuris* spp. (Lodha *et al.*, 1977; Bansal *et al.*, 1989). Anthelmintic resistance has been reported to fenbendazole against *Strongyloides* spp. in camels (Partani *et al.*, 1995b).

Treatment of calves on two occasions i.e. on day 9-11 post calving and on day 25 post calving with larvicidals (pyrantel or levamisole hydrochloride) will be suffice for the complete control of toxocarosis and also to minimize the infection of ascarids to be available for the susceptible animals (Roberts, 1990). Control of this infection and also of strongyloidosis is possible by provision of basic level of hygiene.

(iii) Use of nematophagus fungi: One of the alternatives for the control of GINs in animals is biological control using nematophagous fungi (*Duddingtonia flagrans*) isolated from the faeces of grazing animals in Gujarat (Sanyal, 2000) and Rajasthan (Khan *et al.*, 2009). These fungi have superior predacious capacity and gut survival ability.

(iv) Use of indigenous medicinal plants: Aqueous extracts of *Azadirachta indica* leaf extracts showed significant reduction in egg embryonation and egg hatching at a concentration of 1.25 mg/ml suggesting embryocidal and ovicidal property against *H. contortus* (Singh *et al.*, 2008a). The aqueous extracts of *Buteafrondos* (Palas) seeds have also been shown to cause 90.73% larval mortality of *H.contortus* and needs to be evaluated for their *in vivo* efficacy, dose determination, application and toxicity in animas (Swarnkar *et al.*, 2008).

Conclusions/future projections

Epidemiolocal data on GINs in ruminants from different agro-climatic zones shows that *T. vitulorum* in calves of buffaloes, cows, mithun and yak, *H. contortus* in sheep, goats, cattle and buffaloes, and

H. longistipes in camels are dominant parasites. The presence of other genera of GINs including *Trichostrongylus, Bunostomum, Nematodirella, Nematodirus,Oesophagostomum, Strongyloides, Trichuris, Chabertia,*etc. with dominant nematodes in mixed infections aggravate the clinical signs of PGE and thus, result into economic losses to livestock owners in the form of high morbidity and mortality. *Teladorsagia circumcincta* was also identified in goats from Bareilly (UP) based on morphological and molecular assay by using PCR–RFLP. Season-wise incidence is higher in rainy and post rainy seasons because of suitable environmental conditions for the development of pre-parasitic stages of GINs. The animals of hill regions were found with low infections as compared to tarai regions. Several factors including variations in susceptibility of hosts and their breeds to nematode parasites, genetic resistance of hosts to GINs, anthelmintic resistance, periparturient and spring rise phenomenon, and influence of reproductive stages of reproduction of host(s) influence the intensity of infections. GINs are responsible for damaging the GI mucosa which further leads to decreased absorption of required nutrients and leakage of proteins. The clinical signs produced resulting from these changes results into anorexia, anaemia, progressive weakness, loss in production of milk/ meat/ wool, diarrhoea/ dysentery, bottle jaw condition, etc. The diagnosis of most of these GIN infections is still dependent on gold standard method of faecal examination. Attempts have been made to develop immunological tests to detect some of GINs having longer incubation period/ tissue stages but these studies needs to be carried further to have diagnostic kits to undertake micro epidemiological studies and timely control measures. Though market is flooded with several classes of anthelmintics for the treatment of nematode infections but poor quality of anthelmintics and their misuse led to the development of resistant nematodes. Therefore, there is an urgent need for judicious use of anthelmintics and also for regular monitoring of their efficacy/ resistance with molecular tools developed/ to be developed against dominant GI nematodes of ruminants. Future focus of studies for control of GINs should be based on updating of epidemiological information on economically important GINs and preparation of anthelmintic schedules for animals of each agro-climatic zone. The disease forecast system also needs to be developed for major agro-climatic zones for use in strategic control programmes.

References

Agrawal, N., Sharma, D.K. and Mandal, A. (2010). Susceptibility of Jamunapari and Sirohi goats to natural *Haemonchus contortus* infection. *Parasitology Today-Ecology to Molecular Biology*, Souvenir cum Abstract Compendium, pp.18.

Ahmad, M. and Ansari, J.A. (1987). Prevalence of gastrointestinal nematodes of sheep and goats at Aligarh. *IndianVet. Med. J.*, 11: 165-170.

Anon (2003). Livestock census.Department of Animal Husbandry, Dairying and Fisheries, Ministry of Agriculture, Government of India.

Anon (2004). Annual Progress report (2003-2004) on All India Network Programme on Gastrointestinal Parasitism, ICAR, New Delhi.

Anon (2008). Annual Progress report (2007-2008) on All India Network Programme on Gastrointestinal Parasitism, ICAR, New Delhi.

Bal, M.S.,Mahajan, Verma, S, Alka and Sharma, S. (2007). Outbreaks of parasitic gastrointestinal parasites in sheep and goats.*J. Vet.Parasitol.*, 21: 93-96.

Bandyopadhyay, S., Pal, P., Rehman, H. and Bujarbaruah (2007). Occurrence of gastrointestinal parasites in domestic yaks (*Paephagusgrunniens*) in Sikkim. Proceedings of 18th National Congress of Veterinary Parasitology, pp. 86.

Banerjee, P.S., Bhatia, B.B. and Garg, S.K. (1998). Comparative evaluation of IHA and CIEP in diagnosis of *Toxocara vitulorum* in pregnant cows and buffaloes. *Trop.Anim.Hlth.Prod.*, 30: 253-256.

Bansal, S.R., Bhardwaj, R.M., Tika Ram, S.M. and Bhtanagar, P.K. (1989). Preliminary field studies on the efficacy of albendazole against clinical cases of gastrointestinal nematodiasis in camels in Haryana. *J. Vet. Parasitol.*, 3: 143-44.

Barua, C.C., Chamuah, J.K., Barua, A.G., Salq, A., Hazarika, A. and Biswas, R. (2009). Prevalence of gastrointestinal parasites in ruminants. *Indian Vet.J.*, 86: 747-748.

Basith, S.A., Raman, M. and Bharathi, R.S. (2010). Impact of climatology onpasture larval burdenin North Eastern Zone of Tamil Nadu. *Parasitology Today-Ecology to Molecular Biology*, Souvenir cum Abstract Compendium, pp.8.

Bharkhad, G.P., Deshpande, P.D. and Narladkar, B.W. (1999).Gastrointestinal parasitosis in bovine calves in Marathwada, *J. Vet.Parasitol.*, 13: 143-146.

Bhat, M.S., Sudan, N.A., Shahardar, R.A. and Mir, A.Q. (2007). Prevalence ofgastrointestinal nematodosis in sheep in Kashmir valley. *J. Vet.Parasitol.*, 21: 89-91.

Borthakur, S.K. and Das, M.R. (1998). Epidemiological studies on gastrointestinal helminthes in dairy animals of Assam. *J. Vet. Parasitol.*, 12: 85-88.

Bukhari, S. and Sanyal, P.K. (2011). Epidemiological intelligence for grazing management in strategic control of parasitic gastroenteritis in small ruminants in India– areview. *Vet. World*, 4: 92-96.

Chamuah J.K., Islam, S., Rajkhowa, S., Rajkhowa, C. and Chakraborty, A.K. (2009). Studies on gastrointestinal helminthes of mithun (*Bosfrontalis*). *J.Vet.Parasitol.*, 23: 37-40.

Chandel, B.S., Josh, S. and Vadodaria, V.P. (1992). Levels of certain biochemical estimates in normal and parasite infected camels (*Camelusdromedarius*). *Indian Vet. J.*, 69: 462-64.

Chaudhri, S.S., Bisla, R.S., Bhanot, V. and Singh, H. (2010). Helminthic and haemoprotozoan infections in clinically sick animals of Eastern Haryana. *Parasitology Today-Ecology to Molecular Biology*(eds. Gupta, S.K., Singh, S., Chaudhri, S.S. and Vohra, S), Souvenir cum Abstract Compendium, pp.9-10.

Chauhan, K.K., Rout, P.K., Singh, P.K., Mandal, A., Singh, H. N., Roy, R. and Singh, S.K. (2003). Susceptibility to gastrointestinal nematode infection in different physiological stages in Jamunapari and Barbarigoats in semiarid tropics.*Small Rum. Res.*, 50: 219-223.

Copeman, D.B.(1982). The importance of helminth parasites in animal production system in tropics. In: Animal Production and Health in Tropics, Pertanian University, Pertanian, Malaysia, pp. 911-997.

Croll, N.A.(1973). Behavioural analysis of nematode movement.*Adv. Parasitol.*, 13:113.

Darzi, M.M., Mir, M.S., Pandit, B.A., Nashiruddullah, N. and Bhat, A.S. (2004). A retrospective study of naturally acquired haemonchosis in sheep. *J.Vet.Parasitol.*, 18: 143-145.

Das, K.M. and Singh, G.B. (1955). Calf ascariosis in India.*Br. Vet. J.*, 111: 342-347.

Das, M. and Singh, S. (2005). Anthelmintic resistance to nematodes in sheep andgoat farms in Hisar.*J.Vet.Parasitol.*, 19: 103-106.

Dey,S., Sanyal, P.K., Mukherjee, K., Sarkar, A.K, Patel, N.K., Mandal, S.C. and Pal, S. (2008). Caprine parasitic gastroenteritis in semi-organised farming conditions. *J.Vet.Parasitol.*, 22: 77-78.

Fleming, M.W. (1997). Cortisol as an indicator of severity of parasitic infection of*H.contortus* in lambs (*Ovis aries*). *Comp.Biochem. Physiol.Mol.Biol.*, 116: 41-44.

Gagan, G., Sharma, D.K., Agarwal, R.D. and Raut, P.K. (2003). Epidemiology of *Haemonchus contortus*infection in goats in semi-arid region of India. *J.Vet.Parasitol.*, 17: 57-60.

Ghalsasi, P.P., Ghalsasi, P.M. and Nimbkar, C. (2009). Proceedings of 19th National Congress of Veterinary Parasitology,pp. 31.

Ghosh, J.D. and Banerjee, D.P.(1998). Comparative evaluation of serodiagnostic tests for tissue toxocarosis in buffaloes (*Bubalus bubalis*).*J. Parasitic Dis.*, 2: 121-125.

Godara, R. and Sharma, R.L. (2010). Parasitic infections in livestock at Jaipur.*J. Vet. Parasitol.*, 24: 193-195.

Gordon, H. and M.(1953). The epidemiology of helminthosis in sheep in winter-rainfall regions of Australia- Preliminaryobservations. *Aust. Vet. J.*, 29: 337-348.

Gupta, N.K.and Mathur, S.(1969). On the incidence, morphology and taxonomy of some nematodes of sheep and goats from Chandigarh and Madras. *Res. Bull.PunjabUni. Sci.*,19: 203-291.

Gupta, R.P. and Paul, J.C. (1990). Sequential changes in the worm population in buffalo calves of eastern Haryana. *Haryana Agri. Uni.J. Res.*, 20: 83-87.

Gupta, R.P. and Pruthi, A.K. (1982). Incidence of *Neoascaris vitulorum* in buffaloandcow calvesin Karnal. *Indian J.Anim. Res.*, 16: 1-4.

Gupta, R.P., Ruprah, N.S and Yadav, C.L.(1986). Some observations on spring-rise phenomenon in sheep in Haryana (India). *India Vet. J.*, 63: 449-453.

Gupta, R.P., Yadav, C.L. and Chaudhri, S.S. (1987). Epizootiology of gastrointestinal nematodes of sheep and goats in Haryana, India. *Vet.Parasitol.*,24: 117-127.

Gupta, R.P., Yadav, C.L. and Gosh, J.D.(1985). Epidemiology of helminthic infections in calves of Haryana state. *Agri.Sci.Dig.*, 5: 53-56.

Gupta, R.P., Yadav, C.L. and Ruprah, N.S. (1988). Epidemiology of ovine helminthiasisin Haryana, India. *Trop.Anim.Hlth.Prod.*, 20: 23-29.

Gwendolen, R. (1950). Observations on the vertical migration of third stage larvae of *H. contortus* (Rud,) on experimental plots of Loliumperenne S24, in relation to meteorological and micrometeorological factors.*Parasitol.*, 40: 127-143.

Halmandge, S., Suranagi, M.D., Murugeppa, A., Sudhindra and Kumar, S.P.(2005). Prevalence of ascariosis in buffalo calves in and around Bidar. *J.Vet.Parasitol.*, 19: 149-151.

Hooda, V., Yadav, C.L., Chaudhri, S.S. and Rajpurohit, B.S. (1999). Variations in resistance to haemonchosis: Selection of female sheep resistant to *Haemonchus contortus*. *J.Helminthol.*,73:137-142.

Jacob, N. and Vadodaria, V.P. (2000). Serum cortisol, tri-iodithyronine (T3) and thyroxine (T4) levels at periparturient periods in Patanwadi ewes. *Indian Vet. J.*, 77: 1040-1042.

Jas, R., Datta, S. and Ghosh, J.D. (2007). Impact of naturally occurring gastrointestinal nematodosis on some mineral concentration in Bengal goats. *Environ.Eco.*, 25: 502-505.

Jas, R., Datta, S. and Ghosh, J.D. (2008a). Haemato-biochemical impact of gastrointestinal nematodosis in Bengal goats. *J.Vet.Parasitol.*, 22: 21-26.

Jas, R., Datta, S. and Ghosh, J.D. (2008b). Haemato-biochemical impact of primary infection of *Oesophagostomum columbianum* in goat. *J. Vet. Parasitol.*, 24: 117-120.

Jas, R., Ghosh, J.D. and Das, K.(2010). Diagnosis of *Oesophagostomum columbianum* infection in goats by indirect enzyme linked immunosorbent assay. *Helminthologia*, 47: 83-87.

Jithendran, K.P. (1998). Epidemiology of gastrointestinal parasites in migratorysheep andgoats in northwest humid Himalayan region. *Indian J. Anim. Sci.*, 68: 894-896.

Jithendran, K.P. and Bhat, T.K.(1999). Epidemiology of parasitoses in dairy animals in the North West Humid Himalayan Region of India with particular reference to gastrointestinal nematodes.*Trop.Anim.Hlth.Prod.*, 31: 205-214.

Jyoti, Hague, M. Singh, N.K., Juyal, P.D., Kaur, A. and Rath, S.S.(2011a). Prevalence of gastrointestinal parasites in organized dairy farms. *Indian Vet. J.*, 88:77-78.

Jyoti, Singh, N.K. and Juyal, P.D.(2011b). Identification and characterization of immune-dominant antigen (s) of *T. vitulorum* in buffaloes (*Bubalus bubalis*). *Vet.Arhiv.*, 81: 369-378.

Katoch, R., Chauhan, P.P. and Joshi, D.K.(2000). Seasonal incidence of gastrointestinal nematodosis in goats of Mathura region.*Indian Vet. J.*, 77: 259-260.

Katoch, R., Mittra, S., Agnihotri, R.K. and Sharma, A.K. (1998). Winter strongylosisinsheep and goats at high altitude: A sporadic occurrence. *Indian Vet. J.*,75: 362-363.

Kaur, H. and Kaur, D.(2008). Prevalence of gastrointestinal parasites in domestic animals of Patiala and its adjoining areas.*J. Vet. Parasitol.*, 22: 25-28.

Khajuria, J.K., Yadav, A., Vohra, S., Katoch, R. and Sood, S. (2009). An outbreak of parasitic gastroenteritis in sheep and goats at R.S.Pura, Jammu. Proceedings of 19th National Congress of Veterinary Parasitology,pp. 38.

Khan, F. A., Swarnkar, C. P., Singh, D., Jayasankar, J. and Bhagwan, P. S. K. (1999). Ovine gastrointestinal parasitism in farmers flock under semi-arid conditions of Rajasthan. *Indian J. Small Rum.*, 5: 65-70.

Khan,P., Singh, S., Swarankar, C.P., Tiwari, R. and Tiwari, J. (2009). Control of gastrointestinalnematodes of sheep in Rajasthan (India). *Indian J.Anim.Sci.*, 79: 9-11.

Kumar, S., Ghorai, S.K.,Nagarajan, G. and Pathak, K.M.L.(2010). Epidemiology of gastro- intestinal parasites in camel in different areas of Rajasthan. Proceedings of 20th National Congress of Veterinary Parasitology,pp. 21.

Kumari, S., Sinha, S.R.P., Sinha, S., Hoda, M.Z., Mandal, K.G. and Sharma, S.K.(2010). Incidence of gastrointestinal helminthosis in sheep and goats in Patna (Bihar).*J. Vet.Parasitol.*, 24: 97-99.

Kumar, A. and Verma, S.P. (2006). Prevalence of gastrointestinal helminthes infection in cow-calves. *Indian J. Vet.Med.*, 26: 43-44.

Kumar, R. and Yadav, C.L.(1994). Prevalence of fenbendazole resistance in ovine nematodes in North-West India.*Trop.Anim.Hlth.Prod.*, 26:230-234.

Kumar, R.R., Yadav, C.L., Garg, R, Banerjee, P.S. and Vatsya, S.(2008a). Prevalence of gastro-intestinal nematodes in sheep and goats in some parts of North-West India. *Indian J.Anim.Sci.*, 78: 1244-1246.

Kumar, R.R., Yadav, C.L. and Vatsya, S.(2008b). Biological variations in susceptible and resistant strains of *Haemonchus contortus* in sheep. *Indian J.Anim.Sci.*, 78: 950-952.

Kumar, S. and Yadav, C.L. (1991). Comparative efficacy of ivermectin, fenbendazole and levamisole against gastrointestinal nematodiasis in camels. *Indian Vet. J.*, 68: 787-789.

Laha, R., Das, M., Goswami, A., Bordoloi, R.K. and Kharguria, G.(2010). Prevalence of gastro-intestinal parasitism in Assam hill goats of Meghalaya. Proceedings of 20th National Congress of Veterinary Parasitology,pp. 17.

Lodha, K.R. and Raisinghani, P.M. (1979). Report of *Nematodirelladromedarii* (Nematoda: Trichostrongylidae) on the Indian camel (*Camelusdromedarius*) with remarks on the genus *Nematodirella*,Yorke and Maplestone, *Indian J.Anim.Sci.*, 49: 817-22.

Lodha, K.R., Raisinghani, P.M. and Karwasra, R.S. (1977). Chemotherapeutic trials of some anthelmintics against helminth parasites of camels. *Indian J. Anim.Sci.*, 48: 677-82.

Maharshi, A.K., Swarnkar, C.P., Singh, D. and Manohar, G.S. (2010). Persistent efficacy of moxi dectinagainst benzimidazole resistant strain of ovine *Haemonchus contortus*. *J. Vet.Parasitol.*, 24: 55-58.

Makhdoomi, D.M., Shugufta N., Mandey, S.D and Molve, B. (1995). Incidence of differentovine gastrointestinal parasites in Kashmir. *Indian Vet.J.*,72: 898-900.

Makvana, V.N. and Singh, V.(2009).Emergence of anthelmintic resistance in nematode parasitesof sheep at an organized farm in Gujarat. *J. Vet.Parasitol.*, 23: 171-173.

Mehlhorn, H.(1988). Parasitology in Focus, Springer-Verlog, Berlin, Heidelberg, Germany.

Nasreen, S., Jeelani, S.G. and Hakeem, M.(2005). Incidence of gastrointestinal nematodes in sheep in Kashmir Valley. *J. Vet.Parasitol.*, 19: 27-29.

Ogbourne, C.P.(1972). Observation on free living stages of strongylid nematodes in horses. *Parasitol.*, 64: 461-477.

Pal, P. and Bandyopadhyay, S.(2004). Prevalence of gastrointestinal nematodosisin goats inSikkim. *J. Vet.Parasitol.*, 18: 127-130.

Parsani, H.R., Singh, V. and Momin, R.R.(2008).Common parasitic diseases of Camel. *Vet.World*, 1: 317-318.

Partani, A.K., Kumar, D., Manohar, G.S. and Bhan, A.K.(1996). Epidemiology of gastro- intestinal nematodes of camel (*Camelusdromedarius*) at Bikaner (Rajasthan).*J. Vet.Parasitol.*, 10: 23-32.

Partani, A.K., Kumar, D., Manohar, G.S. and Bhan, A.K.(1998).Clinical manifestations of natural infection with gastrointestinal nematodes in camel.*J.Camel Prac. Res.*, 5:255-256.

Partani, A.K., Rai, A.K., Kumar, D., Kataria, A.K. and Swarnkar, C.P. (1995a). Haematological and biochemical changes in camels naturally infected with gastrointestinal nematodes. *J.Camel Prac.Res.*, 2: 33-36.

Partani, A.K., Rai, A.K., Kumar, D., Kataria, A.K. and Swarnkar, C.P.(1995b). Suspected resistance of gastrointestinal nematodes in camels to tetramisole and fenbendazole. *J. Vet.Parasitol.*, 9: 99-103.

Pradhan, K.B., Thakur, D.K. and Sudhan, N.A.(1991). Incidence of gastrointestinal parasites in suckling calves in Ranchi. *J.Res.Birsa Agri.Uni.*, 3: 123.

Rajkhowa, S., Bujarbaruah, K.M., Rajkhowa, C. and Thong, K. (2005). Incidence of intestinal parasitism in mithun (*Bosfrontalis*). *J. Vet. Parasitol.*, 19: 39-41.

Rajkhowa, S., Rajkhowa, C., Thong, K.and Vupru, K. (2003). Studies on parasitic diseases of mithun calves.In: NRCM Annual Report of ICAR(2002-2003), Jharnapani, Nagaland.

Raman, M., Ananadan, R., Joseph, S.A. and Sanyal, P.K. (1999). Epidemiology of gastrointestinal helminthes in dairy animals in and around Madras.*J. Vet. Parasitol.*, 13: 163-164.

Raman, M., Basith, S.A. and Bharathi, R.S.(2009). Development of forecasting model for helminthic infections in Tamil Nadu. Proceedings of XIXth National Congress of Veterinary Parasitology, pp. 34.

Rao, R.R., Rao, R. and Kumar, U.(2000). Incidence of *Toxocara vitulorum* in buffalo calves around Hyderabad, India. *J. Vet.Parasitol.*, 14: 79-80.

Rewatkar, S.G., Deshmukh, S.K., Deskar, S.K., Maske, D.K., Jumde, P.D., Bhangale, G.N. and Srikhande, G.B. (2009). Gastrointestinal helminthosis in migratory camels. Proceedings of 19th National Congress of Veterinary Parasitology,pp.57.

Roberts, J.A. (1990). The life cycle of *Toxocara vitulorum* in Asian buffalo (*Bubalus bubalis*).*Int.J.Parasitol.*, 20: 833-840.

Roberts, J.A., Fernando, S.T. and Sivanathan, S. (1990). *Toxocara vitulorum* in the milk of the buffalo (*Bubalus bubalis*) cows. *Res. Vet.Sci.*, 49: 289-301.

Sanyal, P.K. (1988). Preliminary studies on hypobiosis diapause phenomenon of *Haemonchus contortus. Indian Vet. Med.J.*,12: 11-14.

Sanyal, P.K. (1989). Seasonal availability of ovine strongyle larvae on pasture sub temperate Tamil Nadu.*Indian J.Anim.Sci.*, 59: 1491-1493.

Sanyal, P.K.(1991). Studies on monitoring of control strategy against ovine parasitic gastroenteritis in sub temperate Tamil Nadu.*Indian Vet. Med.J.*,15: 261-265.

Sanyal, P.K.(1998). Integrated parasite management in ruminants in India: A concept note on biological control of gastro-intestinal parasites of ruminants using predacious fungi. Animal Production and Health Paper 141, FAO, Rome, pp. 54-65.

Sanyal, P.K. (2000). Presence of predacious fungi in fresh faeces of ruminants in western India. *J. Vet.Parasitol.*, 14:133-135.

Sanyal, P.K. and Gour, D. (1984). Studies on pasture sampling on the availability of ovine strongyle larvae in sub temperate Tamil Nadu. *Int. J. Anim.Sci.*, 4: 167-170.

Sanyal, P.K and Singh, D.K. (1995). Parasitic gastroenteritis. *In:* proceedings of workshop on control strategy against gastrointestinal parasites in dairy animals in India using urea molasses blocks. National Dairy Development Board, Anand, Gujarat.

Sanyal, P.K., Swarnkar, C.P., Singh, D., Khan, F.A. and Bhagwan, P.S.K. (2003). Sheep and albendazole for a new approach on judicious use of anthelmintics.*J. Vet.Parasitol.*, 17: 15-19.

Sciacca, J., Ketschek, A., Forbes, W.M., Boston, R., Guerrero, J., Ashton, F.T., Gamble, R.H. and Schad, G.A.(2002). Vertical migration by the infective larvae of three species of parasitic nematodes: is behaviour really a response to gravity? *Parasitol.*, 125: 553-560.

Sena, D. S, Mal, G., Kumar, R. and Sahani, M. S.(2000). Prevalence, haemato-biochemical studies and chemotherapy of gastrointestinal nematode infection in camels.*J. Vet.Parasitol.*, 14:151-153.

Shahoo, N., Mishra, A. and Dey, P.C. (1991). A note on incidence of helminthiasis in buffalo-calves with special reference to ascariasis. *Orissa Vet.J.*, 16: 52-54.

Shankar, D. (1999). Studies on the incidence, chemotherapy and effect of corticosteroids and certain anti-autacoid agents on *T. vitulorum* infection (Thesis abstract). *J. Vet. Parasitol.*, 13: 178.

Shankar, M., Prasad, A., Kumar, M. and Singh, C. (2007). Morphological and molecular identification of *Teladorsagiacircumcincta* from goats. *J. Vet. Parasitol.*, 21: 21-24.

Shankar, D., Tiwari, J. and Sachan, B.(2010). Studies on gastrointestina lhelminthosis indifferent ruminant animalsof Mathura, UP.*Parasitology Today-Ecology to Molecular Biology* (ed. Gupta, S.K., Singh, S., Chaudhri, S.S. and Vohra, S.), Souvenir cum Abstract Compendium, pp.10.

Sharma, L.K. (1991). Efficacy of anthelmintics against gastrointestinal nematodes in camels. *Indian Vet.J.*, 68: 1069-72.

Sharma, R.L. and Godara, R.(2010). Metazoan diseases of livestock in the Greater Himalayan regions of India and their diagnosis: An overview. *J.Vet.Parasitol.*, 24: 1-16.

Singh, D. and Swarnkar, C.P.(2010). Harnessing the advantages of over dispersionin faecal egg counts through targeted selective treatment and breeding for genetic resistance. *Parasitology Today-Ecology to Molecular Biology*, (eds. Gupta, S.K., Singh, S., Chaudhri, S.S. and Vohra, S.), Souvenir cum Abstract Compendium, pp.5.

Singh, D., Swarnkar, C.P and Khan, F.A. (2002). Anthelmintic resistance ingastrointestinal nematodes of livestock in India. *J.Vet.Parasitol.*, 16: 115-130.

Singh, D., Swarnkar, C.P., Khan, F.A.and Bhagwan, P.S.K. (2008a). *In vitro* ovicidal activity of *Azadirachta indica*leaf extract against *H. contortus* eggs.*Indian J.Anim.Sci.*, 78: 1108-10.

Singh, D., Swarnkar, C.P., Khan, F.A., Srivastava, C.P. and Bhagwan, P.S.K.(2008b). Epidemiology of ovine gastrointestinal nematodes at an organized farm in Rajasthan, India. *Small Rum.Res.*, 26: 31-37.

Singh, D., Swarnkar, C.P., Kumar, S., Prince, L.L.L. and Arora, A.L.(2009). Performance of the Avikalin sheep selected for resistance to *H. contortus*. *J.Vet. Parasitol.*, 23: 23-27.

Singh, H., Banerjee, P.S. and Yadav, C.L.(2003). Seroprevalence of *Toxocara vitulorum* in peri-parturient buffaloes and cattle. *Indian J.Anim.Sci.,* 73: 269-270.

Singh, H., Rai, H.S., Singh, N.K.and Kaur, A.(2005). Survey of helminthic infectionsin Ludhiana.*J. Vet.Parasitol.,* 19: 97-101.

Singh, S. and Yadav, C.L. (1997). A survey of anthelmintic resistance by nematodes in gastro-intestinal nematodes of livestock in India. *J. Vet. Parasitol.,* 10: 115-130.

Singh, S., Yadav, C.L. and Banerjee, D.P. (1997). Comparison of the post-parturient rise in faecal egg counts of indigenous and cross bred ewes. *J.Helminthol.,* 71: 249-252.

Singh, V., Kumar, S. and Yadav, C.L. (1993). Establishment of camel isolates of *Haemonchus longistipes* and *Trichostrongylus colubriformis* in goats. *Vet.Parasitol.,*51:69-75.

Soulsby, E.J.L.(1982). Helminths, Arthropods and Protozoa of Domesticated Animals. 7th ed.,ELBS and Baillere Tindal, London, pp. 809.

Swarnkar, C.P., Khan, F.A., Singh, D. and Bhagwan, P.S.K.(2000). Efficacy of closantel in sheep naturally infected with gastrointestinal nematodes. *J. Vet.Parasitol.,* 14: 75-76.

Swarnkar, C.P., Singh, D., Khan, F.A. and Bhagwan, P.S.K.(1999). Multiple anthelmintic resistance in *Haemonchus contortus* of sheep. *Indian J.Anim.Sci.,* 69: 547-549.

Swarnkar, C.P., Singh, D., Khan, F.A., Kumar, M., Bhagwan, P.S.K. and Dubey, S.C. (2008). *In vitro* ovicidal and larvicidal activity of *Buteafrondosa* (Palas) seeds extract in *Haemonchus contortus. J. Vet. Parasitol.,* 22: 45-48.

Swarnkar, C.P., Singh, D., Khan, F.A., Srivastava, C.P. and Bhagwan, P.S.K.(1997). Development and survival of *Haemonchus contortus* larvae on pasture under semi-arid conditions of Rajasthan.*J. Vet. Parasitol.,* 11: 37-41.

Swarnkar, C.P., Singh, D. and Solanki, V.K.(2010). Prevalence of gastrointestinal parasites of sheep in semi-arid Rajasthan-a field study. *Indian J. Sm. Rum.,* 16: 221-27.

Swarnkar, C.P., Singh, D., Srivastava, C.P., Bhagwan, P.S.K. and Dimri, U.(1996).A retro-spective study on ovine gastrointestinal helminthuses under semi-arid conditions. *J. Vet. Parasitol.,*10: 15-21.

Tanwar, R.K., Chahar, A. and Fakhrudin (2005). Prevalence of gastrointestinal nematodes in camel (*Camelusdromedarius*) in and around Bikaner, Rajasthan. *Vet.Pract.,* 6: 133-34.

Tariq, K.A., Chisti, M.Z., Ahmed, F. and Shawl, A.S. (2008). Epidemiology of gastrointestinal nematodes of sheep managed under traditional husbandry system in Kashmir valley. *Vet.Parasitol.*, 158: 138-143.

Taylor, M.A., Coop, R.L. and Wall, R.L. (2007).Veterinary Parasitology. 3rd ed., Blackwell Publications Ltd., pp. 59.

Urquhart, G.M., Armour, J., Duncan, J.L., Dunn, A.M. and Jenings, F.M. (1996). Veterinary Parasitology. 2nd ed., Blackwell Science, London, pp. 307.

Vardharajan, A. (2002). Prevalence of gastrointestinal nematodes in camel and its treatment with fenbendazole. *Intas Polivet*, 3: 10-12.

Woolastan, R.R. and Windon, R.C.(2001). Selection of sheep for response to *Trichostrongylus colubriformis* larvae: genetic parameters. *Anim.Sci.*, 69: 335-344.

Yadav, A., Khajuria, J.K. and Raina, A.K. (2006). Seasonal incidence of gastrointestinal parasites in sheep and goats of Jammu. *J. Vet. Parasitol.*, 20: 65-68.

Yadav, C. L. and Garg, R.(2004). Anthelmintic resistance in gastrointestinal nematodes of sheep in Haryana. *J.Vet.Parasitol.*,18: 39-41.

Yadav, C.L., Grewal, H.S. and Banerjee, D.P.(1993). Susceptibility of two crossbreeds of sheep to *Haemonchus contortus*. *Int.J.Parasitol.*, 23: 819-822.

Yadav, C.L. and Kumar, S.(1990). Trial of albendazole and mebendazole against naturalgastro-intestinal nematodes of camels. *Indian Vet. J.*, 67: 864-866.

Yadav, C.L, Kumar, R.R., Banerjee, P.S., Godara, R., Garg, R. and Vatsya, S.(2009). Epidemiology of gastrointestinal nematodosis in sheep. *Indian Vet.J.*, 86: 1010-1013.

Yadav, C.L, Kumar, R.R., Garg, R., Vatsya, S. and Banerjee, P.S.(2008a). Epidemiology of gastrointestinal nematodosis in goats of Uttrakhand. *Indian J.Anim.Sci.*, 78: 1370-1372.

Yadav, C.L., Kumar, R.R., Vatsya, S, Garg, R. and Banerjee, P.S. (2008b). Epidemiological studies on gastrointestinal nematodosis in cattle and buffaloes. *J.Vet.Parasitol.*, 22:49-52.

Yadav, C.L., Kumar, R., Uppal, R.P. and Verma, S.P. (1995). Multiple anthelmintic resistance in *Haemonchus contortus* on a sheep farm in India. *Vet. Parasitol.*, 60: 355-360.

Yadav, C.L. and Sardana, J.R.(1999). An outbreak of gastrointestinal nematodosisin dairy cattle in Hisar, India. *J.Vet.Parasitol.*, 13: 23-26.

Yadav, C.L. and Singh, V.(1991). Efficacy of thiophanate against *Haemonchus* and *Trichostrongylus* infection in camels.*J.Vet.Parasitol.*,5: 59-60.

Yadav, N.K. (2004). Genetics of resistance to *Haemonchus contortus* in Muzzafarnagar sheep. MSc Thesis, Central Institute for Research on Goats, Makhdoom, Mathura, UP, pp. 55.

Yadav, N.K., Mandal, A., Sharma, D.K., Rout, P.K. and Roy, R. (2008C). Influence of reproductive stages on gastrointestinal nematodes of sheep. *Indian J. Anim. Sci.*, 78: 161-162.

❑❑❑

Chapter 6

Meat-borne Parasitic Zoonoses

Sunil Kumar[1], R. Katoch[2] and Zuhaib F. Bhat[1]

[1] Division of Livestock Products Technology

[2] Division of Veterinary Parasitology

Faculty of Veterinary Sciences and Animal Husbandry

Sher-e-Kashmir University of Agricultural Sciences and Technology-Jammu, R.S. Pura-181 102

Introduction

Although food-borne parasitic diseases are generally under recognized; however, they have received considerable attention in the last few decades. It is known that food-borne parasitic infections such as toxoplasmosis, giardiosis and cysticercosis affect many millions of people worldwide and they are often characterized by having fatal consequences. Although humans may serve as host of around 300 species of parasitic worms and over 70 species of protozoa (Cox, 2002), only around 100 species are known to be food-borne (Orlandi *et al.,* 2002). Changing eating habits, population growth and movements, global trade of foodstuff, changes in food production systems, climate change, increased awareness and better diagnostic tools are some of the main drivers affecting the emergence or re-emergence of many food-borne parasitic diseases in recent years (Broglia and Kapel, 2011). Meat-borne parasitic infections are no exception to it and are becoming more common due to certain factors like globalization of the meat supply, increased consumption and demand of meat and meat products, change in culinary habits, increasing demand for exotic and raw meat cuisines, increase in the population of highly susceptible persons, and increased international travel. Some of these infections are well recognized, but are considered emerging (WHO, 2002) because they have recently become more common and are more detected because of improved diagnostic tools and better communication (Dorny *et al.*, 2009). In the past, the consumption of raw or undercooked meat and fish was associated with specific cultures and practices, but with shifting consumer habits, globalization of meat supplies, cosmopolitan eating habits and increased international travel what once were regarded as rare diseases of discrete geographical distribution are now becoming increasingly more widespread (Slifko *et al.*, 2000). Rapid, refrigerated meat transport which became available to an unprecedented degree at the end of the 20thcentury is one of the major contributing factors for the increased meat-borne parasitic infections (Orlandi *et al.*, 2002).

Furthermore, population growth, urbanization, economic growth and flourishing markets have led to the increasing demand for meat and animal products (Delgado, 2003; Costales *et al.*, 2006; Steinfeld *et al.*, 2006). There is an increased need for livestock products including meat on a global scale because of changing nutritional needs driven by growing incomes and demographic transitions (Rosegrant *et al.*, 1999; Speedy, 2003; Steinfeld *et al.*, 2006). Until 2020, meat demand is expected to increase highly in developing countries and slightly in developed countries (Rosegrant *et al.*, 1999; Delgado, 2003). To meet these increased meat demands of modern society, animals are intensively kept and production is optimized disregarding the well-being of the animals. This increasing global demand for protein of animal origin has also led to certain farming practices (e.g. aquaculture) increasing in developing or emerging countries, where health monitoring may not be sufficiently implemented. This intensification of the production systems in developing countries will lead to the increased risk of zoonotic infections.

There is a wide variety of food products that may be contaminated with one or more parasites and consequently enabling transmission to human beings. The prevalence of specific parasite infective stages in food supplies varies between countries and regions. The sources of food-borne products contaminated with infective stages of parasites are pigs, cattle, fish, crabs, crayfish, snails, frogs, snakes and aquatic plants. The parasites that may be acquired by eating these foods are nematodes, trematodes, cestodes and protozoa. Humans get infected by eating raw or undercooked meat infected with cystic stages of the parasites. Meat of reptiles, amphibians and fish can be infected with a variety of infective stages of parasites, including trematodes (*Opisthorchis* spp., *Clonorchis sinensis* etc), cestodes (*Diphyllobothrium* and *Spirometra* spp.), nematodes (*Gnathostoma* spp., anisakine parasites), and pentastomids that can cause zoonotic infections in humans when consumed raw or not properly cooked meat. Meat-borne parasite infections among the major food-borne parasites are *Toxoplasma gondii, Sarcocystis* spp., *Taenia* spp. and *Trichinella* spp. In most countries measures are taken to prevent humans from becoming infected with meat-borne helminths by inspecting the meat in the slaughterhouses or laboratory. Meat inspection is the principal method applied in the control of *Taenia* spp. and *Trichinella* spp. However, it is often not very sensitive, frequently not practiced, and not done for toxoplasmosis and sarcocystosis. Meat inspection for cysticercosis has a low sensitivity, resulting in a high number of infected carcasses entering the food chain. Furthermore, a large proportion of the carcasses escape meat inspection in developing countries because it is not practiced or because the animals are not slaughtered under official supervision. Cooking is effective in killing the parasites if the appropriate temperature is reached in the core of the meat products. Except for some species of *Trichinella,* which show remarkable resistance, freezing and other meat processing techniques such as smoking, drying, curing, etc. are other effective ways to reduce the risk of infection.

Taenia saginata

Taenia saginata, the beef tapeworm of humans is one of the largest cestodes, with an average length of 4-8 meters, lives exclusively in the small intestine of man whereas the intermediate stage *Cysticercus bovis* is found in cattle. The head or scolex bears four elliptical suckers, has no rostellum or hooks, and is said to be unarmed. *Taenia saginata* possesses about 2000 segments and each gravid segment measures upto 2 cm in length. It contains uterus which is having 15-35 delicate lateral branches and may contain about 80,000-1,00,000 eggs. A person harbouring *T. saginata* infection excretes about 10 million eggs per week. The cosmopolitan distribution of *T. saginata* is due to consumption of raw or undercooked beef and there are estimated 45 million cases worldwide.

The infection in cattle occurs when it feeds on pasture which is contaminated with human faeces infected with *T. saginata*. The chances of infection are more when cattle are grazed on pastures irrigated with inadequately treated sewage and when cattle are fed for extended periods in feedlot. When the eggs are ingested by the cattle, embryo hatch in the duodenum, penetrate the gut wall and the lymphatics or blood vessels of the hepatic portal system and spread to the muscles via general circulation. The embryos that become lodged in the muscles develop into oval cyst (*Cysticercus bovis*)- the so-called "beef measles" a white nodule after 2 weeks of infection but it is clearly visible at 4 weeks. The development of mature infective cyst takes 60-75 days. It appears as a delicate, fluid filled bladder surrounded by fibrous capsule and measures about 8x5 mm. It is pinkish in colour and single scolex is seen as opaque white spot. The cyst may remain viable up to 2 years. Later on, it undergoes degeneration changing from caseation to calcification.

When man consumes raw or inadequately cooked beef, *Cysticercus bovis* reach to small intestine wherein outer covering is lost and the scolex evaginates and attaches to mucosa and grow to sexually mature tapeworms in about 3 months. The adult tapeworms are located in the ileum with their scolex embedded in the mucosa and rest of the organism hanging free in the lumen.

The predilection sites for *Cysticercus bovis* in intermediate host (cattle) are the masseter muscles, heart, tongue, shoulder, diaphragm and oesophagus, and occasionally in fat, liver, lungs and lymph nodes. The viability of cyst can be checked by incubating it at 37°C for 30 minutes in a solution of 30% bile and 70% normal saline. In viable cyst, evagination of head occurs.

In countries where infection of *T. saginata* in man is common and cattle is having frequent access for tapeworm ova, the cattle may develop an active immunity resulting in less incidence of *Cysticercus bovis* cysts in adults as compared to young ones.

Taenia saginata in human beings has less clinical importance as compared to *T. solium*, as it causes only taeniosis and not cysticercosis in humans. Intestinal taeniosis may be manifested by nausea, weight loss, abdominal discomfort and anal pruritis, but occasionally more severe symptoms such as intestinal perforation and peritonitis (Jongwutiwes *et al.*, 2004). In India, the prevalence of *T. saginata* was 1.5% in 1988 (Ahmed *et al.*, 1988). In Western countries, the prevalence rate varies from 0.01 to 10% (Cabaret *et al.*, 2002). Kebede *et al.*(2009) have reported a prevalence of up to 70% from East African countries like Ethiopia.

Many workers have suggested that low sensitivity of meat inspection results in the under estimation of bovine cysticercosis (Geerts *et al.*, 1981; Kyvsgaard *et al.*,1990; Dorny *et al.*,2000). Bovine cysticercosis inflicts serious economic losses to the cattle industry which mainly occurs due to condemnation of valuable carcass, refrigeration and downgrading of infected carcasses (Yoder *et al.*, 1994; Giesecke, 1997; Dorny *et al.*, 2009). In Iran where about 0.02% of cattle carcasses are condemned due to *Cysticercus bovis*, the annual economic losses are to the tune of $4,00,000 (Jahed Khaniki *et al.*, 2010). In highly endemic areas such as many parts of Africa, the prevalence is greater than 20% (Abunna *et al.*, 2007; Opera *et al.*, 2006).

Codex Alimentarius commission prescribes that heavily infected carcasses and viscera must be totally condemned whereas cases of moderate or light infection or small numbers of dead/degenerated *cysticerci* must be subjected to heat treatment. Storage of beef at -5°C for 15 days, at -10°C for 9 days or at -15°C for 6 days kill the *cysticerci* and make the meat safe for human consumption (Hilwig *et al.*, 1978). Many countries suggest that carcasses found to be positive for *cysticerci* must be frozen at -10°C for at least 14 days to render it safe for human consumption.

Taenia solium

Taenia solium has global distribution but incidences are low or negligible in high income countries and in countries where pork is not utilized as a food animal. The main endemic area includes Latin America, China, South-East Asia and Sub Saharan Africa.

In humans, *T. solium* is responsible for neurocysticercosis which may be fatal and is considered as the most common cause of acquired epilepsy (Gajadhar *et al.*, 2006). The studies suggest that in low or middle income endemic countries approximately 30% cases of epilepsy are due to neurocysticercosis (Ndimubanzi *et al.*, 2010). Neurocys ticercosis has been recognized as an emerging global disease causing an estimated 50,000 deaths annually (Roman *et al.*, 2000). It is less widely distributed than *T. saginata* with an estimated 3 million cases.

The estimated global burden of epilepsy is about 7.8 million DALYS (Disability Adjusted Life Years) and out of this about 6.5 million DALYS occur in Sub Saharan Africa, Latin America, South Asia and Western Pacific (including China); where *T. solium* is highly endemic.

Taenia solium occurs in the small intestine of man and measures 3-8 meters in length and is composed of 800-900 segments. The head of *T. solium* is globular and less than 1 mm in diameter and is having a double row of 26-28 hooks that's why it is also known as armed tapeworm of man. *Taenia solium* generally occurs singly in man's intestine but in endemic areas its number may vary up to 25. Incidence of *T. solium* is associated with poverty, illiteracy and poor hygiene, allowing pigs to have access to human faeces. Increased immigration and travelling has made this parasitic infection an important import disease particularly in non-endemic regions such as US (Sorvillo *et al.*, 2007). Due to rapid expansion of small scale pig industry by masses in Africa, a significant increase in cases of cysticercosis in pigs and man has been noticed, however, in most industrialized countries the infections of *T. solium* has almost been eradicated due to socio-economic upliftment and intensification of pig husbandry system. The individual gravid segment of *T. solium* can be differentiated from *T. saginata* on the basis of gravid uterus which is having 7-16 tree like lateral branches on each side as compared to 14-32 of *T. saginata* and is also smaller in size.

The person harbouring *T. solium* excretes 2,00,000-3,00,000 ova daily as it passes 7-10 segments daily with stool and each segment containing about 30,000-40,000 ova. The infection of adult worm shows nervousness, loss of weight, anorexia, abdominal pain and digestive upsets.

The cystic stage of *T. solium* is known as *Cysticercus cellulosae* and is most commonly found in pigs though it can also occur in the wild boar and less commonly in the cat, rat, monkey, cattle, sheep and deer while man and dog can also act as an intermediate host. The size of *Cysticercus cellulosae* varies according to developmental stage which may vary from pin head size to 15x10 mm. At 20 days, the size of cyst is of pin head, at 60 days pea size with visible head and at 110 days all the cysts are of approximately same size with scolex invaginated. Young pigs are more susceptible than older ones. The cyst are elliptical in form and have a predilection for subcutaneous tissue, brain, muscle particularly the heart, diaphragm, internal masseters, tongue, neck, shoulder, intercostals and abdominal muscles although, they can occur in the viscera also but at lesser rate particularly in liver, lung, kidney and eyes. The cysts in the pig muscles (measly pork) are generally scattered and few in number. Cysticercosis in man is not acquired by eating meat but through accidental ingestion of eggs in vegetables, salads, fast foods, etc., wherein raw or undercooked vegetables are used. Alternatively, humans may be infected by the ingestion of *T. solium* ova from an infected person (carrier) or due to auto infections which may occur due to retrograde movements of the intestinal contents, resulting in a more severe disease than that produced by *T. saginata* as the embryo may release form the eggs by successive exposure to the acid stomach and alkaline intestinal juices. Cysticercosis in man also occur due to transfer of ova to the mouth by unclean fingers after defaecation but the ingestion of soil, water or unclean vegetables is the most likely source of human infections. *Cysticercus cellulosae* cysts can remain viable for some years and with time cysts tend to degenerate and become caseated and calcified. Caseated or calcified cysts are not viable. In pigs cyst may be detected after 8 weeks of infection during post mortem examination.

Humans are commonly infected by the consumption of inadequately cooked pork containing *cysticerci*, resulting in the development of *T. solium* tapeworms in human intestine. The presence of adult tape worm in the small intestine is manifested by the abdominal pain, digestive disturbances, diarrhoea/constipation, nervousness and loss of weight but most of cases are asymptomatic except irritation which occurs due to passage of segments from the anus.

The cystic manifestation of disease in human beings with *cysticerci* invading muscles throughout the body may result in heart failure when myocardium is involved. Brain involvement (neurocysticercosis) usually results in severe neurological disorders and may be fatal. In the endemic areas, the brain surgery is a common phenomenon for removal of *cysticerci*.

The diagnosis for the infection of adult tapeworm in man can be made on the basis of morphology of gravid proglottids and scolex in the faeces or on anal swabs. The scolex of all tapeworms has four suckers but the scolex of *T. solium* is armed with hooks. Subcutaneous *cysticerci* in man may be visible or palpated. Confirmed diagnosis can be made on microscopic examination of excised part. The presence of *cysticerci* in brain, spinal cord or visceral organs can be made by X-rays, computerized axial tomography or ultrasound. Serodiagnosis can be used to confirm the diagnosis.

In pigs, detection of *cysticerci* usually occurs on postmortem; however, heavily infected pigs may be diagnosed ante-mortem by palpation of cysts in the tongue. Saini *et al.* (1997) reported that such type of screening is insensitive particularly in lightly infected carcasses. Rodriguez-del-Rosal *et al.* (1989) reported that infected pigs can be diagnosed by detection of products of *T. solium* in the serum by using double homologous monoclonal antibody based enzyme immunoassay.

This technique may be very helpful in detecting the swine cysticercosis during ante-mortem. Commercially available enzyme-linked immunosorbent (ELISA) and enzyme-linked immuno-transfer blot (EITB) assays have high sensitivity and specificity and may be used as epidemiological tools for screening herds for cysticercosis but not for assessing individual animals (Sciutto *et al.*, 1998; Van Kerckhoven *et al.*, 1998). During post mortem the detection of *Cysticercus cellulosae* generally involves splitting of pig carcasses into two sides and inspection of intercostal and cervical muscles and those of the diaphragm, abdomen and thigh. The heart, tongue and larynx should also be examined. In African countries, the shoulder muscles of pigs are frequently inspected whereas in some countries triceps brachii muscle is exposed by making a deep incision about 2.5 cm above the elbow joint. Affected carcasses must be condemned or treated properly by cooking or freezing to kill the parasite. In the endemic area, before slaughter treatment of pig with praziquantel at the rate of 50 mg per kg body for 15 days may reduce the incidence of *Cysticercus cellulosae* by 80% and can prevent huge losses due to high condemnation rates.

Heating of meat to a temperature of 56°C ensure the destruction of *Cysticercus bovis* and *Cysticercus cellulosae* (Allen, 1947; Hird and Pullen, 1979), although the cysts have been found alive in the center of a large joint in pork even after roasting. Pickling in brine solution is a reliable method for destruction of cysts. The cyst may remain alive for 5-6 weeks even after the death of its host. Even decomposition of carcasses does not guarantee death of cyst. Affected carcasses and organs must be condemned.

The control of *T. solium* is based on improving the living standards, health education, improved hygiene and pig husbandry system, efficient meat inspection and mass treatment of pigs and humans. Novel approaches include single dose treatment with oxfendazole of pigs and vaccination of pigs with recombinant antigens (Gonzales *et al.*, 1996; Lightowlers *et al.*, 2000). In experimental models, recombinant vaccines have been found very effective in protecting the pigs from *T. solium* (Gonzalez *et al.*, 2005). A synthetic peptide vaccine has been found to be very effective in reducing the prevalence and intensity against natural infection (Huerta *et al.*, 2002).

Public must be educated about the personnel hygiene. Persons must wash the hand with soap or liquid detergent after defaecation and before eating. Proper toilet facilities must be provided to prevent the contamination of soil, water and food. The use of effluent for soil irrigation or fertilization must be prohibited. Livestock must be prevented to get access to human faeces and latrines. Effective meat inspection procedure must be adopted in the slaughter houses and condemned carcasses must be disposed of or rendered properly. Consumption of raw meat must be prohibited and it must be properly cooked before consumption. Affected persons must be treated with effective taenidicidal drugs such as praziquantel, niclosamide, etc.

Toxoplasmosis

Toxoplasmosis, caused by the protozoan parasite *Toxoplasma gondii* is a neglected and under reported disease, despite having a high disease burden similar to that of salmonellosis and campylobacteriosis. *Toxoplasma gondii* is a crescent-shaped minute (16µmx3µm) intracellular parasite belonging to the sporozoa, a subphylum of the Protozoa. The parasite possess no locomotor organs or flagella in the adult stage and have complex life cycle involving a tissue phase (tachyzoites, bradyzoites in cyst) found in many host species and an intestinal phase (oocysts shed in faeces) recognized only in fields. *T. gondii* has a wide distribution in domestic and wild animals, and was first described in an African rodent, the *gondii*, in 1908. The prevalence of infection differs between wild and farm animals. Among wild carnivores, the rate of infection mainly depends on predator-prey behavior and scavenging activity, whereas animal husbandry practices influence the rate of infection in farm animals. Pigs, sheep and goats are more commonly infected than other livestock and represent a significant source of *T. gondii* for humans and other animals. *T. gondii* infection in cattle and buffalo occurs rarely (Tenter *et al.,* 2000). Cats and small wild animals have high prevalence of infection and probably contribute significantly in *T. gondii* infection in food animals.

The infection rates in pig are generally higher in breeding populations than in market pigs, reflecting that the time of exposure is a key factor in acquiring the infection. In 1983-84, the prevalence of infection in USA was 23.9% in pigs with higher rate in breeder (42%) than in market (23%) pigs (Dubey, 1990; Dubey *et al.,* 1991). In 1992, the infection from same area was reduced to 20.8% in breeders and 3.1% in finisher pigs due to confinement of animals (Weigel *et al.,* 1995). Intensive managemental practices for raising pigs has decreased the prevalence of infection from 75% to less than 10% in many civilized countries and less than 1% in few European countries (Tenter *et al.,* 2000). In a nationwide survey carried out in retail stores of US, a prevalence of only 0.38% was observed in pork (Dubey *et al.,* 2005). However, a re-emergence of toxoplasmosis has been noticed in pigs raised in organic farms with outdoor access (Kijlstra *et al.,* 2004).

The parasite is usually transmitted by the accidental ingestion of sporulated oocysts shed in the faeces of felids or by ingestion of raw or undercooked meat of infected animals or unwashed vegetables contaminated by the cat faeces. In Western and Asian countries, the consumption of undercooked meat is the most likely source of infections (Fallah *et al.,* 2008; Han *et al.,* 2008).

The disease causes abortion in sheep and goats. The fetal cotyledons show numerous characteristic white flecks or nodules and are bright to dark red as compared to deep purple colour in normal conditions.

Toxoplasmosis is a major zoonosis with global distribution. A large proportion of the world's population has serological evidence of infection. The global burden of disease attributable to toxoplasmosis is presently not known, but there is evidence to suggest that it is considerable. Human infection with *T. gondii* is relatively high as compared to most other diseases. Dubey and Beattie (1988) have reported that 100% of the population is infected in many countries. Dubey (1994) has reported that in a survey carried out in USA, about 30% of the population was found either infected or exposed to infection. In France, the prevalence rate of *T. gondii* infection ranged from 42-84% (Dubey and Beattie, 1988).

Toxoplasmosis is especially dangerous to pregnant females where it may cause miscarriage or may pass the infection to the foetus resulting in foetal death, neonatal death or various congenital defects such as hydrocephalus, other CNS abnormalities and choriorenitis, blindness or mental retardation. Toxoplasmosis is also a serious problem in immune suppressed individuals such as HIV patients and transplant patients. A serological survey carried out on pregnant women in Chile suggested that 43% of the seropositive women were also seropositive for oocyst antigen suggesting that 57% acquired the infection through meat (Munoz-Zanzi *et al.,* 2010). In adult immune competent persons the infections is usually mild or unapparent with no significant health effects. Certain individuals may show symptoms of flu, swollen lymph glands, fatigue, joint and muscle pain. *Toxoplasma gondii* is considered the most common cause of retinochoriodítis worldwide and it has been shown that 24% of the people with ocular disease due to infection with *Toxoplasma* eventually become legally blind (Bosch-Driessen *et al.*, 2002). Recent studies showed that most cases of ocular *toxoplasmosis* are attributed to acquired disease, which means that prevention should be directed not only to pregnant women and immune compromised persons, but also towards the general population (Kijlstra and Jongert, 2009). In immune suppressed individual infection may be life threatening (Gajadhar *et al.*,2006).

The global seroprevalence of toxoplasmosis in pregnant women or women of child bearing age varies between 5.3% and 78% and is increasing with age (Pappas *et al.*, 2009). Such variability illustrates differences in exposure across the globe. Singh and Pandit (2004) have reported that the seroprevalence rate among pregnant women in first four month of pregnancy was 45% for *Toxoplasma* IgG antibodies and only 3.3 percent for IgM. Yashodhara *et al.* (2004) in a similar study found a seroprevalence of 33% IgG in women of lower income group as compared to 22% in those of higher socio-economic group. Sundar *et al.* (2007) on the basis of high seroprevalence among 1000 serum samples collected from apparently healthy voluntary blood donors from urban area in Karnataka have concluded that screening for *T. gondii* should be included in blood testing schedule before transfusion. The seroprevalence of *T. gondii* is lower in strict vegetarians (Hall *et al.*, 1999; Roghmann *et al.*, 1999).

In India, the transmission of *T. gondii* to humans through meat of pig, chicken, sheep and goat seems to be of low importance since these meats are properly cooked before consumption. Transmission of *T. gondii* through oocysts shed by infected cats appears to be a more viable source of *Toxoplasma* infection for humans and animals in India (Dubey, 1986). These oocysts can be found virtually anywhere including pig feed and pig barns where cats are resident (Dubey *et al.*, 1995). Chhabra *et al.* (1985) reported that 9.7 to 33.7% cases of sheep, goats, pigs, cattle, buffaloes, camels, horses, cats and dogs were found positive for antibodies to *T. gondii*. A few cases of abortions were, however, seen in goats with titers of 1:64 or above and a neonatal mortality was seen in goat born to dams with titers from 1:8 to 1:256 from Parbhani (Singh and Msolla, 1986). Carcasses affected with toxoplasmosis generally lose their infectivity very shortly after death. Freezing, heating, curing or smoking quickly inactivates the parasites. Cooking is considered as the effective means for destroying the trophozoites and cysts. Infected carcasses and feed stuff also considered as the important sources of infection through ingestion but respiratory infection may also occur. Since felines are rarely kept as pet/companion animal in the Indian families and the prevalence of *Toxoplasma* cyst in sheep, goat and poultry is quite high. Probably adoption of international cuisines and use of meat of these animals in fast food may become important source of infection in years to come.

Several techniques have been developed for the detection of *T. gondii* in the animals and environments but their reliability is questionable. Diagnostic approach may include serological tests, isolation of parasites using traditional methods, bioassays and PCR (Dubey, 2004). Serological tests include various forms of agglutination tests and ELISA. Modified agglutination test using preserved whole tachyzoites has been suggested as the most sensitive and specific test method (Dubey *et al.*, 1995). However, this test is not suitable for use in the slaughterhouse or under field conditions. To prevent the spread of disease public must be educated not to consume raw or undercooked meat and to wash and peel fruit and vegetables before consuming them raw. Tachyzoites and bradyzoites can be destroyed by the usual disinfectants and by desiccation but oocysts are very resistant and can remain infective for more than one year. Pregnant women without *T. gondii* antibody should avoid cleaning litter pans and avoid contact with cats of unknown feeding history. Hand should be washed after handling raw meat and before eating, especially after doing work in the garden as there may be possibility of contact with cat faeces. Affected organs and carcasses, if their condition is poor, should be condemned. Some livestock species infection with *T. gondii* can be prevented by elimination of cat from the environment. Organic farming and outdoor housing of the livestock presents additional difficulties in control of *T. gondii* (Kijlstra *et al.*, 2004). The cooking temperature required for the destruction of *T. gondii* is lesser than the required for *T. spiralis*. Dubey *et al.* (1990) have reported that *T. gondii* can be killed by heating the pork at 49°C for 336 seconds or at 55°C for 44 seconds or at 61°C for 6 seconds after attaining the uniform temperature. Microwave cooking has produced inconsistent results with regards to *T. gondii* destruction probably due to uneven heating. The cyst of *T. gondii* has been found alive even after freezing of tissue at -6.7°C for 11.2 days and at -3.9°C for 22.4 days but the parasites were inactivated instantaneously at a temperature of -9.4°C and lower (Kotula *et al.*, 1991). Irradiation of tissue at a dose rate of $4\text{-}5\times10^4$ rads with Cs^{137} make the cyst non infective.

Trichinosis

Trichinella, a nematode parasite, is one of the most widespread zoonotic pathogens in the world. Till date, eight species and four genotypes within two clades (encapsulated and non-encapsulated) have been recognized in this genus (Pozio and Murrel, 2006; Zarlenga *et al.,* 2006; Krivokapich *et al.,* 2008). In addition to the species found in the domestic pig (*Trichinella spiralis* or *T-1*), several other species (*T. nativa* or *T-2, T. britovi* or *T-3* and *T. pseudospiralis* or T-4) and types (*T-5, T-6, T-7* and *T-8*) are found in wildlife (Pozio *et al.,* 1992). Till date, all *Trichinella* infections occurring in animals and humans have been attributed to *T. spiralis. Trichinella spiralis* is a small nematode parasite of carnivorous and omnivorous animals. The adult worm lives in the intestine of mammals and the larval form in the muscular tissues of same host. In humans parasite causes a serious disease called trichinosis or trichinellosis. The sexes are distinct, the male being 1.5 mm and the female 3-4 mm long. The mouth of the worm is round and unarmed. The male possess a pair of flaps on either side of cloaca. Trichinellosis in humans occurs with the ingestion of *Trichinella* larvae that are encysted in muscular tissue of domestic or wild animal meat. Infection in man worldwide usually occurs through the ingestion of raw or undercooked meat usually pork. However, meats of wild boars and horses have played a significant role during outbreaks within the past decades (Gottstein *et al.,* 2009). The first symptom of disease is observed when embryo worm invade the muscular tissue and are usually those of enteritis.

Infection by *Trichinella* spp. has been reported in domestic and wild animals of all the continents, with the exception of Antarctica (Pozio and Murrel, 2006). Trichinellosis is more prevalent in the temperate northern hemisphere and Arctic than in the tropics and southern hemisphere. *Trichinella spiralis* is found in the intestine and muscular tissue of the pig, rat, mouse, dog, cat, bear, wild boar, man and other mammals. In East Africa, it has been recovered from a number of wild carnivores including leopard, jackal and hyena. In Germany, trichinellosis is wide spread in foxes and is considered as more common than pig. Many people in the Arctic, especially in Greenland are infected by eating the flesh of infected polar bears, walruses, seals, etc.

Cattle, sheep and horses possess certain degree of natural immunity against *Trichinella.* If trichinosed meat is fed to them, the adult worms develop in the intestines but only rarely larvae are found in the muscles. Similarly birds harbor the intestinal form of *Trichinella* after artificial infection but larvae are only occasionally found in the muscles and are usually degenerated (Gracey and Collins, 1992).

In 1981, 46 cases of trichinellosis were detected in New York due to the consumption of ethnic dishes that contained raw or partially cooked pork particularly homemade pork sausage.

Adult worms are only found in the small intestines of animals that have recently eaten *trichinosed* flesh i.e. muscle containing larvae. The gastric juice dissolves the cyst walls and larvae are liberated. They develop into sexually mature adults in the intestine and mate within two days. The males die soon after mating and after two weeks of infection only females are present. These females live for 5-8 weeks, penetrate the intestinal mucous membrane and reach the lymph space where each gives to about 1,350-1,500 larvae. The larvae enter the lymph stream and then moves to the systemic blood circulatory system via thoracic duct. Further development of larvae occurs in the muscle only. Now larvae are widespread via arterial blood supply. The larvae are motile and have a predilection for striped muscle particularly those having low glycogen content. The larvae enter the muscle fibers. After entering the muscle fiber, larvae become quiescent and increase in size. About two weeks after infection they become about 8 times their original size and then curl up within the muscle fibers into a typical spiral coil. On the basis of this unique shape the worm has got its name. After three weeks of infection, the embryo becomes 3 mm long and growth ceases. Two months after infection tissue reaction occurs due to irritation of embryo, and the embryo becomes enclosed in an oval muscle cyst whose long axis remains parallel to the long axis of muscle fiber. The cyst becomes fully developed at three months and measure about 0.5x0.25 mm. Initially these cysts are structure less, made up of hyaline material and translucent and not easy to detect upto 2-3 months. 6-8 months later cyst becomes infiltrated with fat and lime salts are deposited. The cysts tend to become calcified but can remain alive for many years. Encapsulation is a prerequisite if parasite wants to survive within the muscular tissue. Calcified *Trichinella* has been known to remain alive in man for upto 31 years and in pig for 12 years (Gracey and Collins, 1992).

The cysts are found in the striped muscles and the actual site depends on the species of animal. In pig, the majority of cysts are found in the skeletal muscles of respiratory tract particularly in pillars of diaphragm, muscles of tongue and larynx and the abdominal and intercostal muscles. In rodents, the muscles of mastication are most frequently involved.

In most of the domestic and wild animals, infection remains undiagnosed. Severe infection causes enteritis which is manifested by diarrhoea. The presence of larvae in muscles is associated with fever, stiffness, muscular spasm, dyspnoea, facial oedema and hoarseness. Death may occur in heavily infected animals due to respiratory failure.

Incubation period of *Trichinella spiralis* in man is 7-14 days after ingestion of infected meat. Most of the infection remains subclinical but in some cases disease may be fatal. Most of the mild cases are misdiagnosed as influenza or other viral infections. Persons feel muscular pain and oedema of the upper eyelids in early stages followed by conjunctival and retinal haemorrhage and photophobia. In prolonged cases remittent fever, weakness, anorexia, sweating, chills and diarrhoea occur. In severe conditions, cardiac and respiratory complications occurs leading to death due to myocardial failure. Human cases of trichinellosis have been documented in 55 countries (Torgerson and Macpherson, 2011). It has been estimated that about 11 million people are infected worldwide and it is recognized that significant underreporting occurs for reasons relating to test methodology and health care infrastructure (Dupouy-Camet, 2000). Pozio (2011) has reported that approximately 10,000 cases occur annually with 0.2% of these cases being fatal. Even a few larvae (1-50/g) in human muscle are considered heavy infection and 1000/g is considered critical.

In India, there are few reports of the occurrence of *T. spiralis* in some mammalian hosts, namely from a civet cat in Kolkata (Schad and Chowdhury, 1967); a Bandicota bengalensis in Mumbai (Niphadkar, 1973) and in 3 of 500 domestic pigs examined in Bombay (Niphadkar *et al.*, 1979). Mohan *et al.* (2002) reported a case of human trichinellosis. The cysts were found in psoas muscle during drainage of an abscess.

In China, epidemics of trichinosis have been reported. In Henan Province, one third of 3630 pigs examined were found infected with larvae of *Trichinella* spp. (Wu, 1986). In Hong Kong, barbecue and "steam boat seasons" in summer and winter are the source of trichinellosis. Besides eating habits, socio-environmental factors also contribute to this infection (Ko, 1991). About 3% of pigs slaughtered in Hong Kong which were imported from China were found positive for *T. spiralis* (Ko, 1991). In Thailand, during 1967-73, 3,55,820 pig diaphragms were collected from different slaughterhouses of Northern Province. These samples were examined by trichinoscope and out of these, 19 samples were found positive for *T. spiralis* larvae and the number of larvae varied from 2-800 per gram of samples (Khamboonruang, 1991).

Disposal of infected carcasses of pigs or hunted wild boars, wolves and foxes in nature or waste disposal sites might be a driving force in spreading *T. spiralis* infections in wild rat populations (Neghina, 2010). Jovic *et al.* (2001) showed by bioassay using rats that *T. spiralis* larvae in artificially infected pork meat that had been buried in the ground at a depth of 30-100 cm, remain infective for rats for more than 91 days. Rats were shown to be a potential reservoir host species of *Trichinella* using mathematical models, provided that cannibalism occurs (Takumi, 2010).

The oldest but still frequently used method for detection of *Trichinella* cysts is the compression method. In this method grain sized portion of muscles are collected from diaphragm, tongue and pharyngeal muscles and are compressed between two thick glass slides (a compressorium) and examined under a magnification of 15-40 in the trichinoscope. Digestion methods provide better efficiency for the direct detection of trichinae in pork. In this method, tissue samples are collected from the predilection sites of parasites. These samples are subjected to digestion in acidified pepsin. Larvae, freed from their muscle cell capsules can be recovered by a series of sedimentation steps, then visualized and enumerated under a microscope (Gamble, 1997). In pork, the diaphragm and tongue muscle have more numbers of larvae as compared to other muscles. Sample size may vary from one gm (as per EU) to five gm (as per USDA) or even larger to increase sensitivity. The sensitivity of the former sample size is approximately three larvae per gm (LPG) and latter is one LPG or less. The details of digestion test can be seen in the Directives of European Economic Community (EEC, 1977, 1984), in USDA Code of Federal Regulations (1994) and in OIE Manual of Standards (Gamble and Murrel, 1996).

In practice, the compression method using the trichinoscope has an approximate sensitivity of more than 5 LPG of tissue (Borowka and Ring, 1993) while the sensitivity of digestion method is approximately 3 LPG. Generally it is considered that pork having more than one LPG pose a significant public health risk.

An alternative method of testing pigs for trichinellosis is the detection of antibodies of parasites in the serum sample. This method is generally considered reliable for herd testing but it cannot detect all infected animals particularly animals in the early stages of infection (Gazadhar *et al.*, 2006). ELISA can be used for testing of pigs for *Trichinella* in both pre and post slaughter applications (Gamble *et al.*, 1988). This has been proved highly sensitive and specific and no cross reaction occurs during this test.

Trichinellosis is not only a public health hazard but also an economic problem in pig production and food safety. Because of the high importance of the disease efforts must be focused on the elimination of *Trichinella* from the food chain. Side by side efforts should be made to prevent the exposure of human beings from infected pork products. To achieve this, inspection programme may be implemented at the slaughter places for the detection of trichinellosis in pigs. The incidences of trichinellosis can be reduced by effective public education, prevention of garbage feeding to pigs, rodent control and improved farming and managemental practices (Gamble *et al.*, 2000). Methods for detection of trichinellosis include digestion of muscles to free larvae, compression technique to visualize cysts in muscles (trichinoscopy), direct or indirect serological tests, PCR, histology and bioassay (Gajadhar *et al.*, 2006). The digestion assay allows the intensity of infection to be quantified and is the most sensitive technique for testing individual animal carcasses (Gamble *et al.*, 2000). Where inspection of pork carcass is not possible alternate methods may be carried out to prevent exposure of humans to potentially contaminated pork products. These methods may include cooking, freezing, curing, irradiation, etc. which make the pork products *T. spiralis* larvae free.

Proper cooking of pork and pork products may destroy all stages of *Trichinella*. *Trichinella spiralis* has been shown to be killed in 47minutes at 52°C, in 6 minutes at 55°C and in less than a minute at 60°C (Kotula *et al.*, 1983). These time-temperature combinations are effective only when product reaches and maintains the temperature evenly distributed throughout the meat. Inconsistent results have been obtained from the alternative methods of cooking e.g. microwaves, in which all parasites were not completely inactivated when the products were heated to the prescribed end point temperature (Kotula *et al.*,

1983). The USDA Code of Federal Regulations describes that pork products must be cooked for 2 hours at 52.2°C, one hour at 53.4°C, 30 minutes at 54.5°C, 15 minutes at 55.6°C, 1 minute at 60°C and instant at 62.2°C to inactivate the parasites. However, USDA recommends that fresh pork products must be cooked to an internal temperature of 77°C to provide safety margin.

Freezing of pork products for longer duration may destroy all stages of *T. spiralis*. The time required to kill trichinae by freezing were 4 days at -10°C, 64 minutes at -15°C, 8 minutes at -20°C and instantly at -23.3°C. The USDA Code of Federal Regulation states that pork to be used in processed meat products must be frozen at -37.2°C for 30 minutes, at -34.5°C for 8 hours, at -31.7°C for 22 hours, at -28.9°C for 35 hours, at -26.1°C for 48 hours, at -23.3°C for 63 hours, at -20.6°C for 82 hours or at -17.8°C for 106 hours. The extra time has been recommended for freezing to equalize the temperature within the meat along with the margin of safety. Some species of *Trichinella* e.g. T_2 (*T. nativa*) and T_6 can survive and remains infective at normal freezing temperature. Freeze resistant species of *Trichinella* has resulted in several outbreaks of human trichinellosis (Dworkin *et al.*, 1996; Margolis *et al.*, 1979).

During curing, the meat product is covered/coated/sprinkled or mixed with salt mixture or brine solution is injected into it and kept at refrigeration temperature to achieve uniform distribution. Several pork products like ham, sausages, pork shoulders and other ready to eat products can be prepared by application of curing technique. In the presence of salt, the cysts become dehydrated by osmosis. Generally the combined effect of time temperature, amount of salt and thickness of the product interact to destroy any trichinae that may be present. Small products and products containing salt that are heated to a high temperature take less processing time to become safe from trichinae. Unfortunately, no single or even combination of parameters achieved by curing has been shown to correlate definitely with trichinae inactivation.

An irradiation dose level of 0.2-0.3 kGy prevents the maturation of encysted larvae in meat. Treatment by one kGy makes the pork carcass safe from trichinae and is approved by Food and Drug Administration in USA. Spent fuel rods are used to provide gamma radiation from Cs^{135} and Co^{60}.

Sarcocystosis

Sarcocystosis has been recognized as a disease in animals and man, and has received the attention of scientists all over the world. With the global attention, work on this protozoan parasite has also been initiated in domestic animals in India. The parasite has an obligatory two host life cycle having pre-predator relationships. Herbivores and omnivores act as the intermediate hosts; acquire infection by ingesting the sporocysts which are shed in the faeces of carnivores/omnivores, known to act as definitive hosts. On the other hand definitive hosts become infected with *Sarcocystis* spp. by ingesting the sarcocysts in the muscles of intermediate hosts. The main established definitive hosts of *Sarcocystis* spp. in domestic animals are dogs and cats. A variety of species of *Sarcocystis* have been found in India in cattle, buffaloes, sheep, goats, horses and pigs and have been reported from various parts of the country (Shah, 1983). The distribution of *Sarcocystis* is recorded in various organs, i.e. heart, oesophagus, diaphragm, tongue, ocular, thigh and tail muscles.

The zoonotic significance has been recognized with the establishment of two species, i.e. *S. hominis* (cattle origin) and *S. suihominis* (pig origin) as cause of disease in humans. Humans get infected by eating raw or undercooked meat infected with cyst stages of this parasite. Man is acting as the definitive host for *S. suihominis* and *S. hominis* but clinical disease in humans has not been reported in the country. The microcysts of *S. suihominis* have been recentlyidentified and differentiated from species of S. *miescheriana* in striated muscles of different organs of pigs in India (Solanki *et al.*, 1991) and the prevalence of *S. suihominis* had been found surprisingly higher (47.11%) than S. *miescheriana*(43.14%). It is established that *S. suihominis* and *S. hominis* cause digestive disturbances and, at times, life threatening symptoms in human beings who eat undercooked meat of these animals (Shah, 1984; Juyal and Bhatia, 1989). *Sarcocystis suihominis* causes more severe digestive troubles in humans than *S. hominis*. There is only one report on the occurrence of *S. hominis* in India in muscles of cattle in Madhya Pradesh (Jain and Shah, 1987) and the cysts have been reported in two clinical reports in human beings at Lucknow in Uttar Pradesh (Gupta *et al.*, 1973; Aggarwal and Srivastava, 1983). *Sarcocystis suihominis* infection had been reported by Banerjee *et al.* (1994) in humans at Pantnagar (Uttarakhand). These workers found positivity in stool samples of 14 out of 20 children belonging to families who slaughter pigs without any meat inspection procedure. Further these children had the history of consuming raw pork and passed typical sporocysts in stools. Despite the reported high prevalence of porcine *S. suihominis* in India, there does not appear to be any other report of human sarcocystosis. Clearly, this is a lacuna in our information that calls for attention (Chhabra and Singla, 2009).

In most countries measures are taken to prevent humans from becoming infected with meat-borne helminths by inspecting the meat in the slaughterhouse or laboratory but for sarcocystosis no specific meat inspection is done. In addition, in developing countries, like India, a large proportion of the carcasses escape meat inspection because it is not practiced or because the animals are not slaughtered in abattoirs. Stray dogs play a main role in the transmission of the infection, as they can be easily seen eating meat offal outside the slaughter houses.

One of the principal sources of infection to man in India is through consumption of raw or uncooked pork or improperly cooked pork products like sausages. Pigs are mostly reared by the economically depressed class in India in rural areas which mainly live under unhygienic and unsanitary conditions. They are generally fed on garbag and human refuge, including night soil. The oprophagic nature of pigs exposes them to infective materials of all kinds. Their slaughtering is not held in regular abattoirs and generally slaughtered in the backyard of the slums and houses of the owners in many parts of the country without official supervision and the offals are carelessly discarded. Humans particularly children get infected by eating either raw meat infected with cyst stages of this parasite or undercooked meat after a little bit of roasting in the fire. Half-roasted pork is considered a delicacy in some communities, particularly on the occasion of a ceremony.

The effective steps should be taken to control this infection in animals and man by avoiding the exposure of dogs and cats to raw meat and offals and by avoiding the contamination of feed and water with the sporocysts. Cooking is effective in killing the parasites if the appropriate temperature is reached in the core of the meat product (70°C for 15 minutes) (Saleque *et al.*, 1990). Freezing and other meat processing techniques such as drying, smoking, curing, etc. are other effective ways to reduce the risk of infection.

Conclusion

Globalization of the meat supply, increased consumption and demand of meat and meat products, change in culinary habits, increasing demand for exotic and raw meat cuisines, climatic change associated with global warming, increased vector populations, changing socio-economic conditions, poverty, the lack of safe drinking water, the large number of stray animals, certain cooking practices, defecating outdoors, poor personal hygiene, high population density and increased international travel are responsible for the rising prevalence of meat-borne parasitic zoonoses in India. In this changing scenario, food safety is of the utmost importance. There is an increasing risk to consumers of acquiring the infections in non-endemic areas because of an increasing availability and interest in ethnic foods. Health education, controlled slaughter, control of animal movements, vector control, higher socio-economic development and improved risk assessments can help to control meat-borne parasitic zoonoses in the country. Strict meat inspection and condemnation of the carcasses by the appropriate authorities can prevent the establishment of important parasitic zoonotic infections. However, in remote rural areas where animals are slaughtered locally and meat inspection is not available, people are at risk of obtaining unsafe food and eating only properly cooked food is the only wayout. Overall, there is an urgent need for better monitoring and control of meat-borne parasites using new technologies.

References

Abunna, F., Tilahun, G., Megersa, B., Regassa, A. and Kumsa, B. (2007). Bovine cysticercosis in cattle slaughtered at A wassa municipal a battoir, Ethiopia: prevalence, cyst viability, distribution and its public health implication. *Zoo. Pub. Hlth.*, 55: 83–88.

Aggarwal, P.K. and Srivastava, A.N. (1983). Sarcocystosis in man. A report of two cases. *Histopath.*, 7: 783-7.

Ahmed, M., Zutshi, M.L. and Ahmad Shah, S.N. (1988). Intestinal parasites in Kashmiris (rural study). *Ind. J. Parasitol.*, 12: 41-44.

Allen, R.W. (1947). The thermal death point of *cysticerci* of *Taenia saginata*. *J. Parasitol.*, 33: 331-338.

Banerjee, P.S., Bhatia, B.B. and Pandit, B.A. (1994). *Sarcocystis hominis* infection in human beings in India. *J. Vet. Parasitol.*, 8: 57-58.

Borowka, H.J. and Ring, C. (1993). *Trichinenfreie* Region - eine realistis che Prämisefür den Verbraucherschutz. *Fleischwirtsch*, 73(12): 1362-1366.

Bosch-Driessen, L.E., Berendschot, T.T., Ongkosuwito, J.V. and Rothova, A. (2002). Ocular toxoplasmosis: clinical features and prognosis of 154 patients. *Ophthalmol.*, 109: 869-878.

Broglia, A. and Kapel, C. (2011). Changing dietary habits in a changing world: Emerging drivers for the transmission of foodborne parasitic zoonoses. *Vet. Parasitol.,* 182: 2-13.

Cabaret, J., Geerts, S., Madeline, M., Bellandonne, C. and Barbier, D. (2002). The use of urban sludge on pastures: the cysticercosis threat. *Vet. Res.,* 33: 575-597.

Chhabra, M.B. and Singla, L.D. (2009). Food borne parasitic zoonosis in India: Review of recent reports of human infections. *J. Vet. Parasitol.,* 23(2): 103-110.

Chhabra, M.B., Gupta, S.L. and Gautum, O.P. (1985). *Toxoplasma* seroprevalence in animals in Northern India. *Int. J. Zoon.,* 12: 136-42.

Costales, A., Gerber, P. and Steinfeld, H. (2006). Underneath the livestock revolution. Livestock report, Rome, Italy: Food and Agriculture Organization of the United Nations.

Cox, F.E. (2002). History of human parasitology.*Clin. Microbiol. Rev.,* 15: 595-612.

Delgado, C.L. (2003). Rising consumption of meat and milk in developing countries has created a new food revolution. *J.Nutr.,* 133: 3907-3910.

Dorny, P., Praet, N., Deckers, N. and Gabriel, S. (2009). Emerging food-borne parasites. *Vet. Parasitol.,* 163: 196-206.

Dorny, P., Vercammen, F., Brandt, J., Vansteenkiste, W., Berkvens, D. and Geerts, S. (2000). Sero-epidemiological study of *Taenia saginata cysticercosis* in Belgian cattle. *Vet. Parasitol.,* 88: 43-49.

Dubey, J.P. (1987). Toxoplasmosis in domestic animals in India.Present and future. *J. Vet. Parasitol.,* 1: 13-18.

Dubey, J.P., Rotula, A.W., Sharar, A., Andrews, C.D. and Lindsay, D.S. (1990). Effect of high temperature on infectivity of *Toxoplasma gondii* tissue cysts in pork. *J. Parasitol.,* 76: 201-204.

Dubey, J.P., Thulliez, P., Weigel, R.M., Andrews, C.D., Lind, P. and Powell, E.C. (1995). Sensitivity and specificity of various serologic tests for detection of *Toxoplasma gondii* infection in naturally infected sows. *Am. J. Vet. Res.,* 56 (8): 1030-1036.

Dubey, J.P. (1986). A review of toxoplasmosis in cattle. *Vet. Parasitol.,* 22: 177-202.

Dubey, J.P. (1990). Status of toxoplasmosis in pigs in the United States. *J. Am. Vet. Med. Assoc.,*196 (2): 270-274.

Dubey, J.P. (1994). Toxoplasmosis. *J. Am. Vet. Med. Assoc.,* 205: 1593-1598.

Dubey, J.P. (2004). Toxoplasmosis-a water borne zoonosis. *Vet. Parasitol.,* 126: 57-72.

Dubey, J.P. and Beattie, C.P. (1988). Toxoplasmosis in man (*Homo sapiens*). In: Toxoplasmosis of animals and man. Boca Raton, FL: CRC Press Inc., pp. 41-60.

Dubey, J.P., Hill, D.E., Jones, J.L., Hightower, A.W., Kirkland, E., Roberts, J.M., Marcet, P.L., Lehmann, T., Vianna, M.C., Miska, K., Sreekumar, C., Kwok, O.C., Shen, S.K. and Gamble, H.R. (2005). Prevalence of viable *Toxoplasma gondii* in beef, chicken, and pork from retail meat stores in the United States: risk assessment to consumers. *J. Parasitol.*, 91: 1082-1093.

Dubey, J.P., Leighty, J.C., Beal, V.C., Anderson, W.R., Andrews, C.D. and Thulliez, P. (1991). National seroprevalence of *Toxoplasma gondii* in pigs. *J. Parasitol.*, 77 (4): 517-521.

Dupouy-Camet, J. (2000). Trichinellosis: a worldwide zoonosis. In:*Trichinella* and Trichinellosis (A.A. Gajadhar and H.R. Gamble, eds.). *Vet. Parasitol.*, 93: 191-200.

Dworkin, M.S., Gamble, H.A., Zarlenga, D.S. and Tennican, P.J. (1996). Outbreak of trichinellosis associated with eating cougar jelly. *J. Infect. Dis.*,174: 663-666.

European Economic Community (1977). Council Directive 77/96/EEC of 21 December 1976 on the examination for trichinae (*Trichinella spiralis*) upon importation from third countries of fresh meat derived from domestic swine. *Off. J. Eur. Communities*, No. L. 26/67 of 31.01.77.

European Economic Community (1984). Council Directive 84/319/EEC of 7 June 1984 amending the Annexes to Council Directive 77/96/EEC on the examination for trichinae (*Trichinella spiralis*) upon importation from third countries of fresh meat derived from domestic swine. *Off. J. Eur. Communities*, No. L. 167/34 of 27.06.84.

Fallah, M., Rabiee, S., Matini, M. and Taherkhani, H. (2008). Seroepidemiology of Toxoplasmosis in primi gravida women in Hamadan, Islamic Republic of Iran, 2004. *East Medit. Hlth. J.*, 14: 163-171.

Frits, F.J., Franssen, Manoj Fonville, Katsuhisa Takumi, Isabelle Vallée, Aurélie Grasset, Marie A. Koedam, Piet W. Wester, Pascal Boireau and Joke W.B. Van der Giessen (2011). Antibody response against *Trichinella spiralis* in experimentally infected rats is dose dependent. *Vet. Res.*, 42: 113-123.

Gajadhar, A.A., Scandrett, W.B. and Forbes, L.B. (2006). Overview of food- and water-borne zoonotic parasites at the farm level. *Rev. Sci. Tech. Off. Int.Epiz.*, 25 (2): 595-606.

Gamble, H.R. (1997). Parasites associated with pork and pork products. *Rev. Sci. Tech. Off. Int.Epiz.*,16(2): 496-506.

Gamble, H.R. and Murrell, K.D. (1996). Trichinellosis. In: Manual of standards for diagnostic tests and vaccines, 3rd ed., Office International des Epizooties, Paris, 477-480.

Gamble, H.R., Bessonov, A.S., Cuperlovic, K., Gajadhar, A.A., Van Knapen, F., Noeckler, K., Schenone, H. and Zhu, X. (2000). International Commission on Trichinellosis: recommendations on methods for the control of *Trichinella* in domestic and wild animals intended for human consumption. In: *Trichinella* and Trichinellosis (A.A. Gajadhar and H.R. Gamble, eds.). *Vet. Parasitol.*, 93: 393-408.

Gamble, H.R., Rapic, D., Marinculic, A. and Murrell, K.D. (1988). Influence of cultivation conditions on specificity of excretory-secretory antigens for the immunodiagnosis of Trichinellosis. *Vet. Parasitol.*, 30: 131-137.

Geerts, S., Kumar, V., Aerts, N. and Ceulemans, F. (1981). Comparative evaluation of immunoelectrophoresis, counter immunoelectrophoresis and ELISA for the diagnosis of *Taenia saginata cysticercosis.Vet.Parasitol.*, 8: 299-307.

Giesecke, W.H. (1997). Prevalence and economic implications of taeniasis/ *cysticercosis* in South Africa. In: Cysticercosis. Report on a workshop held at the Onderstepoort Veterinary Institute, Onderstepoort, South Africa, 18-19 August, 1997, pp. 19-70.

Gonzales, A.E., Garcia, H.H., Gilman, R.H., Gavidia, C.M., Tsang, V.C., Bernal, T., Falcon, N., Romero, M. and Lopez-Urbina, M.T. (1996). Effective, single dose treatment or porcine *cysticercosis* with oxfendazole. *Am. J. Trop. Med. Hyg.*, 54: 391-394.

Gonzalez, A.E., Gauci, C.G., Barber, D., Gilman, R.H., Tsang, V.C.W., Garcia, H.H., Verastegui, M. and Lightowlers, M.W. (2005). Vaccination of pigs to control human neurocysticercosis. *Am. J. Trop. Med.Hyg.*, 72(6): 837-839.

Gottstein, B., Pozio, E. and No'ckler, K. (2009). Epidemiology, diagnosis, treatment and control of Trichinellosis.*Clin.Microbiol. Rev.*, 22: 127-145.

Gracey, J.F. and Collins, D.S. (1992). Parasitic diseases. In: Meat Hygiene. Ninth ed., Bailliere Tindall, London.

Gupta, O.K., Nath, P., Bhatia, K.B. and Mehrotra, R.M.L. (1973). *Sarcocystis* infection in man. *Ind. J. Path. Bact.*,16: 73-5.

Hall, S.M., Pandit, A., Golwilkar, A. and Williams, T.S. (1999). How do Jains get *Toxoplasma* infection? *Lancet*, 354: 486-487.

Han, K., Shin, D.W., Lee, T.Y. and Lee, Y.H. (2008). Seroprevalence of *Toxoplasma gondii* infection and risk factors associated with seropositivity of pregnant women in Korea. *J. Parasitol.*, 94: 963-965.

Hilwig, R.W., Cramer, J.D. and Forsyth, K.S. (1978). Freezing times and temperatures required to kill *cysticerci* of *Taenia Saginata* in beef. *Vet. Parasitol.*, 4: 215-219.

Hird, D.W. and Pullen, M.M. (1979). Tapeworms, meat and man: a brief review and update of cysticercosis caused by *Taenia saginata* and *Taenia solium*. *J. Food. Protec.*, 42(1): 58-64.

Huerta, M., De Aluga, A.S., Fragoso, G., Toledo, A., Villalobos, N., Hernandez, M., Gevorkian, G., Acero, G., Diaz, A., Alvarez, I., Avila, R., Beltran, C., Garcia, G., Martinez, J.J., Larralde, C. and Sciutto, E. (2002). Synthetic peptide vaccine against *Taenia solium* pig cysticercosis: successful vaccination in a controlled field trial in rural Mexico. *Vaccine*, 20: 262-266.

Jahed Khaniki, G.R., Raei, M., Kia, E.B., Motevalli Haghi, A. and Selseleh, M. (2010). Prevalence of bovine cysticercosis in slaughtered cattle in Iran. *Trop. Anim. Hlth. Prod.*, 42: 141-143.

Jain, P.C. and Shah, H.L. (1987). *Sarcocystis hominis* in cattle in Madhya Pradesh and its public health importance. *Ind. Vet. J.*, 64: 650-654.

Jongwutiwes, S., Putaporntip, C., Chantachum, N. and Sampatanukul, P. (2004). Jejunal perforation caused by morphologically abnormal *Taenia saginata saginata* infection. *J. Infect.*, 49: 324-328.

Jovic, S., Djordjevic, M., Kulisic, Z., Pavlovic., S. and Radenkovic, B. (2001). Infectivity of *Trichinella spiralis* larvae in pork buried in the ground. *Parasite*, 8: S213-215.

Juyal, P.D. and Bhatia, B.B. (1989). *Sarcocystosis*: an emerging zoonosis. *Ind. Vet. Med. J.*, 13:66-69.

Kebede, N., Tilahu, G. and Hailu, A. (2009). Current status of bovine cysticercosis of slaughtered cattle in Addis Ababa Abattoir, Ethiopia. *Trop. Anim. Hlth. Prod.*, 41: 291-294.

Khamboonruang, C. (1991). On emerging problems in foodborne parasitic zoonosis: impact on agriculture and public health. In: Cross JH, ed. Emerging problems in food-borne parasitic zoonosis: impact on agriculture and public health. Proceedings of the 33rd SEAMEO-TROPMED Regional Seminar. *Southeast Asian J. Trop. Med. Pub. Hlth.*,22:1-7.

Kijlstra, A. and Jongert, E. (2009). *Toxoplasma*-safe meat: close to reality? *Trends Parasitol.*, 25: 18-22.

Kijlstra, A., Eissen, O., Cornelissen, A., Munniksma, J., Eijck, K. and Kortbeek, I.T. (2004). *Toxoplasma gondii* infection in animal-friendly pig production systems. *Invest. Ophthalmol. Vis. Sci.*, 45: 3165-3169.

Ko, R.C. (1991). Current status of food-borne parasitic zoonoses in Hong Kong (1991). In: Cross JH, ed. Emerging problems in food-borne parasitic zoonosis:

impact on agriculture and public health. Proceedings of the 33rd SEAMEO-TROPMED Regional Seminar. *Southeast Asian J. Trop. Med. Pub.Hlth.*, 22: 42-47.

Kotula A.W., Dubey J.P., Sharar A.K., Andrews C.D., Shen S.K. and Lindsay D.S. (1991). Effect of freezing on infectivityof *Toxoplasma gondii* tissue cysts in pork. *J.Food Protec.*, 54 (9): 687-690.

Kotula, A.W., Murrell, K.D., Acosta-Stein, L., Lamb, L. and Douglass, L. (1983). Destruction of *Trichinella spiralis* during cooking. *J. Food. Sci.*, 48: 765-768.

Kotula, A.W., Murrell, K.D., Acosta-Stein, L., Lamb, L. and Douglass, L. (1983). *Trichinella spiralis*: effect of high temperature on infectivity in pork. *Expl. Parasitol.*, 56: 15-19.

Krivokapich, S.J., Prous, C.L., Gatti, G.M., Confalonieri, V., Molina, V., Matarasso, H. and Guarnera, E. (2008). Molecular evidence for a novel encapsulated genotype of *Trichinella* from Patagonia, Argentina. *Vet.Parasitol.*, 156: 234-240.

Krivokapich, S.J., Prous, C.L., Gatti, G.M., Confalonieri, V., Molina, V., C Mikkonen, T, Valkama, J., Wihiman, H. and Sukura, A. (2005). Spatial variation of *Trichinella* prevalence in rats in Finnish waste disposal sites. *J. Parasitol.*, 91: 210-213.

Kyvsgaard, N.C., Ilsøe, B., Henriksen, S.A. and Nansen, P., (1990). Distribution of *Taenia saginata* cysts in carcasses of experimentally infected calves and its significance for routine meat inspection. *Res. Vet. Sci.*, 49: 29-33.

Lightowlers, M.W., Flisser, A., Gauci, C.G., Heath, D.D., Jensen, O. and Rolfe, R. (2000).Vaccination against cysticercosis and hydati disease.*Parasitol.Today*, 16: 191-196.

Lunden, A. and Uggia, A. (1992). Infectivity of *Toxoplasma gondii* in mutton following curing, smoking, freezing or microwave cooking. *Int. J. Parasitol.*, 15: 357-363.

Margolis, H.S., Middaugh, J.P. and Burgees, R.D. (1979). Arctic Trichinosis: two Alaskan outbreaks from walrus meat. *J. Infect. Dis.*,139: 102-105.

Mohan, H., Aggarwal, R., Nada, R., Punia, R.P.S. and Ahluwalia, M. (2002).Trichinosis of psoas muscle. *J. Assoc. Physicians India*, 50: 729-730.

Munoz-Zanzi, C.A., Fry, P., Lesina, B. and Hill, D. (2010). *Toxoplasma gondii* oocyst specific antibodies and source of infection. *Emerg. Infect. Dis.*, 16: 1591-1593.

Ndimubanzi, P.C., Carabin, H., Budke, C.M., Nguyen, H., Qian, Y.J., Rainwater, E., Dickey, M., Reynolds, S. and Stoner, J.A. (2010). A systematic review of the frequency of neurocysticercosis with a focus on people with epilepsy. *PLoS.Negl. Trop. Dis.*, 4(11): e870.

Neghina, R. (2010). Trichinellosis, a Romanian never-ending story. An overview of traditions, culinary customs, and public health conditions. *Foodborne Pathog. Dis.*,7: 999-1003.

Niphadkar, S.M. (1973). *Trichinella spiralis* (Owen, 1833) in Bandicota bengalensis (Gray) in Bombay.*Curr. Sci.*, 42: 135-136.

Niphadkar, S.M., Pradhan, M.H. and Deshpande, V.S. (1979). Rediscovery of *Trichinella spiralis* (Owen, 1835) in domestic pigs in India. *Curr. Sci.*, 48: 372-373.

Opara, M.N., Ukpong, U.M., Okoli, I.C. and Anosike, J. (2006). Cysticercosis of slaughter cattle in southeastern Nigeria. *Ann. N. Y. Acad. Sci.*, 1081: 339-346.

Orlandi, P.A., Chu, D.M.T., Bier, J.W. and Jackson, G.J. (2002). Parasites and the food supply. *Food Technol.*, 56: 72–81.

Pappas, G., Roussos, N. and Falagas, M.E. (2009). Toxoplasmosis snapshots:global status of *Toxoplasma gondii* seroprevalence and implication for pregnancy and congenital toxoplasmosis. *Int. J. Parasitol.*, 39: 1385-1394.

Paul, R.T. and Calum, N.L.M. (2011). The socioeconomic burden of parasitic zoonoses: Global trends. *Vet. Parasitol.*, 182: 79- 95.

Pozio, E. (2011). Trichinellosis. In: Palmer, S., Soulsby, E.J.L., Torgerson, P., Brown, D. (eds.), Zoonoses,Oxford University Press, Oxford.

Pozio, E. and Murrell, K.D. (2006). Systematics and epidemiology of *Trichinella*. *Adv. Parasitol.*, 63: 367-439.

Pozio, E., La Rosa, G., Murrell, K.D. and Lichtenfels, J.R. (1992). Taxonomic revision of the genus *Trichinella*. *J. Parasitol.*, 78: 654-659.

Rodriguez-del-Rosal, E., Correa, D. and Flisser, A. (1989). *Vet. Rec.*, 124: 488.

Roghmann, M.C., Faulkner, C.T., Lefkowitz, A., Patton, S. and Zimmerman, J. (1999). Decreased seroprevalence for *Toxoplasma gondii* in Seventh DayAdventists in Maryland. *Am. J. Trop. Med. Hyg.*, 60: 790-792.

Roman, G., Sotelo, J., Brutto, O.D., Flisser, A., Dumas, M., Wadia, N., Botero, D., Cruz, M., Garcia, H., De Bittencourt, P.R.M., Trelles, L., Arriagada, C., Lorenzana, P., Nash, T.E. and Spina-Franca, A. (2000). A proposal to declare neurocysticercosis an international reportable disease. *Bull. WHO*, 78(3): 399-406.

Rosegrant, M., Leach, N. and Gerpacio, R. (1999). Alternative futures for world cereal and meat consumption. *Proc. Nutr. Soc.*, 58(2): 219-234.

Saini, P.K., Webert, D.W. and McCaskey, P.C. (1997). Food safety and regulatory aspects of cattle and swine cysticercosis. *J. Food Protec.*, 60 (4): 447-453.

Saleque, A., Juyal, P.D. and Bhatia, B.B. (1990). *Spirometra* spp. in a domestic cat in India. *Vet. Parasitol.*, 35: 273-276.

Schad, G.A. and Chowdhury, A.N. (1967). *Trichinella spiralis* in India.Rediscovery in Calcutta and the ecology of its maintenance in nature.*Trans. R. Soc. Trop. Med. Hyg.*, 61: 244-248.

Sciutto, E., Martinez, J.J., Villalobos, N.M., Hernandez, M., Jose, M.V., Beltran, C., Rodarte, F., Flores, I., Bobadilla, J.R., Fragoso, G., Parkhouse, M.E., Harrison, L.J.S. and De Aluja,A.S. (1998).Limitations of current diagnostic procedures for the diagnosis of *Taenia solium* cysticercosis in rural pigs. *Vet.Parasitol.*, 79: 299-313.

Shah, H.L. (1983). Epidemiology of *Sarcocystis* in domestic animals. *Haryana Vet.*, 22:59-73.

Shah, H.L. (1984). *Sarcocystis*as zoonosis. In: Compendium of lectures. Summer Institute on animal parasitic infections of public health importance at APAU, Tirupati.

Singh, B. and Msolla, P. (1986). Seroprevalence and pathogenesis of *Toxoplasma gondii* in sheep and goats in tropical regions. *Bull. Anim. Hlth. Prod. Afr.*, 34: 236-240.

Singh, S. and Pandit, A.J. (2004). Incidence and prevalence of toxoplasmosis in Indian pregnant women: a prospective study. *Am. J. Reprod. Immunol.*, 52: 276-283.

Slifko, T.R., Smith, H.V. and Rose, J.B. (2000). Emerging parasite zoonoses associated with water and food. *Int. J. Parasitol.*, 30: 1379-1393.

Solanki, P.K., Srivastava, H.O.P. and Shah, H.L. (1991). Prevalence of *Sarcocystis* in naturally infected pigs in Madhya Pradesh with an epidemiological explanation for the higher prevalence of *Sarcocystis suihominis*. *Ind. J. Anim. Sci.*, 67(8): 820-821.

Sorvillo, F.J., DeGiorgio, C. and Waterman, S.H. (2007). Deaths from cysticercosis, United States. *Emerg. Infect. Dis.*, 13: 230-235.

Speedy, A.W. (2003). Global production and consumption of animal source food. *J. Nutr.*, 133: 4048-4053.

Steinfeld, H., Gerber, P., Wassenaar, T., Castel, V., Rosales, M. and De Haan, C. (2006). Livestock's long shadow: environmental issues and options (Rome: Food and Agriculture Organization of the United Nations, p. xxi). Available at: www.virtualcentre.org/en/library/ key pub/longshad/A0701E00.

Sundar, P., Mahadevan, A., Jayshree, R.S., Subbakrishna, D. and Shankar, S.K. (2007). *Toxoplasma* seroprevalence in healthy voluntary blood donors from urban Karnataka. *Ind. J. Med. Res.*, 126: 50-55.

Takumi, K., Franssen, F., Fonville, M., Grasset, A., Vallee, I., Boireau, P., Teunis, P. and Van der Giessen, J. (2010). Within-host dynamics of *Trichinella spiralis* predict persistent parasite transmission in rat populations. *Int. J. Parasitol.*, 40: 1317-1324.

Tenter, A., Heckeroth, A. and Weiss, L. (2000). *Toxoplasma gondii*: from animals to humans. *Int. J. Parasitol.*, 30: 1217-1258.

Torgerson, P.R. and Macpherson, C.N.L. (2011). The socioeconomic burden of parasitic zoonoses: global trends. *Vet.Parasitol.*, 182: 79-95.

United States Department of Agriculture (1994). Code of Federal Regulations: animals and animal products. Federal Register, Title 9, Chapter III, Paragraph 318.10.

Van Kerckhoven, I., Vansteenkiste, W., Claes, M., Geerts, S. and Brandt, J. (1998). Improved detection of circulating antigen in cattle infected with *Taenia saginata* metacestodes. *Vet.Parasitol.*, 76: 269-274.

Weigel, R.M., Dubey, J.P., Siegel, A.M., Hoefling, D., Reynolds, D., Herr, L., Kitron, U.D., Shen, S.K., Thulliez, P., Fayer, R. and Todd, K.S. (1995). Prevalence of antibodies to *Toxoplasma gondii* in swine in Illinois in 1992. *J. Am. Vet. Med. Assoc.*, 206(11): 1747-1751.

WHO (2002). Foodborne Diseases, Emerging. Fact sheet no. 124.

Wu, A.H. (1986). An investigation on trichinosis in Dengxian County, Henan. *J. Parasitol. Parasit. Dis.*, 4: 66.

Yashodhara, P., Ramalakshmi, B.A., Lakshmi, V. and Krishna, T.P. (2004). Socio-economic status and prevalence of toxoplasmosis during pregnancy. *Ind. J. Med. Microbiol.*, 22: 241-243.

Yoder, D.R., Ebel, E.D., Hancock, D.D. and Combs, B.A. (1994). Epidemiologic findings from an outbreak of cysticercosis in feedlot cattle. *J. Am. Vet. Med. Assoc.*, 205: 45-50.

Zarlenga, D.S., Rosenthal, B., La Rosa, G., Pozio, E. and Hoberg, E.P. (2006). An old genus learns new tricks: late Tertiary colonization and speciation of *Trichinella* nematodes among Eutheria. *Proc. Natl. Acad.Sci.*, USA, 103: 7354-7359.

□□□

Chapter 7

An Overview of Myiasis in Domestic Animals of India

R. Katoch, Anish Yadav and R. Godara
Division of Veterinary Parasitology
Faculty of Veterinary Sciences and Animal Husbandry
Sher-e-Kashmir University of Agricultural Sciences and Technology-Jammu,
R.S. Pura-181 102

Introduction

The terms myiasis has been derived from the Greek word, myia, meaning fly and it was proposed by the Hope (1840) to refer to diseases originating specifically with dipterous larvae. However, as per Zumpt (1965) myiasis is defined as "The infestation of live human and vertebrate animals with dipterous larvae, which at least for a certain period, feed on the host's dead or living tissue, liquid body substances or ingested food". The myiasis causing flies have reduced mouth parts as they belong to suborder-Cyclorrhapha wherein mandibles and maxillae are absent. Majority of myiasis causing flies exist for a very small period in nature and their maximum period is passed in host as a larval stage, which is probably a way of adaptability. Thus, the prevalence of myiasis causing flies depends upon availability of susceptible host and proper environmental conditions like temperature, humidity, nectar, etc. The larvae of myiasis causing flies have been successfully used to improve necrotic healing in humans (Courtenay *et al.*, 2000). These flies have also been successfully used as pollinators without much maintenance, on mango trees (Sharma *et al.*, 1998).

Myiasis has been classified by various workers on basis of various aspects. Based on anatomical position in or on the host or according to the parasitic relationship of the Diptera with the host, it can be classified as obligatory or facultative or accidental or pseudomyiasis

(James, 1947; Zumpt, 1965; Kettle, 1984). Anatomical myiasis is divided into nasal (caused by larvae of *Oestrus ovis*), visceral (caused by larvae of *Hypoderma* and *Gasterophilus* spp.) and cutaneous (caused by larvae of subfamily *Calliphorinae* spp.). Cutaneous form is also termed as facultative form in literature because these flies can continue their life cycle without live vertebrate host, whereas visceral and nasal form are termed as obligatory type as they cannot complete their life cycle without live vertebrate host. Patton (1922) defined a third group of myiasis causing species, those that cause accidental myiasis when their eggs or larvae are ingested by the host. Zumpt (1965) termed these as pseudomyiasis.

Myiasis in domestic animals is a worldwide problem and causes huge economic losses in terms of production and tissue damage to animal husbandry sector. Economic losses due to myiasis from screw worm in Central America were calculated to be $650 million annually (Snow *et al.*, 1985). Simple control of new world screw worm fly using sterile insect technique has annual producer benefits of $796 million, $292 million and $77.9 million in USA, Mexico and Central America, respectively (Vargas-Teran *et al.*, 2005). *Lucilia cuprina* alone causes average annual loss of 280 million to Australia sheep industry (Urech *et al.*, 2009). The present write up highlight all aspects of myiasis in livestock in India.

Oestrosis / Nasal myiasis

Nasal myiasis is caused by larvae of *Oestrus ovis*. The fly is dark grey in colour with small black spots which are prominent on thorax (Soulsby, 1982). They lay their larvae around nostrils of the host. The larvae migrate upwards, moult and then either get attached to the nasal mucous membrane or reach the nasal sinuses (frontal and maxillary) and turbinate bones where they remain for several months. The majority of larvae is eventually sneezed out and pupates on the ground. A few of them who have grown up and are not able to come out from small openings of frontal sinuses or turbinate bones, erode into the cranial cavity and injure brain leading to development of nervous symptoms like incoordination of movement and high step gait similar to that of gid. Thus, the disease produced by *O. ovis* larvae is also called as false gid. These larvae may often be found in unusual situations such as trachea and, rarely, even over brain (Chhabra and Ruprah, 1976), trachea and bronchi of sheep (Shahardar *et al.*, 2001), mandibular spongy bones of goat associated with very deep erosions

(Godara *et al.*, 2010) and rumen of sheep (Muraleedharan *et al.*, 1999). The infestation of *O. ovis* larvae causes weight and production loss. These losses ranged from 1.1 to 4.6 kg of meat, 200-500 gm of wool and up to 10% of milk (Ilchmann *et al.*, 1986). In addition, it also predisposes host to pleuropneumonia (Rantunga and Rajamahendran, 1972), lung abscess and interstitial pneumonia (Dorchies *et al.*, 1993). This infestation was reported to be more common in lambs as compared to adults in causing brain congestion (Narladkar *et al.*, 1977). Nasal bots are wide spread in Mediterranean and tropical areas and in infected animals they induce sneezing and nasal discharge which may become caked with dust making breathing very difficult. The larvae of Oestridae family are host-specific but sometimes they may be deposited in human eyes including a painful opthalmomyiasis of short duration (Carlos *et al.*, 2010). The infected animal firstly suffer form fly strike when fly eject with larvae (terror stricken look), secondly suffer with myiasis with typical nasal discharge and sneezing related to sinusitis.

In South India, Jagannath *et al.* (1989a, b) revealed *O. ovis* larvae in 69.03, 41.93, 48.28 and 36.96% heads of sheep, lambs, goats and kids of Karnataka, respectively. Infestation were most common in cold weather (January-February), followed by north- eastern monsoon (October-December), hot weather (March-May) and south west monsoon (June-September). The infestation rates increased as temperature, rainfall and relative humidity decreased. Nasal myiasis has been reported in Karnataka (Jagannath *et al.*, 1989c) and Tamil Nadu (Joseph and Karunamoorthy, 1991; Ramprabhu *et al.*, 2002). It has also been recorded from goats of Pondicherry (Sreekrishnan and Das, 1999) and Kerala (Rajamohanan and Pailt, 1971). Jeyathilkan *et al.* (2008) has reported *O. ovis* infestation in Macheri sheep of Tamil Nadu organized farm. In Central India, Hiware (2006) when examined 321 sheep reported *O. ovis* larvae in 158 animals. It was observed that higher infection during colder months may be due to life cycle of *O. ovis* i.e. the fly deposits larvae during this period and also due to inactiveness of the larvae during this season. A checklist and key to Indian Oestridae has been given by Pal and Datta (1989).

Oestrus ovis infection has been reported in sheep and goats from North Western Himalayan region. In Jammu region, Katoch *et al.* (2006) revealed prevalence of 43.79 and 28.89% prevalence of *O. ovis* larvae in 306 sheep and 433 goats during one year slaughter house study. The mean year round infestation per animal (all instars) was 32.6 and

18.4 in sheep and goats, respectively in the month of December. The highest infestation was during winter (December to February) and the lowest in August. Recently, Saleem (2012) have reported high prevalence rate of larvae of *O. ovis* (99 and 89%, respectively in sheep and goats) from Jammu district. The different larval stages of *O. ovis* were found all throughout the year and fly was active during February to August when average temperature was 33.4^{0}C and relative humidity was 65%. The older animals suffer more with larvae of *O. ovis* as compared to young animals below one year of age. The animals of rain fed region (Kandi area) showed higher prevalence rate as compared to irrigated plain area of Jammu district. The overall mean intensity of *O. ovis* larvae in sheep and goats was observed to be 16.9 and 7.34%, respectively. Nasal myiasis has also been observed in Kashmir region. Shahardar and Rashid (1998) observed larvae of *O. ovis* in nasal passage and adjoining frontal sinuses of a goat whereas Shahardar *et al.* (2001) recovered second stage larvae of *O. ovis* from unusual sites (trachea and primary bronchus) of Corriedale sheep. Oestrosis has been observed in sheep of Himachal Pradesh (Singh *et al.*, 1990), In Haryana, Gupta *et al.* (1985) examined 670 heads of sheep and recorded *O.ovis* larvae in 72% heads. The average year round infestation rate was 7.6 larvae/sheep and the highest monthly average was 10.3 larvae/sheep in December month. Low prevalence (4%) of *O. ovis* larvae were observed in sheep at Hisar (Singh and Chhabra, 1974). In Rajasthan, Pathak (1992) examined 384 goats and 466 sheep at Bikaner abattoir. It was found that 81.3% sheep and 53.4% goats were harboring *O. ovis* larvae. Like other studies, it was observed that infestation was highest in cold weather and the lowest in August. It was also proposed that in India, 3 generations of flies occur during the year, around June- July, September and November.

Tanwani and Jain (1986) have reported its presence in a dog. Similarly, the rare occurrence in man has been reported by Joseph and Karunamoorthy (1991). Sen and Fletcher (1962) have also mentioned zoonotic potential of *O. ovis* larvae particularly in children of shepherds with nasal discharge.

Majority of workers have reported nasal myiasis infection based on post slaughter examination as ante mortem diagnosis is difficult. Cozab (1988) and Jagannath *et al.* (1989d) have employed indirect hemaglutination (IHA) and intra dermal test (ID) and found IHA to be more sensitive in diagnosis of oestrosis. Furthermore, L_2 antigen detected a higher percentage of positive animals (59%) than L_3 (30%), indicating it to be more immunogenic.

Pathological lesions of oestrosis have been characterised in acute stages by increased goblet cell activity in the lining mucosa, excessive mucous secretion from submucosal glands, submucosal edema and infiltration of neutrophils and eosinophils in nasal passages. In subacute cases, the catarrhal inflammation was moderate and infiltrating cells consisted of an admixture of mononuclear cells and eosinophils whereas in chronic cases there was diffuse infiltration of mononuclear cells and connective tissue proliferation with minimal catarrhal changes (Jagannath *et al.*, 1989e). The cerebral cortex of infected animals showed degeneration of neurons with increased perineuronal space and softening of brain. The other pathological changes observed were engorgement of blood vessel and vacuolation of brain substance with increased number of glial cells and mild perivascular cuffing by mononuclear cells (Saleem, 2012). In goats, pleuropneumonia due to larvae of *O. ovis* is also on records (Chhabra and Ruprah, 1976). Angulo *et al.* (2007) have reported seven positive enzymatic activities in salivary gland products of *O. ovis* larvae i.e. acid phosphatase, naphthol, AS-BI- phosphohydrolase, esterase (C_4), esterase lipase (C_8) Leucine arylamidase, a- glucosidase and N-acetyl-ß-glucosamindase. Optimum pH for proteolytic activity was 8.0; proteolytic activity increases with temperature (10-15°C) and then drastically decreased at 60°C. Proteases belonged to serine subclass which is likely involved in larval nutrition and host immuno modulation. Proteolytic activity was detected in the 20–63 kDa range.

Oral or parenteral administration of rafoxanide @ 7.5mg/kg and Oxyclozanide @ 15 mg/Kg have been reported to be highly efficacious in treatment of nasal myiasis (Maru *et al.*, 1986; Sanyal *et al.*, 1986; D'Souza *et al.*, 1992; Muraleedharan, 1999). Single application of ivermectin has shown high efficacy against gastrointestinal nematodes and nasal bot (Singh *et al.*, 1990; Sharma and Siddiqui, 1991; Singh and Gill, 1995). Singh and Gill (1995) have also observed Nitroxynil @ 20mg/Kg body weight to be highly efficacious against nasal myiasis. Gupta *et al.* (1983) observed that single drench of trichlorophen reduces 88.4% larval counts in lambs as compared to control group.

Visceral myiasis

Hypodermosis : Hypoderma fly usually lays its eggs on hairs of forelegs (singly in case of *H. bovis* and more than five in case of *H.*

lineatum) and rarely on the body. Eggs are fixed to hairs by means of terminal clasps. Larva hatch and crawl down the hair to the skin, through which it penetrates. The larvae of *Hypoderma* spp. live as subcutaneous parasites and are host-specific. *Hypoderma bovis* migrate below the skin along nerves to the spinal cord and finally reach epidural fat of spine in thoracic and lumber vertebrae. *H.lineatum* moves between fascial planes of muscles and along connective tissue and reach to submucosa of the oesophagus (Colebrook and Wall, 2004). Finally in both cases it forms warbles on the back and drops on the ground to pupate (Zumpt, 1965). *Hypoderma* spp. in goats do not show migratory phase, all stages are found in the subcutaneous tissues (Otranto *et al.*, 2004; Yadav *et al.*, 2011). The larval migration in cattle results in licked beef formation and dropping of larva from back results in formation of holes in skin leading to heavy economic losses to meat and hide industry. Sometimes, the treatment of migratory phase may cause partial or complete paralysis and blocking of oesophagus. In goats, it hampers body weight gain, milk production and reduces quality of meat and hides (Yadav *et al.*, 2006). *Hypoderma* have been recorded from cattle of Himachal Pradesh (Sharma *et al.*, 1999; Katoch *et al.*, 2004), Jammu (Yadav *et al.*, 2006), Haryana (Singh and Chhabra, 1974) and Rajasthan (Kumar *et al.*, 1990). Sen and Fletcher (1962) reported *H. lineatum* infection from all hill stations of the country and Punjab (50-90%), except Kashmir valley. Yadav *et al* (2006) have reported that *H. lineatum* Fly is active from mid June to August in Jammu region and infestation of warbles is more animals feeding on open grazing system as compared to stall fed animals. In goats, *Hypoderma* from Himachal Pradesh has been reported from Kullu region (Soni, 1942), whereas high incidence of *Hypoderma* spp. larvae has been reported from goats of Jammu and Kashmir (Yadav *et al.*, 2006, 2011). Katoch *et al.* (2004) reported 50-75% loss in milk production due to *Hypoderma* spp. infestation in cattle in Himachal Pradesh, India.

The prevalence of larval stages of warble fly infestation at Jammu abattoir was recorded from July 2003 to June 2005 in 5556 goats brought from five districts of Jammu province and slaughtered at Jammu abattoir. The overall infestation was recorded to be 36.34%. District wise prevalence in decreasing order was Udhampur (40.53%), Kathua (40.27%), Rajouri (34.47%), Jammu (33.79%) and Doda (11.88%). Yadav *et al.* (2012) have estimated approximately a loss of rupees 200 million due to *Przhevalskiana silenus* in goats in the Jammu region of Jammu and Kashmir state of India.

Gasterophilosis : Gasterophilus fly lays its eggs on the hairs of face and foreleg region in equines. Post hatching, their larvae migrate through cheek or tongue mucosa and finally settle in stomach. They are found attached to stomach and small intestine of equines, elephant and rhinoceros (Soulsby, 1982; Colebrook and Wall, 2004). At the site of larval attachment, erosions, ulcers, mucosal proliferation, gastric abscesses and stomach perforation may occur which may lead to peritonitis, general debilitation and rectal prolapse (Zumpt, 1965; Soulsby, 1982; Colebrook and Wall, 2004). It has been reported to occur in equines of Jammu and Kashmir (Sharma *et al.*, 2005), Himachal Pradesh (Chahota and Katoch, 1999; Katoch *et al.*, 2003) and Haryana (Singh and Chhabra, 1974; Tripathi *et al.*, 1994). Rao *et al.* (1990) recorded its occurrence in a wild ass (*Equinus hemionus pollas*) in Andhra Pradesh.

On control aspect not much work has been conducted in India. Singh *et al.* (2007) have reported high efficacy of injectable ivermectin against *Gasterophilus* spp. in Kathiawari equines maintained at Veterinary College, Mathura.

Cutaneous myiasis

Cutaneous myiasis is caused by the larvae belonging to subfamily-Calliphorinae. In sheep, calliphorinae myiasis is also called as strike. It is caused by larvae of various species of *Lucilia, Phormia, Calliphora* and *Chrysomyia*. The flies lay cluster of eggs on soiled wool or wounds and then larvae hatch. Larvae moult twice to become maggots and mature larvae fall on ground to pupate and give rise to imago. These flies are of three types: primary, secondary and tertiary flies. The primary flies are the ones which can initiate strike by laying eggs on living sheep and create favourable conditions for larvae of secondary flies. They secrete proteolytic enzymes, digest and liquefy tissues of host and feed on it. Eggs laid by secondary flies then develop into larvae and increase the wound by making tunnels in it. They also compete for food with larvae of primary flies and do not allow primary larvae to develop further in these wounds. Literature also reveals that larvae of secondary flies release specific odour because of which primary flies do not come near to the wound. The other important feature of secondary flies is that they cannot initiate strike but attack those sheep which have already been struck by primary flies. Tertiary flies like *Musca* and *Fannia* come in the last and cannot cause much damage. This preference for fly attack does not hold well on wounds of other domestic animals and man. The primary flies are widely prevalent in India and have been reported in different states.

Bionomics, distribution and seasonal occurrence of *Lucilia cuprina* is well studied in Calcutta and Kerala (Subramanian and Mohan, 1980, 1982; Das and Dasgupta, 1982; Nandi, 1994, 2002). *Lucilia* spp. has also been recorded from Punjab (Singh and Bharti, 2000) and Karnataka (Valandikar and Hiregoudar, 1996). Sharma *et al.* (1978) have reported different varieties of *L. cuprina* within the same species. These green bottle flies do exist in Himachal Pradesh and Jammu and Kashmir and are responsible for cutaneous myiasis in sheep (personal observation; Kour, 2011). The fly takes about fortnight at 26-27^{0}C to complete its whole life cycle (Sen and Fletcher, 1962). Kour (2011) reported that in Jammu *Lucilia* spp. are more common in summer and monsoon seasons and are abundant in open fields as compared to farms. It may be due to the fact that females prefer to oviposit on fresh meat and carcass which is mostly seen out doors (Sen and fletcher, 1962). Breeding of *Lucilia* spp. on meat and sweets shops in Indian markets is already on records (Sen and Fletcher, 1962).

Some other aspects like developmental study of thermotolerance and heat shock response, chromosomes of salivary glands and its response to diverse environmental stresses like heat and heavy metal toxicity and midgut as the main site for cholesterol absorption in *Lucilia* have been studied in India (Joshi and Agarwal, 1977; Sharma *et al.*, 1978; Tiwari *et al.*, 1995; Joshi and Tiwari, 2000). The research pertaining to control of *Lucilia* spp. in India suggest that hatch rate of eggs decreases with increased gamma radiation and at 7000 rads both male and female flies are sterilized without any effect on their behaviour (Karunamoorthy and Lalitha, 1987). They are repelled in decreasing order by using chemicals biphenyl, phenyl phenol, phenol and acetone (Shamsi *et al.*, 1990). Diflubenzuron inhibits chitin production leading to insect mortality (Subramanium, 2003). Sheep strike by *Lucilia cuprina* can lead to rapid increase in temperature and respiration accompanied by loss of weight and appetite (Broad meadow *et al.*, 1984).

The prevalence of *Calliphora* spp. has been reported from West Bengal (Paul *et al.*, 1990; Nandi, 2002), Punjab, Haryana, Himachal, Delhi, Uttarakhand and Rajasthan (Singh and Bharti, 2000; Bharti and Singh, 2002; Sidhu and Singh, 2002), Karnataka (Valandikar and Hiregoudar, 1996) and Orissa (Das *et al.*, 2002). Patnaik and Mishra (1977) have reported *Calliphora vicina* to be the only species responsible for cutaneous myiasis in cattle of Orissa. They reported that its highest incidence was during rainy season and vulvo-vaginal myiasis was commonest due to lack of post parturient care. Khan (1986) also collected larvae of *C. vicina* (*C. erythrocephala*) from body lesions and hooves of cattle and buffaloes in Andaman. Kumar and Joshi (1995) have also reported myiasis by larvae of *Calliphora* spp. in water buffaloes, cows, calves, goats and dogs of Mathura region. The larvae of *Calliphora* spp. have also been recorded from wounds of different livestock of Himachal Pradesh while evaluating efficacy of negashunt (Bayer) against maggots. They are also common in Jammu and Kashmir and are found on decomposing carcasses as well as on wounds (Kour, 2011). Like *Lucilia* they were also found abundant in open field as compared to farms. The studies pertaining to control suggest that thiourea causes inhibition of development, irregularity of follicle epithelial nuclei, clumping of chromatin material of follicle epithelial and nurse cell nuclei, vacuolation of nurse cell and oocyte cytoplasm and delayed and poor synthesis of yolk in the oocyte of these flies (Deepak and Chaudhary, 1978). Colchine arrested the development of nurse cell and oocytes in *C. vicina* (Shukla and Singh, 1979). Singh (1981) reported that certain microorganisms like *Bacillus, Micrococcus, Proteus* and *Streptococcus* spp. play important role in metabolism of topically applied dieldrin and pretreatment of flies with Gentamycin and Amphoterecin-B blocked dieldrin metabolism to a certain extent.

Kumar and Joshi (1995) successfully treated cutaneous myiasis predominantly caused by *Calliphora* spp. among domestic animals by topical and systemic application of ivermectin. Pattanayak and Mishra (1977) reported turpentine oil to be completely effective in treating cutaneous myiasis caused by *Calliphora* spp. in bovines.

Chrysomyia flies are secondary flies in strike. Paul *et al.* (1988, 1990) have reported its occurrence in rural, urban and forested areas of West Bengal. They have also reported its relative harmful effects on domestic animals in West Bengal. Its presence has also been reported from Punjab (Singh and Bharti, 2000). Its distribution, bionomics have also been studied in and around Calcutta (Nandi, 1994) and Kerala (Subramanian and Mohan, 1980). *Chrysomyia megacephala* has been reported most common during the rainy season (Valandikar and Hiregauda, 1996). The larvae of *C. bezziana* have been reported from buffaloes of Madras (Thilagar *et al.*, 1991; Senthilvel and Raman, 1999) and Karnataka (Reddy and Krishna, 1995), yaks of northeast (Biswas, 1994), leprosy patients (Sreevatsa *et al.*, 1990) and humans suffering from filarial lympadema (Radhakrishnan *et al.*, 1994). In Chennai, it has been observed in pressure and traumatic wounds of intensively housed cattle and buffaloes (Thilagar *et al.*, 1991). Devinder *et al.* (1991) have made morphological studies on the maggots belonging to two Indian species of *Chrysomyia*.

On control aspect of *Chrysomyia* literature is scanty. Subramaniam (2002, 2003) have reported that higher concentration of diflubenzuron is larvicidal while its lower concentration reduces longevity and fecundity of flies, number of eggs laid, percentage of egg hatch and development of adults. It also inhibits chitin production in *C. bezziana.* Shamsi *et al.* (1990) reported repellent action in decreasing order of biphenyl, phenyl phenol, phenol and acetone against *C. rufifacies.* Jamil (1988) have recorded sensitivity of *C. rufifacies* to toxic baits. Ivermectin has been reported to be highly efficacious against maggot wounds caused by *C. bezziana* in dogs (Reddy *et al.*, 1993), lion (Sharma, 1994) and buffaloes (Reddy and Krishna, 1995; Senthilvel and Raman, 1999) without any side effects. Katoch *et al.*, (2013) reported larvae of *C. bezziana* in buffalo of five years with traumatic wound in the abnormal growth at the base of tail in Jammu. The larval burrow into healthy tissues adjacent to wound and could also penetrale in to bones sorrounding the wound. (Prasad *et al.*, 2000). Myiasis irrespective of fly particularly on wounds has been recorded to be 11.9% in sheep and goats of Haryana (Verma *et al.*, 2004). Similarly, Panda and Pattanaik (2003) found that a combination of maggiticide and dressol was generally effective in controlling maggots in wound and promoting wound healing.

Lastly, it is concluded that myiasis is a major problem of livestock in India. Visceral myiasis causes huge economic losses in terms of reduced body weight gain, decreased milk, meat and wool production, lowering the quality of hide and rupture of intestine leading to death of animal. *Oestrus ovis* also has zoonotic potential. Thus, the epidemiology of various myiasis causing flies in different agro-climatic zones of India must be determined, so that suitable control measures may be adopted for reducing its incidence in livestock.

Literature pertaining to cutaneous myiasis suggests that surgical interventions if not of prime need, should be delayed during rainy season so as to reduce the incidence of cutaneous myiasis. Fly trap placement in animal sheds should be made mandatory. Additionally, netting may also be adopted in stall fed animals to reduce the prevalence of myiasis. Fast faecal disposal, application of fly repellants and removal of organic wastes from sheds reduce the incidence of myiasis in farm animals.

References

Bharti, M. and Singh, D. (2002). Occurrence of different larval stages of blow flies (Diptera: Calliphoridae) on decaying rabbit carcasses. *J. Entomol. Res.*, 26(4): 343-350.

Biswas, D., Barari, S.K. and Pal, R.N. (1994). Parasitic infections in yaks (*Poephagus grunniens*). National symposium on advances in veterinary research and their impact on animal health and production, held at the Indian Veterinary Research Institute, Izatnagar, February 10-11, 1994, pp. 36.

Chahota, R and Katoch, R.C. (1999). Caecal impaction due to bots infestation leading to gastric rupture - a case report. *Centaur*, 16(2): 30-31

Chhabra, M.B. and Ruprah, N.S. (1976). Observations on incidence and biology of *Oestrus ovis* L. *Indian Vet. J.*, 53:180-184

Colebrook, E. and Wall, R. (2004). Ectoparasites of livestock in Europe and the Mediterranean region. *Vet. Parasitol.*, 120: 251-274

Courtenay, M., Church, J.C. and Ryan, T.J. (2000). Larva therapy in wound management. *J. Royal Soci. Med.*, 93(2): 72-74

Cozab, N. (1988). Studies on the incidence, biology and serodiagnosis of *Oestrus ovis* Linnaeus, 1761 (Diptera: Oestridae) in Karnataka State. *Mysore J. Agri. Sci..*, 22(2): 290

Das, A.K., Panda, D.N. and Panda, M.R. (2002). Prevalence of myiasis causing fly larvae in organic baits in Bhubaneswar. *J. Vet. Parasitol.*, 16(1): 73-74

Das, S.K. and Dasgupta, B. (1982). Seasonal occurrence of blow-flies and flesh-flies in Calcutta. *Oriental-Insects*, 16(1): 119-128

Deepak, V. and Chaudhry, H.S. (1978). Histopathological effects of thiourea on the ovarian development of *Calliphora erythrocephala*. *App. Entomol. Zool.*, 13(1): 34-37

Devinder, S. and Kaur, H. (1991). Comparative morphological studies on the maggots belonging to two Indian species of *Chrysomyia* (Diptera: Calliphoridae). Entomology for Defense Services Proceedings of the Symposium held on12-14 September (eds. Ramachandran, P.K., Sukumaran, D. and Rao, S.S.), pp. 193-200

D'Souza, P.E., Satyanarayana, K., Jagannath, M.S., Rajeswari, Y.B., Rahman, S.A and Govindaiah, M.G. (1992). Control of nasal myiasis in sheep with rafoxanide. *Indian Vet. Med. J.*, 16(1): 34-36

Dorchies, P., Yilma, J.M. and Savey, J. (1993). Prevalence of lung abscesses and interstitial pneumonia in ovine oestrosis. *Vet. Rec.*, 133: 325.

Godara, R., Sharma, R.L. and Sharma, C.S. (2010). Aberrant infestation of goat mandibles with *Oestrus ovis* larvae. *Trop. Anim. Hlth. Prod.*, 42: 137-139.

Gupta, S.K., Ruprah, N.S. and Chhabra, M.B. (1985). Bionomics of *Oestrus ovis* (sheep nasal fly). *Indian Vet. Med. J.*, 9(2): 71-75

Gupta, S.K., Ruprah, N.S. and Chhabra, M.B. (1983). Comparative efficacy of some chemotherapeutic agents against *Oestrus ovis* larvae in sheep. *Indian Vet. J.*, 60: 795-798

Hiware, C.L. (2006). Population dynamics of *Oestrus ovis* from sheep. *J. Vet. Parasitol.*, 20(2) : 187-188

Ilchmann, G., Betke, P. and Grafe, D. (1986). Studies on oestrosis and its control in the Mongolian Perples Republic. *Vet. Med.*, 41: 128-132.

Jagannath, M.S., Cozab, N., Rahman, S.A. and Honnappa, T.G. (1989a). Studies on the biology of *Oestrus ovis* Linnaeus, 1761 (Diptera: Oestridae). *Indian Vet. J.*, 66(7): 677-679

Jagannath, M.S., Cozab, N., Rahman, S.A. and Honnappa, T.G. (1989b). Factors influencing *Oestrus ovis* infestation in sheep and goats. *Curr. Res. Uni. Agri. Sci.*, 28(8): 118-119

Jagannath, M.S., Cozab, N., Rahman, S.A. and Honnappa, T.G. (1989c). Incidence of *Oestrus ovis* in sheep and goats. *Indian J. Anim. Sci.*, 59(10): 1216-1219

Jagannath, M.S., Cozab, N., Rahman, S.A. and Honnappa, T.G. (1989d). Serodiagnosis of *Oestrus ovis* infestation in sheep and goats. *Indian J. Anim. Sci.*, 59(10): 1220-1224

Jagannath, M.S., Cozab, N. and Vijayasarathi, S.K. (1989e). Histopathological changes in the nasal passage of sheep and goats infested with *Oestrus ovis* (Diptera: Oestridae). *Indian J. Anim. Sci.*, 59(1): 87-91

James, M.T. (1947). The flies that cause myiasis in man. USDA Misc. Pub. No. 631, pp. 175

Jamil, N. (1988). Sensitivity of *Chrysomyia rufifacies* to toxic baits. *Indian J. Entomol.*, 48(1): 82-84

Joseph, S.A. and Karunamoorthy, G. (1991). Studies on the haematophagous arthropods of zoonotic importance in Tamil Nadu. Entomology for Defense Services Proceedings of the Symposium held on 12-14 September, 1990 (eds. Ramachandran, P.K., Sukumaran, D. and Rao, S.S.), pp. 185-192

Joshi, A. and Tiwari, P.K. (2000). Chromosomal responses of blowfly *Lucilia cuprina* to heat and heavy metal stress. *Genetica*, 109(3): 211-218

Joshi, M. and Agarwal, H.C. (1977). Site of cholesterol absorption in some insects. *J. Insect Physiol.*, 23(3): 403-404

Karunamoorthy, G. and Lalitha, C.M. (1987). Effects of gamma radiation on sheep blowfly *Lucilia cuprina* (Wiedemann, 1830) irradiated as pupae. *Indian J. Anim. Sci.*, 57(7): 654-658

Katoch, R., Agnihotri, R.K., Singh, M.M., Panda, A.K. and Mitra, S. (2004). Increasing incidence of hypodermosis in Kanga Valley of Himachal Pradesh. *J. Vet. Parasitol.*, 19 (1): 67-68

Katoch, R., Bhardwaj, R.L., Rajput, R., Panda, A.K., Sharma, A., Rajesh, R. and Sharma, A. (2003). Incidence of bots in equines of North Western Himalayas .*Centaur*, **20**(4): 66-67

Katoch, R: Godara, R., Yadav, A., Sharma, S. and Ahmad. I, Occurrence of *Chrysomya bezziana* in buffalo in Jammu. *Journal of Parasit Dis. Doi* 10. 1007/s 12639-013-02632.

Katoch, R., Yadav, A., Khajuria, J.K., Vohra, S. and Srivastava, A.K. (2006). Epidemiology of *Oestrus ovis* infestation in sheep and goats in Jammu district. Presented at XVII Annual Convention of IAAVP (2006) at Pondicherry.

Kour, P (2011) Seasonal Prevalence of cutaneous myiasis in animals in Jammu. MVSc thesis Submiitted to Sher-e-Kashmir University of Agricultural Sciences and Technology of Jammu, pp 32-52.

Kettle, D.S. (1984). Medical and Veterinary Entomology. London and Sydney, Cross Helm., pp. 658

Khan, M.H. (1986). Fly problem on animals in Andaman's. *Indian J. Anim. Hlth.*, 25(2): 141-143

Kumar, D., Jatkar, P.R., Raisinghani, P.M., Gahlot, G.C., Abdulkayum and Jairath, L.K. (1990). Implications of warbles (*Hypoderma lineatum*) infection in draught affected cattle at Bikaner, Rajasthan. *Indian J. Anim. Sci.*, 60 (4): 433-435

Kumar, A and Joshi, B.P. (1995). Studies on the clinical efficacy of ivermectin against cutaneous myiasis in domestic animals. *Indian Vet. J.*, 72(3): 277-280

Maru, A., Sanyal, P.K., Arora, A.L. (1986). Ingestible rafoxanide in treatment of sheep flocks affected with nasal myiasis. *Indian Vet. J.*, 63(2): 153-155

Muraleedharan, K., Murthy, H.K.S. and Sahadev, A. (1999). Some observations on nasal myiasis in sheep and goats and its treatment with rafoxanide and oxyclozanide. *J. Vet. Parasitol.*, 13(1): 57-58

Nandi, B.C. (1994). Studies on calliphorid flies (Diptera: Calliphoridae) from Calcutta and adjoining areas. *J. Bengal Natural History Soc.*, 13(2): 37-47

Nandi, B.C. (2002). Blow flies (Diptera: Calliphoridae) of West Bengal, India with a note on their biodiversity. *Rec. Zoologi. Sur. India*, 100(1/2): 117-129

Narladkar, B.W., Kulkarni, D. and Shastri, U.V. (1977). *Oestrus ovis* infestation in Deccani sheep. *J. Vet. Parasitol.*, 11: 81-82

Otranto, D. and Traversa, D. (2004). Molecular evidence indicating that *Przhevalskiana silenus, Przhevalskiana aegagri* and *Przhevalskiana crossii* (Diptera: Oestridae) are one species. *Acta Parasitol.*, 49:173-176

Pal, T.K. and Datta, M. (1989). The Oestridae (Diptera) of India: a synopsis. *J. Bengal Natural History Soc.*, 8(1): 5-21

Panda, D.N. and Pattanaik, T.K. (2003). Efficacy of Maggoticite lotion and Dressol ointment and lotion in the treatment of maggoted and surgical wounds. *Indian Vet. J.*, 80(5): 441-442.

Pathak, K.M.L. (1992). Incidence of *Oestrus ovis* in sheep and goats in Rajasthan state of India. *Indian J. Anim. Sci.*, 62(1): 50

Pattanayak, P.C. and Misra, S.C. (1977). Studies on the epidemiology, biology and control of bovine cutaneous myiasis flies. *Orissa Vet. J.*, 11(2): 52-57

Patton, W.S. (1922). Notes on the myiasis producing Diptera of man and animals. *Bull. Entomol. Res.*, 12: 239-261

Paul, A., Roy, P. and Dasgupta, B. (1988). Altitudinal distribution of sarco-saprophagous flies in selected urban and rural areas of Jalpaiguri district, West Bengal, India. *J. Bengal Natural History Soc.*, 6(1): 49-57

Paul, A.K., Roy, P. and Dasgupta, B. (1990). Studies on the degree of domestication and relative dangerousness of flies (Diptera: Calliphoridae, Muscidae and Sarcophagidae) of Jalpaiguri district, West Bengal, India. *J. Bengal Natural History Soc.*, 9(2): 41-53

Prased, S., Kumarasinghe, N., Karunaweera, N.D. and Ihalamulla, R.L. (2000) A study of cutaneous myiasis in Sri Lanka. *Int. J. Dermatol* 39: 689-694.

Radhakrishnan, R., Srinivasan, R., Krishnamoorthy, K., Sabesan, S. and Pani, S.P. (1994). Myiasis in filarial lymphoedema due to *Chrysomyia bezziana*. *Nat. Med. J. India.* 7(3):117-118

Rajamohanan, K. and Pailt, E.P. (1971). Nasal myiasis in goats in Kerala. *Kerala J. Vet. Sci.* 2(2): 91-93

Ramprabhu, R., Anna, T., Subramanian, M. and Dhanapalan, P. (2002). *Oestrus ovis* in a goat - a case report. *Indian J. Sm. Rum.*, 8(1): 76-77

Ranatunga, P. and Rajamahendran, P. (1972). Observations on the occurrence of *Oestrus ovis* L (Diptera: Oestridae) and pleuropneumonia in goats on dry zone farm in Ceylon. *Bull. Entomol. Res.*, 61: 657-659.

Rao, P.B., Rao, D., Kumar, N. and Madhekar, D.R. (1990). Occurrence of bots in a wild ass (*Equinus hemionus pollas*). *Indian Vet. J.*, 67(12): 1171.

Reddy, N.R.J., Setty, D.R.L., Ranganath, L., D'Souza, P.E. and Jagannath, M.S. (1993). Ivermectin in cutaneous myiasis of dogs. *Indian Vet. J.*, 70 (6): 557-558.

Reddy, P.M.T and Krishna, B.V.M. (1995). Ivermectin in cutaneous myiasis of buffaloes. *Buff. Bull.* 14(4): 75.

Saleem, T. (2012). Epidemiology of *Oestrus ovis* in sheep and goats. M.V.Sc thesis submitted to Sher-e-Kashmir University of Agricultural Sciences and Technology of Jammu, pp. 41.

Sanyal, P.K., Maru, A. and Gupta, A.K. (1986). The use of injectable rafoxanide against natural ovine nasal myiasis. *Vet. Parasitol.*, 19(1/2): 127-131.

Sen, S.K and Fletcher, T.B. (1962). Veterinary Entomology and Acarology in India. Indian Council of Agricultural Research Press, New Delhi, pp. 1-688.

Senthilvel, K. and Raman, M. (1999). Efficacy of ivermectin against cutaneous myiasis (caused by *Chrysomyia bezziana*) in buffalo. *Indian J. Vet. Med.*, 19(1): 82.

Shahardar, R.A., Darzi, M.M. and Pandit, B.A. (2001). Recovery of larvae of *Oestrus ovis* from trachea and bronchi of sheep. *J. Vet. Parasitol.*, 15(1): 85.

Shahardar, R.A. and Rashid, A. (1998).Occurrence of larvae of *Oestrus ovis* in a goat in Kashmir valley- a note. *J. Vet. Parasitol.*, 12(2): 147.

Shamsi, S.P., Khan, N.H. and Rizvi, S.S.A. (1990). Repellency effects of phenol, phenyl phenol, biphenyl and acetone on *Chrysomyia rufifacies* (Macq.) and *Lucilia cuprina* (Wide.). *Indian J. Entomol.*, 52(4): 669-674.

Sharma, G.P., Handa, S.M., Kaur, P. and Kaur, S. (1978). Salivary gland chromosomes of *Lucilia cuprina* (Diptera- Calliphoridae). *Cytobios.*, 17 (67-68): 183-194.

Sharma, S.K., Katoch, R. and Sharma, A. (1999). *Hypoderma* infestation in a cow: A case report. *Indian Vet. J.*, 76: 1105.

Sharma, S.P. and Siddiqui, A.A. (1991). Therapeutic evaluation of ivermectin against nasal bots in sheep. *Indian J. Vet. Med.*, 11(1-2): 75.

Sharma, S.K., Yadav, A., Sudan, J.S. and Gupta, A. (2005). Bot infestation in equine- A case report. *Intas Polivet*, 6: 364-365.

Sharma, T.R. (1994). Efficacy of ivermectin in treating maggot wounds in lions. *Indian Vet. J.*, 71(3): 275-276.

Sharma, S., Abbas, S.R. and Shukia, R.P. (1998). An easy and quick method of breeding flies for pollination of mango blossoms. *Insect Environment*, 4(3): 76-77.

Shukla, G.S. and Singh, R.N. (1979). Effect of colchicine on the nucleocytoplasmic relations of nurse cells and developing oocyte in the blow fly, *Calliphora erythrocephala* (Meig.). *J. Entomol. Res.*, 1(1): 108-110.

Sidhu, I.S. and Singh, D. (2002). Blow flies (Diptera: Calliphoridae) collected from north-western region including two new records from India. *Uttar Pradesh J. Zool.*, 22: 93-95.

Singh, A. and Chhabra, R.C. (1974). Incidence of arthropod pests of domesticated animals and birds. *Indian J. Anim. Sci.*, 43(5): 393-397.

Singh, D. and Bharti, M. (2000). Forensically important blow flies (Diptera: Calliphoridae) of Punjab (India). *Uttar Pradesh J. Zool.*, 20(3): 249-251.

Singh, D., Gulyani, R. and Solanki, V.K. (1990). Efficacy of ivermectin in the treatment of gastro-intestinal nematodiasis and nasal myiasis in sheep. *Indian Vet. Med. J.*, 14:198-200.

Singh, G.J.P. (1981). Studies on the role of microorganisms in the metabolism of dieldrin in the epicuticular wax layer of blowflies *Calliphora erythrocephala*. *Pesticide Bioch. Physiol.*, 16(3): 256-266.

Singh, J. and Gill, B.S. (1995). Efficacy of ivermectin and nitroxinil against *Oestrus ovis* in sheep. *J. Vet. Parasitol.*, 9(2): 131-132.

Singh, Y., Dayashankar and Katoch, R. (2007). Efficacy of ivermectin against strongyles in Kathiawari horses. *Vet. Pract.*, 8(2): 157-158.

Snow, J.W., Whitten, C.J., Salinas, A., Ferrer, J. and Sudlow, W.H. (1985). The screwworm *Cochliomyia hominivorax* (Diptera: Calliphoridae) in Central America and proposed plans for its eradication south to the Darien Gap in Panama. *J. Med. Entomol.*, 22: 353-360

Soni, B.N. (1942). Eggs of the goat warble fly (*Hypoderma crossii,* Patton). *Curr. Sci.*, 11: 280-281

Soulsby, E.J.L. (1982). Helminths, Arthropods and Protozoa of Domesticated Animals. 7th ed., ELBS, London, pp. 432-437

Sreekrishnan, R. and Das, S.S. (1999). *Oestrus ovis* infestation in goats in Pondicherry- a report. *J. Vet. Parasitol.*, 13(1): 71-72

Sreevatsa, M., G.N., Husain, S., Girdhar, A., Bhat, H.R. and Girdhar, B.K. (1990). Preliminary observations on myiasis in leprosy patients. *Leprosy Review*, 61(4): 375-378

Subramanian, H. (2002). Effect of diflubenzuron on the developmental stages of *Chrysomyia bezziana*. *J. Vet. Parasitol.*, 16(2): 181-182

Subramanian, H. (2003). Effect of diflubenzuron on chitin production inhibition in larvae of myiasis producing flies. *Indian J. Anim. Sci.*, 73(7): 753-754

Subramanian, H. and Mohan, K.R. (1980). Biology of the blowflies *Chrysomyia megacephala, Chrysomyia rufifacies* and *Lucilia cuprina*. *Kerala J. Vet. Sci.*, 11(2): 252-261

Subramanian, H. and Monahan, K.R. (1982). Incidence and etiology of cutaneous myiasis in domestic animals in Trichur. *Kerala J. Vet. Sci.*, 11(1): 80-84

Tanwani, S.K. and Jain, P.C. (1986). *Oestrus ovis* larva in the nasal cavity of a dog. *Haryana Veterinarian*, 25(1): 37-38

Thilagar, S., Ayyappan, S., Richard, M.G, Balasubramanian, S., Dewan, M.S. and Mohammed, M. (1991). A note on clinical survey of myiasis in bovines. *Indian J. Vet. Surgery*, 12: 124

Tiwari, P.K., Mohan, D.R.K. and Joshi, A. (1995). Developmental study of thermotolerance and the heat shock response in *Lucilia cuprina* (Weidemann). *J. Biosciences*, 20(3): 341-354

Tripathi, B.N., Singh, B.K and Yadav, M.P. (1994). Parasitic gastritis in Indian Equidae with *Gasterophilus intestinalis* larvae and *Draschia megastoma* infestation. *J. App. Anim. Res.*, 5(1): 73-76

Valandikar, S.C. and Hiregoudar, L.S. (1996). Occurrence of calliphorid, sarcophagid and muscid flies at Bangalore. *Curr. Res. Uni. Agri. Sci. Bangalore,* 25(1): 1-2

Vargas-Teran, M., Hofman, H.C. and Tweddle, N.E. (2005). Impact of screwworm eradication programmes using the sterile insect technique. In: Sterile insect Technique. Principles and Practice in Area-wide Integrated Pest Management (By, V.A. Dyck, J. Hendrichs and A.S. Robinson).

Verma, S.C., Mahajan, N.K., Dahiya, J.P. and Gita-Malik (2004). Survey on the incidence of various health problems affecting sheep and goats in Haryana. *Indian Vet. J.*, 81: 349-351

Yadav, A., Katoch, R., Khajuria, J.K., Katoch, M. and Rastogi, A. (2012). Economic impact of *Przhevalskiana silenus* infestation in native goats of northern India. *Trop. Anim. Hlth Prod.*, 44: 581-587

Yadav, A., Katoch, R., Khajuria, J.K., Katoch, M. and Agrawal, R. (2011). Prevalence and biology of goat warble fly infestation by *Przhevalskiana silenus* in Jammu province, India. *Trop. Anim. Hlth Prod.*, 43: 1487-1492

Yadav, A., Katoch, R., Khajuria, J.K. and Vohra, S. (2006). Epidemiology, economic losses and control of warble fly (*Przhevalskiana silenus* Brauer, 1858) infestation in goats of Jammu region. Presented at XVII Annual Convention of IAAVP 2006 at Pondicherry.

Zumpt, F. (1965). Myiasis in man and animals of the Old World. A textbook for Physicians, Veterinarians and Zoologists. Butterworths & Co. London, pp. 1-267.

❑❑❑

Chapter 8

Taeniid Cysticercosis- An Emerging and Re-emerging Cyclozoonoses

Placid E. D'Souza
Centre of Advanced Faculty Training,
Department of Parasitology, Veterinary College, KVAFSU,
Hebbal, Bangalore – 560 024, India

Cysticercosis of domestic and wild animals is caused by the larval stages of taeniid tapeworms, the adult stages of which occur in the intestine of humans and dogs or wild canids. Bovine and porcine cysticercosis is caused by the larval forms of human tapeworms, *Taenia saginata* and *Taenia solium,* respectively. Cysticercosis of sheep and goats is caused by adult tapeworms that occur in the intestine of dogs and wild canids throughout the world. Cysticerci of *Taenia ovis* occur in the muscles, those of *T. hydatigena* in the peritoneal cavity and on the liver of sheep. The most dangerous cysticercosis is attributed to *T. solium,* because it is a perfect zoonosis or euzoonosis because humans can act as both definitive and intermediate hosts.

Aristophanes a comedian referred to the bladders of cysticerci by comparing their appearance to that of hailstones in 380 and 375 B.C. Aristotle (384-322 B.C.) in his "History of Animals", opined that pig meat which is tender have bladders which are like hailstones in the region of the thigh, neck and loin where they generally appear. If they are few in number, the meat is leaner; if they are many, the meat becomes soft and filled with serous fluid. Pigs affected with this disease are easily recognized; in effect, the bladders can be seen on the inferior surface of the tongue where they are particularly abundant. Furthermore, the sick animals cannot keep their hind legs still. However, pigs do not suffer from this disease while they are nursing. The bladders can be made to disappear with "spelt wheat" (a species of wheat from cold, poor land) which at the same time serves as fodder. Paranoli (1550) was the first to describe the presence of round, white bladders full of a clear fluid in the corpus callosum of man.

The name "cysticercosis" was given by Laennec derived from the Greek words "kystic" meaning bladder and "kercos" signifying tail. In 1809, believing that cysticerci constituted a species of animal, Rudolphi gave them the surname of "cellulosae" due to their great affinity for connective tissue.

About 2 million years ago, Hoberg believes, African hominids, which scavenged for food or preyed on antelope and other bovids, were exposed to colonization by these tapeworms. The worms were using hyena and large cats as definitive host and bovids as intermediate hosts. Humans gave tapeworms to domestic animals because they were established in man before the domestication and explained that *T. saginata* and *T. saginata asiatica* were human - parasitic sister species and the divergence between them occurred at least 1, 60,000 years ago. It occurred with the migration of early humans from Africa to Asia. There the worms continued to parasitize their hosts and an isolated group evolved to become *T. saginata asiatica.*

Taenia saginata cysticercosis occurs worldwide, but is at particularly high prevalence in Africa, less so in Caucasian and South/ Central Asian and eastern Mediterranean countries. *T. solium* is largely confined to Central and South America, southern Africa, parts of the Common Wealth of Independent States (CIS), the people's Republic of China and non-Islamic countries of Asia where there are free range scavenging pigs.

Taenia saginata, the beef tapeworm has a cosmopolitan distribution and occurs in developing countries due to poor hygienic habits and consumption of raw or insufficiently cooked meat. It is also a great problem in developed nations due to difficulty in detection and also due to consumption of certain preparations involving improper cooking of beef even though the standard of meat inspection is high. The eggs of this tapeworm have been shown to survive almost all stages of sewage treatment as indicated in the Table 1 (Burger, 1984).

Table1: *Taenia saginata* : survival of eggs in sewage and sludge

Medium	Conditions	Survival (days)	Infectivity remaining
Sewage	Laboratory, 18°C	16	Yes
Sewage	Exp. plant, trickling filter	42	No
Sewage	Septic tank	40	Not tested
Sewage	Plant, raw waste water	Yes	Yes
Sludge	Lab, anaerobic digestion, 25-29°C	200	Not tested
Sludge	Lab, anaerobic digestion 35°C	<5	No
Sludge	Plant, anaerobic digestion 26-28°C	56	Not tested
Sludge	Plant, anaerobic digestion, Cold	38	Not tested
Sludge	Exp. plant, activated sludge	42	Not tested
Effluent	Plant, activated sludge	Yes	Yes
Effluent	Plant, trickling filter + lagoon	No	No
Effluent	Plant, lagoons	No	No

An infected individual is able to excrete daily up to 5 million oncospheres into the environment and the average number of excreted oncospheres constitutes 1.5 million. Therefore, intensive environmental contamination can occur. In Great Britain and USA, cattle are the normal intermediate hosts but in tropical countries other ruminants such as goats, sheep, llama, giraffe, etc. may also be involved.

In human beings in a single worm infection, the worm develops to 3 meters in length and can produce 600 proglottids. The effect on human health is indicated by diarrhoea, abdominal pain, headache and increased appetite and sometimes may be asymptomatic and mainly objectionable on aesthetic grounds. The gravid proglottides are spontaneously discharged and are usually motile. They may creep out of the anus onto the perianal skin and may migrate over the clothes or on the ground shedding eggs as they go. This has a psychological effect on the patients. In cattle, the larval stage *Cysticercus bovis,* which is about 1.0 cm in diameter filled with fluid and a clearly visible scolex is located in the striated muscles especially the tongue, masseter, intercostal muscles and heart. Symptoms are not serious but heavy infections with eggs leads to fever, anorexia, debilitation and muscle stiffness. Calves given massive doses of *T. saginata* eggs experimentally were found to develop severe myocarditis and heart failure. Cysticerci remain viable up to 8 months in cattle, whereas the worm can survive in human beings for many years.

In Great Britain and Australia, 'Cysticercosis storms' have been reported to occur in cattle on some farms after grazing on pastures where human sewage was used as fertilizer in the forms of sludge. *T. saginata* ova can survive for more than 200 days in sludge. The other causes for prevalence of cysticercosis include access of cattle to water contaminated with sewage effluents and dispersal of *T. saginata* ova by birds which frequent sewage works or feed on effluent discharged into the river or sea and to occasional contamination of pasture by infected individuals.

Taenia solium, the pork tapeworm infection is regarded as an obligatory cyclozoonosis, an anthropozoonotic helminthiasis or euzoonosis. These terms imply that man is one of the essential or usual hosts involved in the life cycle. So far, apart from man, the adult tapeworm has been experimentally found to develop in the lar gibbon and golden hamsters and to some extent in the dog (Varma and Ahluwalia, 1985). This zoonotic parasite is of special interest and is unique because man can also act as an intermediate host in which case the manifestations can have serious implications to health. The usual intermediate hosts include domestic and wild pigs which are very commonly infected and act as an important source of infection to human beings and other animals such as dogs, monkeys, sheep, goats and rodents.

Humans acquire the tapeworm when eating raw or undercooked pork infected with cysticerci, the larval form of *T. solium*. The cysticerci migrate to the small intestine of humans where they evaginate, attach to the mucosa and within approximately two months develop into adult tapeworms, which can grow to more than 3 meters long. *T. solium* has a head (scolex) armed with a double row of hooks and four suckers. Its body (strobila) consists of several hundred segments or proglottids each containing about 50,000–60,000 eggs. It has generally been accepted that a person is only parasitized by a single *T. solium* at any given time, hence the parasite's name, however, surveys involving treatment of tapeworm carriers and collection of their worms indicate that infections with multiple *T. solium* worms is possible (Jeri *et al.,* 2004).

The most distal proglottids (usually 1–5 daily) detach often in groups from the worm when their eggs have matured and pass out into the environment with the human host's faeces. These eggs can then in turn infect the same (autoinfection) or other humans as well as pigs if they are ingested following direct contact with tapeworm carriers or from consuming water or food contaminated with human faeces. In developing countries, pigs are often allowed to roam and eat human faeces that may contain tapeworm eggs though in some countries human faeces are fed directly to pigs (Flisser, 1988; Pouedet *et al.*, 2002; Shey-Njila *et al.*, 2003). Ingested eggs result in larval worms that migrate to different parts of the human and pig body (e.g. muscles, eyes and brain) via the circulatory system and form cysts resulting in cysticercosis.

Taenia solium is commonly found in Central and southern Latin American, American and Asian countries and occurs in the hyper endemic form. It is also reported from USA and some European countries in previously infected immigrants. Environmental conditions common to most communities where taeniosis and cysticercosis are endemic include inadequate mechanisms for disposal of human faeces together with swine husbandry practices which give the animal access to infected faeces. Pigs reared on free-range system with easy access to human faecal material are commonly infected. Mature proglottids are frequently shed in non-motile ribbons and hence massive infections are common in pigs. Each proglottid may contain as many as 100,000 eggs. Flisser *et al.* (1979) reported low efficiency of establishment of *T. solium* in normal and immune hosts. *Cysticercus cellulosae,* the larval stage of this tapeworm develops in about 10 weeks in pigs. The *Cysticerci* measure 5-20 x 5-10 mm, are milky white in colour and contain fluid rich in albumin and salts and has an invaginated scolex. They infect muscular tissue and are common in the lingual, masseter, diaphragmatic, cardiac muscles and muscles of thigh, shoulder and neck. All the parenchymatous organs, especially brain and eye are commonly infected. Clinical symptoms are usually absent in pigs except when cysticerci are lodged in the eye and brain, however, cysticercosis or measly pork infection in pigs has been found to significantly affect growth, weight gain and causes economic loss. Cysticercosis in pigs occurs very commonly in India because pigs are reared on the free range system in villages, towns and cities with free access to human faeces and sewage. The infection rate ranges from 1.7 to 20.8 % in different states (D'Souza, 2004).

People who neither raise pigs nor consume pork are also at risk of cysticercosis if they ingest *T. solium* eggs after coming into direct or indirect contact with tapeworm carriers. For example, there have been reports of orthodox Jews in North America and Muslims in the Middle

East, all banned from eating pork for religious reasons, being infected from their domestic helpers who were tapeworm carriers originally from endemic countries (Schantz *et al.*, 1992; Al-Shahrani *et al.*, 2003; Hira *et al.*, 2004). Vegetarians in India have been found to be at high risk of infection from tapeworm-infected food preparers (Rajshekhar *et al.*, 2003), while in Vietnam, there have been reports suggesting a link between cysticercosis and the use of human faeces and 'wastewater' for fertilizing crops (Willingham *et al.*, 2003). *Taenia* spp. eggs have also been recovered from several varieties of vegetables and fruits available in local markets in endemic areas (Sorvillo *et al.*, 2004). Everyone in endemic areas should thus be concerned about cysticercosis irrespective of cultural, religious and/or consumption practices. Development workers from non-endemic countries sent to work in endemic countries have also become infected. Although the life cycle of *T. solium* is generally considered to only involve humans and pigs, dogs have been found to harbour *T. solium* cysts and may possibly play a role in transmission in areas of the world where dog meat consumption is practiced. The larval form or bladder worm of *T. solium* infecting people and pigs is effective at avoiding complement activation and thus evading the hosts' immune system such that viable cysts with little or no inflammatory reaction are usually not associated with symptoms (White *et al.*, 1997). It is when cysts are recognized by the host following spontaneous degeneration or after drug treatment that an inflammatory reaction occurs usually resulting in clinical symptoms. Oedema around calcified cysticercal granulomas has also been found to cause symptoms (Nash and Patronas, 1999; Nash *et al.*, 2001, 2004). Unlike cysticercosis, taeniosis causes little if any disability and morbidity.

Cysticercosis the widely prevalent parasitic infection in man caused by the larval form afflicting the central nervous system/brain is termed neurocysticercosis (NCC). It is prevalent in South American, Central American and South East Asian countries. NCC is being reported in many developed nations too. It is not a new problem or a new disease epidemic. It appears as a new disease as the recently introduced brain imaging techniques such as Computerized scans (CT) and Magnetic resonance imaging (MRI) have increased the rates of detection. The routine testing of certain important biological samples by special immunological testing have also increased the detection rate of NCC. NCC the most common form of Cysticercosis clinically presents in a varied manifestation, hence this disease has become a common differential diagnosis in developed countries. The actual incidence of the disease is very difficult to determine. At the National Institute of Mental Health and Neurosciences, Bangalore, the incidence in Neuromicrobiology department among the autopsies is reported to be 4-5%, in the Neuroradiology department it is 10-12 cases per week by imaging studies. The cases of NCC are presented to the neurologist, neurosurgeon or to the psychiatrist (Chandramuki, 2006).

Generally the cysts have a neurotropism (affinity to the nervous system) to settle in the brain. The cysts in the brain may or may not produce symptoms. The symptoms depend on the location of the cyst in the brain, the viability of the cyst (live, dying or dead) and the tissue host reaction around. The most common symptom is seizures/fits. In a study in Nimhans, 30% of patients with seizures especially of adult onset are due to NCC. The other modes of presentation are headaches and increased intracranial tension, space occupying lesions/tumor like syndromes and abnormal behavior.

Cysticercosis can be classified into localized and generalized forms. It can also manifest as disseminated forms. They can be typed as NCC, muscular cysticercosis, ophthalmic cysticercosis, visceral cysticercosis (afflicting deep organs) and many more forms. Most of the cysts in the body can establish a symbiotic relationship with man. The time for expression may vary from host to host or it may be completely asymptomatic. The factors for these differences are yet to be understood.

There is a lack of information on the disease burden due to *T. solium* taeniosis and its associated risk factors in pig farming communities throughout the world. A study was conducted in a rural pig farming community of North India to estimate the prevalence of *T. solium* taeniosis and associated factors based on 1181 subjects in 210 households in 30 villages. Stool specimens from 924 subjects were examined for eggs of *Taenia* and other parasites. Identification of *T. solium* was confirmed by morphological features of segments and species-specific DNA detection from segments and stool. The prevalence of *T. solium* taeniosis was 18.6% (172/924); factors associated with taeniosis on multivariate analysis were age above 15 years, history of passage of *Taenia* segments in stool, undercooked pork consumption and poor hand hygiene (hand-washing with clay/water after defecation). Seventy-eight subjects (6.6%) with epilepsy were identified. The study showed alarmingly high rates of epilepsy and *T.*

solium taeniosis in the study community; it highlights the need for large-scale imaging-based surveys to identify the factors associated with epilepsy including neurocysticercosis. Health education, mass anthelmintic therapy and other preventive measures are required to control the menace of the disease (Kashi *et al.*, 2007).

The World Health Organization estimates that at least 50 million people in the world suffer from epilepsy with more than 80% of epileptics living in developing countries (WHO, 2000, 2001; Del Brutto *et al.*, 2001). NCC is considered to be the most frequent preventable cause of epilepsy in the developing world and the most common parasitic infection of the human nervous system (Roman *et al.*, 2000; Del Brutto *et al.*, 2001). The disease is reported to cause between 20% and 50% of all late-onset epilepsy cases globally and is also reported to be a common cause of juvenile epilepsy.

The clinical manifestations of NCC vary and include asymptomatic infections, blindness from ophthalmic infections, brain parenchymal involvement mostly presenting as seizures, subarachnoid and ventricular involvement resulting in hydrocephalus, chronic meningitis and infarcts, and massive infection and encephalitis, resulting in substantial health care costs in relation to diagnosis and management. Epilepsy is a syndrome with considerable social, psychological, economic and social impact on a community, and patients with epilepsy suffer from a decreasing quality of life according to the frequency of their seizures.

Cysticercosis is considered to be one of the major parasitic diseases known to pose a serious public health threat, impairing development as well as the quality of life in endemic countries by being both a result of and contributor to poverty in endemic areas exacting a triple price by: (i) infection of humans affecting their health, social and family life and productivity, (ii) causing protein-energy malnutrition in nutritionally constrained settings due to poor pork quality and condemnation of pig carcasses, and (iii) seriously reducing the household income of farmers, many of whom are women, as an obstacle to marketing of pigs and pork (Colley, 2000; Carbin *et al.*, 2005). The studies in India indicate that persons with epilepsy have an annual reduction in work productivity of up to 30% (Krishnan *et al.*, 2004). Cysticercosis causes significant economic losses due to downgrading of cattle and pig carcasses. Cysticercosis in pigs has been estimated to cause a loss of half a million dollars from 6 abattoirs in Central America and Panama (Acha and Aguilar, 1964) and up to 81 percent from

Mexico (Antonio, 1982; Cruz *et al.*, 1993). Annual economic loss estimated due to *T. saginata asiatica* was found to be $1,86,73,495 in Taiwan, $1,36,41,021 on Chegu Island and $24,25,500 on Samosir Island and Indonesia.

In India a loss of 64,600 rupees due to 3.8 percent infection in pigs in UP (Pathak and Gaur, 1989) and 2,61,661 out of 61,86,102 rupees due to 4.22% infection in an organised abattoir in Andhra Pradesh (D'Souza, 1996) has been reported. In Africa, losses of 1000 to 2000 million US dollars have been attributed to bovine cysticercosis. Cysticercosis is generally underdiagnosed and under reported.

Taenia saginata asiatica-the emerging zoonotic parasite

This sub species was first recorded in Asian countries and hence given different names such as Asian *Taenia*, Taiwan *Taenia*, Thailand *Taenia*, Korea *Taenia*, Indonesia *Taenia*, *Taeniaasiatica*, etc. Morphological characteristics are presented in Table 2. Fan *et al.* (1990b) and Eom and Rim (1992) experimentally proved pig as the intermediate host for the new parasite. According to their study the clinical manifestations in humans were gastrointestinal and neurological symptoms. Passing proglottids in the faeces was the most frequent sign (95%), followed by anal pruritis (77%), nausea (46%), abdominal pain (45%), dizziness (42%), increased appetite (30%), headache (26%) etc. and the annual economic loss was estimated to be $1,86,73,495 in Taiwan, $1,36,41,021 on Chegu island and Republic of Korea and $24,25,500 in Indonesia.

Further the studies by Fan and coworkers (1990b) and Eom and Rim (1992) established pig as the intermediate host for this subspecies. Clinical manifestations in humans included gastrointestinal and neurological symptoms. Passing proglottids in the faeces was the most frequent sign (95%), followed by anal pruritis (77%), nausea (46%), abdominal pain (45%), dizziness (42%), increased appetite (30%) and headache (26%).

Based on the morphology and PCR-RFLP, scientists have come to the conclusion that this is a subspecies of *T. saginata,* the beef tapeworm. The prevalence of this subspecies was reported for the first time from the Indian subcontinent in a study on porcine cysticercosis at Bangalore by Dhanalakshmi (2003).

Table 2: Differential features of the three zoonotic species of *Taenia*

	Taenia saginata asiatica	*Taenia saginata*	*T. solium*
Intermediate host	Pig, cattle, goat, wild boar, monkey	Cattle, reindeer	Pig, man, monkey, wild boar, dog
Source of infection	Liver	Muscle, viscera	Muscle, brain, viscera
Adult worm			
Length (m)	6(4-8)	4-12	1.5-8
Number of proglottids	674 (260-1016)	2000	700-1000
Scolex	unarmed	unarmed	armed
Way of leaving host	single and spontaneous	single and spontaneous	in groups and passively
Cysticercus			
Period of development	4 weeks	10-12 weeks	7-9 weeks
Length (µm)	1290(450-2000)	3410(1650-5720)	4430(2040-8600)
Width (µm)	1160(580-1850)	2240(1160-3580)	2610(1650-3800)
Ratio (L/W)	1.1:1	1.5:1	1.7:1
Protoscolex (µm)	640 (580-1850)	1720(590-3410)	2440(1650-3520)
Scolex	armed	unarmed	armed
Hooklet	present	absent	present

Diagnosis of taeniosis and cysticercosis in Man

Identification of *Taenia* spp. infecting humans is usually based on a combination of comparative morphology as well as immunological and molecular diagnostic approaches.Routine stool microscopy used for detecting parasite ova is known to have poor specificity and sensitivity for detecting *T. solium* taeniosis with yields ranging from 22.5% to 56% (Allan *et al.*, 1990, 1993; Willingham *et al.*, 2003). This method underestimates the prevalence of taeniosis because *Taenia* eggs are excreted intermittently (Allan *et al.*, 1996). The test's efficacy can thus be improved by repeating it on different days (Hall *et al.*, 1981). Eggs of *T. solium, T. saginata* and*T. saginata asiatica* are morphologically similar so it is necessary to collect complete adult tapeworms or proglottids to determine the infecting species based on morphological characteristics. Mature or gravid proglottids of the tapeworm species can be differentiated on the basis of reproductive organs but need to be fixed and stained correctly to identify the species. Identification of *T. solium* is based on the observation of three ovarian lobes and the absence of a vaginal sphincter in mature proglottids and the presence of 7–16 unilateral uterine branches in gravid proglottids. Counting of the uterine branches can be facilitated by longitudinally sectioning the gravid proglottid, staining it with hematoxylin-eosin and then gently squashing it between glass slides or between the underside and the cover of a petri dish before microscopic evaluation. Unfortunately some overlapping in the number of uterine branches may occur between *Taenia* spp. thus collection of the tapeworm to examine its scolex or molecular assays may be needed to differentiate the infecting species.

*Copro-Antigen Detection ELISA :*The ability to parasitologically detect tapeworm carriers increased dramatically with the development of a test for *Taenia*-specific molecules in faecal samples (copro-antigens). The test is a polyclonal antibody-based sandwich enzyme-linked immunosorbent assay (ELISA) using antibodies obtained from hyperimmune rabbit sera against *T. solium* adult worm somatic antigens (Allan *et al.*, 1990). It has been found to have a sensitivity of about 95% and specificity greater than 99% (Allan *et al.*, 1996). A more rapid dipstick ELISA form of the copro-antigen test has been developed which requires minimal facilities making it a more appropriate option for epidemiological studies though it is less sensitive than the micro-plate assay (Allan *et al.*, 1993). Copro-antigens are detectable prior to patency and cease to be detectable within a week following treatment. They are stable for weeks in unfixed faecal samples kept at room temperature and for years in frozen samples or in chemically fixed samples (e.g. formalin) kept at room temperature (Dorny *et al.*, 2005). The copro-antigen ELISA is only genus specific, making it impossible to differentiate *T. solium* from *T. saginata* or *T. s. asiatica*.

*Copro-DNA Assays :*Various molecular approaches have been developed to detect DNA of *Taenia* spp. in human faeces for diagnosis of taeniosis. These techniques are highly sensitive and species-specific thus overcoming the limitations of differentiation of *Taenia* spp. based on morphology, however, the expense and lack of capacity for utilizing these techniques currently limits their use in *T. solium* endemic countries. Molecular approaches for detecting taeniosis include PCR, PCR coupled to RFLP (Gonzalez *et al.*, 2002; Hidalgo *et al.*, 2002) and multiplex-PCR (Yamasaki *et al.*, 2004). PCR with oligonucleotide primers derived from species-specific DNA probes provides a rapid and sensitive method of taeniosis diagnosis (Gonzalez *et al.*, 2002). PCR–RFLP and multiplex PCR permit differential diagnosis of the *Taenia* spp. without relying on the availability of intact mature or gravid proglottids. Multiplex PCR is an easy and time-saving technique for use on faeces and parasite specimens, does not require DNA sequencing and permits differential diagnosis of *Taenia* species by using a combination of different primer pairs in the same amplification reaction to produce species-specific sequences of mitochondrial DNA that can then be distinguished (Gonzalez *et al.*, 2003; Yamasaki *et al.*, 2002, 2004, 2006). In addition to differentiating between *Taenia* spp. infections, it is valuable for molecular epidemiological studies concerning the genotypic variation in *T. solium* around the world (Okamoto *et al.*, 2001; Nakao *et al.*, 2002).

A fingerstick *T. solium* taeniosis immunoblot assay (EITB-T) was developed using copro-antigens of adult *T. solium* tapeworms for detection of human taeniosis (Wilkins *et al.*, 1999). The new serum *T. solium* taeniosis immunoblot is reported to be highly sensitive (95%) and specific (100%) compared to microscopy and copro-antigen detection (Wilkins *et al.*, 1999;Degiorgio *et al.*, 2005). A limitation of the EITB-T test is that since it detects antibodies to adult *T. solium* worms; it indicates the history of tapeworm infection and not necessarily active infection and thus may result in false positives (Degiorgio *et al.*, 2005). Combination of the EITB-T and the copro-antigen ELISA may be a way of specifically detecting *T. solium* tapeworm carriers while avoiding the need for collecting and identifying the tapeworms from those identified.

Detection of human cysticercosis is based on biopsy of subcutaneous nodules, imaging and immunodiagnosis. The presence of locally secreted specific IgA antibodies in tear specimen from persons with ophthalmic cysticercosis has been reported. The ELISA using *T. solium* larval excretory secretory (ES) antigen demonstrated a diagnostic level of IgA antibodies in tears with 100% sensitivity (6 out of 6 confirmed cases of ophthalmic cysticercosis) whereas, 25 of 34 (73.52%) clinically suspected cases were diagnosed positive. The ELISA using *T. solium* bladder worm somatic antigen detected a diagnostic titre of IgA antibody in tears with a sensitivity of 50% (3 out of 6 confirmed cases). The specificity of the tear IgA ELISA using *T. solium* larval somatic and ES antigens was observed to be 94.87% and 92.3%, respectively. Overall in tears, the ELISA with ES antigens for detection of IgA antibodies showed a higher diagnostic efficiency (93.33%)

compared to somatic antigen (88.88%). The sensitivities of the ELISA for detection of IgA antibodies in tears was observed to be higher than that for detection of IgG antibodies in serum using either somatic or ES antigens of the parasite (Priyadarshi *et al.*, 2008).

Diagnosis of cysticercosis is primarily based on imaging techniques. These imaging techniques are sometimes limited by the small size of visualized lesions and atypical images, which are difficult to be distinguished from abscesses or neoplasms. Therefore, efforts have been directed toward identification and characterization of specific antigens of parasites for development of serodiagnostic method that can detect specific antibody. The glycoproteins of 10–26 kDa in cyst fluid of *T. solium* consisting of a very closely related family of 8-kDa proteins have been widely accepted for serodiagnostic purpose. Four genes (designated Ag1, Ag1V1, Ag2 and Ag2V1) have been identified encoding the 7- and 10-kDa polypeptides. Based on the antigenicities of these clones, Ag1V1 and Ag2 were chosen as ELISA antigens and the Ag1V1/Ag2 chimeric protein was expressed. The Ag1V1/Ag2 chimeric protein showed similar sensitivity and specificity as the native glycoproteins (Yasuhitosako *et al.*, 2006).

DNA-based differential diagnosis for human taeniid cestodes has become a very powerful tool not only for routine identification but also for taeniosis/cysticercosis control programs that aim to detect tapeworm carriers and treat them. It is also indispensable for definitive diagnosis of cysticercosis cases in which histopathological findings are not confirmatory.

Porcine Cysticercosis

Detection of porcine cysticercosis cases is important for determining whether a cysticercosis/taeniosis endemic situation exists and for monitoring any interventions undertaken. Methods for detecting cysticercosis in live pigs include tongue examination and serological testing as well as inspection of carcasses at slaughter.

Lingual Examination: Visual inspection and palpation for cysts on the ventral surface of the tongue is used by farmers and pig traders in endemic countries as an inexpensive and quick way of identifying pigs infected with *T. solium* cysticercosis. The specificity of the technique can be 100% if conducted by a person with experience (Gonzalez *et al.*, 1990; Dorny *et al.*, 2005).

The sensitivity of the technique depends very much on the intensity of infection of the animals and is reported to be as high as 71% in heavily infected pigs though considerably less in pigs with low intensities of infection (Gonzalez *et al.*, 1990; Sciutto *et al.*, 1998; Sato *et al.*, 2003; Dorny *et al.*, 2004, 2005). Thus, this method of detection generally underestimates the prevalence of porcine cysticercosis. However, it can be a useful tool for rapid assessment of sites to determine and monitor endemic 'hot spots' and in countries where official meat inspection is minimal and capacity and/or funding for conducting immunodiagnosis is absent it may be the only method available for detecting porcine cysticercosis.

Pig Carcass Inspection : Official guidelines and practices for the detection of *T. solium* cysticercosis during inspection of pig carcasses vary widely from one country to another. In some countries only visual inspection is carried out on one or several selected muscle and organ sites, while in others incisions in some of these muscle groups may be required. The effectiveness of this method for detecting cases of porcine cysticercosis may be low depending on its thoroughness especially for pigs with low intensities of infection (Sciutto *et al.*, 1998; Boa *et al.*, 2002; Dorny *et al.*, 2004). Records from meat inspection while providing evidence on the presence of porcine cysticercosis are generally considered to underestimate the status of cysticercosis in the pig population due to low sensitivity as well as the fact that farmers and pig traders may avoid taking pigs to official slaughter establishments if they suspect that they are infected with *T. solium* (Gonzalez *et al.*, 1990). Meat inspection when conducted properly provides a useful tool for validating diagnostic methods and intervention strategies. Comparison of meat inspection, CIEP and ELISA in the detection of *T. solium* cysticercosis in pigs amply demonstrated that serodiagnosis is more reliable than meat inspection for detection of the disease (D'Souza and Hafeez, 1999).

Immunodiagnosis : Immunodiagnosis in pigs provides an ante-mortem detection method more sensitive than lingual examination for use in prevalence and community-based surveys as well as intervention studies. Techniques developed for the diagnosis of cysticercosis in humans have also been adapted for use in detecting *T. solium* infection of pigs, including both antibody (EITB and antibody-ELISA) and antigen detection (antigen-ELISA). It has been reported that the sensitivity of these available immunodiagnostic techniques is reduced in pigs with low intensities of infection (Sciutto *et al.*, 1998).

Although the EITB and the newer formulations of antibody-ELISA are popular tests for detecting porcine cysticercosis for both epidemiological studies and monitoring interventions, care should be taken with regard to the overestimation of infection due to the presence of antibodies in pigs in the absence of infection. Anti-cysticercal antibodies (IgG) are passively transferred from sows via colostrum to piglets and have been found to persist for more than six months after weaning (Gonzalez *et al.,* 1999). Considering that most pigs are taken to market at about 9–12 months they will maintain these antibodies for most of their lives whether infected or not. In addition, pigs may also develop a transient antibody response to *T. solium* infection without the establishment of a patent infection as seen in humans (Dorny *et al.,* 2003).

The Antigen-ELISA would be a more appropriate immunodiagnostic test for detecting porcine cysticercosis since pigs usually do not live long enough for the *T. solium* larval stages to die and thus would be expected to have active infection. It has been reported that the Antigen-ELISA is highly specific and sensitive, even detecting pigs harbouring one single *T. solium* cyst (Erhart *et al.,* 2002; Nguekam *et al.,* 2003; Dorny *et al.,* 2004). The circulating antigens can be detected as early as two to six weeks post infection (Nguekam *et al.,* 2003). However, the genus specificity of the Antigen-ELISA test does not allow differentiation of larval *T. solium* infections from larval infections of other *Taenia* spp. such as *T. hydatigena* and possibly *T. s. asiatica,* which becomes problematic in areas where these parasites co-exist (Dorny *et al.,* 2003, 2005). This species specificity problem does not appear to be a problem of the Antibody-ELISA since pigs naturally infected with the bladder worms of *T. hydatigena* are negative by that test (Sato *et al.,* 2003).

The serodiagnostic tests with different antigens standardized in the CAFT in Veterinary Parasitology at Veterinary College, Bangalore include Dot ELISA, CIEP, protein A ELISA; plate ELISA, EITB, latex agglutination test, coagglutination test, IHAT and BFT. The PCR-RFLP was used to demonstrate the prevalence of *T. s. asiatica* in pigs from Bangalore for the first time (D'Souza, 2007).

Treatment and control of porcine cysticercosis

The two commonly used drugs viz. praziquantel and albendazole given orally have been found effective for treating porcine cysticercosis but involve multiple dosing making them impractical for large-scale control programs (Flisser *et al.*, 1990; Torres *et al.*, 1992; Gonzalez *et al.*, 1995; Kaur *et al.*, 1995).

A newer benzimidazole viz. oxfendazole was found to be more than 95% effective in killing cysts in pigs when given in a single dose of 30 mg/kg and pigs may remain resistant to re-infection for at least three months after treatment (Gonzalez *et al.*, 2001). Infected meat in oxfendazole treated pigs needs at least eight weeks for all the cysts to degenerate and up to 12 weeks to achieve a clear, acceptable appearance of the pork for human consumption thereby greatly increasing the meat's commercial value (Gonzalez *et al.*, 1998; Gonzalez, 2002). Oxfendazole has not yet been tested for treating human cysticercosis but has been found to be very effective for reducing the infectivity of larval forms of *Echinococcus granulosus* infecting small ruminants (Blaton *et al.*, 1998; Dueger *et al.*, 1999; Erica *et al.*, 1999; Njoroge *et al.*, 2005).

Vaccination

Several approaches have been examined towards the development of vaccines against *T. solium*, including the application of recombinant oncosphere antigens and peptides (Sciutto *et al.*, 2002; Lightowlers, 2003, 2004, 2006).

Host-protective immune responses to taeniid cestodes are known to be directed towards the egg (oncosphere) in the early developing embryo (Rickard and Williams, 1982). Specific native oncosphere antigens have now been identified as a source of these host-protective responses and recombinant DNA techniques have been used to clone and express the genes encoding these antigens leading to vaccine candidate recombinant antigens (Gauci *et al.*, 1998; Gauci and Lightowlers, 2001). Two of the most promising recombinant *T. solium* oncosphere antigens, designated TSOL 18 and TSOL 45, have been evaluated in experimental vaccine trials in different countries and by groups in Latin America and Africa and have been shown to induce complete or near complete protection against experimental challenge infection in pigs (99.5–99.9% and 97–98.6%, respectively) (Flisser *et al.*, 2004; Gonzalez *et al.*, 2005). Various aspects of this oncosphere antigen subunit vaccine are currently being investigated before proceeding with controlled field trials.

A synthetic vaccine composed of three peptides has been developed in Mexico (Sciutto *et al.*, 2002), which is reported to be both preventative and therapeutic,reducing the parasite load as well as the viability of cysticerci in pigs (Huerta *et al.*, 2000, 2002; de Aluja *et al.*, 2005). It apparently has a cysticidal effect on established bladder worms in vaccinated pigs thus lowering the number of viable cysticerci capable of transforming into tapeworms suggesting that people who ingest cysticerci in the meat of vaccinated pigs will be less at risk to develop intestinal taeniosis. In a field trial conducted in two rural endemic communities it was found that the peptide vaccine reduced by 52.6% the prevalence of naturally acquired porcine cysticercosis and reduced by 97.9% the total number of recovered cysticerci, with 80% of the cysts established in vaccinated pigs found damaged (Huerta *et al.*, 2002). Preliminary results thus suggest that immunization of pigs with the peptide vaccine can confer a high level of protection against an egg challenge while also inducing an immune response against the larvae, which are either destroyed or rendered non-infective. Different methods of antigen production and delivery of the peptide vaccine are being explored to reduce the production costs of synthetic peptides and also improve their immunogenicity in order to increase the possibility of extensive application of the vaccine (Manoutcharian *et al.*, 2004).

DNA vaccination is a new approach. It is an exciting new strategy for the development of non-living sub-unit vaccines because of the generic nature of the production and purification processes required. Recombinant DNA plasmids encoding specific antigens are directly injected into the muscle, skin or other tissues of the host to elicit antigen-specific humoral and cellular immune responses to the gene products. This technique has been actively developed in the past few years against a variety of infectious agents including virus, bacteria and parasites.

Paramyosin, also known as B antigen, was identified as a candidate antigen for helminth vaccines. B antigen is expressed specifically in the larval stage of *T. solium*. The protection rate in pigs with the DNA vaccine B-PV93 was up to 99.5%, substantially higher than that in the control. In a study to improve the effectiveness of protection induced by using a different vector, pcDNA3-B and dosages, the pcDNA3-B was constructed by cloning the nucleotide sequence of B antigen into the pcDNA3.1 plasmid downstream of the CMV promoter. Growing pigs were vaccinated only once. It was observed that pcDNA3-B antigen could induce antigen-specific immune responses that prevent the pigs from cysticercosis.

The use of transgenic plants as new antigen-delivery systems for subunit vaccines has been increasingly explored. Studies have been conducted to develop a papaya-based vaccine against cysticercosis. Synthetic peptides (KETc1, KETc12, and KETc7) were successfully expressed in 19 different transgenic papaya clones and found to be immunogenic. Complete protection against cysticercosis was induced with the soluble extract of the clones that expressed the higher levels of transcripts in up to 90% of the immunized mice. This study represents a key step towards the development of a more effective, sustainable and affordable oral subunit vaccine against human and pig cysticercosis.

To explore ways to lower vaccine production costs and to approach an oral vaccine, an embryogenic papaya cell line, was transformed because it is easily amenable for genetic transformation and because it can be propagated in low-cost cell cultures systems. The use of cell cultures avoids non-desirable environmental effects due to the release of transgenic plants into the environment, and embryogenic papaya callus can be eaten raw with additional side-benefits considering its immunomodulatory properties (Marisela Hernandez *et al.*, 2007).

Recently, a porcine-cysticercosis vaccine has developed, based on three synthetic-peptides (S3Pvac) (KETc1, KETc12 and (GK1) KETc7 of 12, 8 and 18 amino acids, respectively), originally identified in *T. crassiceps*. Its protective capacity was demonstrated (50% reduction in prevalence levels and 98% reduction of infection intensity) in piglets under endemic field conditions, i.e. exposed to the natural infection pressure. Moreover, S3Pvac immunization of previously infected pigs reduced cysticercus viability, and exhibited additional therapeutic properties. Thus, S3Pvac represents a powerful means of controlling cysticercosis. In the case of cysticercosis, oral vaccination seems to be an optimal choice for pigs and human vaccination since both acquire the cysticerci by ingestion of *T. solium* eggs. Thus, a local immune response could avoid parasite entrance through the gut, and the elicited systemic immunity could destroy the parasites that managed to elude mucosal defenses.

In order to reduce vaccine production costs,a recombinant M13 phage version of the anti-cysticercosis tripeptide vaccine (S3Pvac) was developed. The efficacy of S3Pvac-Phage vs. placebo was evaluated in a randomized trial that included 1047 rural pigs in 16 villages of Central Mexico. Three to five months after vaccination 530 pigs were examined by tongue inspection. At 5–27 months of age, 331 pigs (197 vaccinated/

134 controls) were inspected at necropsy. Vaccination reduced 70% the frequency of tongue cysticercosis and, based on necropsy, 54% of muscle-cysticercosis and by 87% the number of cysticerci (Julio Morales *et al.*, 2008).

Conclusions

Taeniid cysticercosis is thus considered as an emerging and re-emerging cyclozoonosis because it has continued to prevail through the ages. The status of *T. solium* cysticercosis in endemic countries of the world has not changed, as it should have considering the advancement in science and technology in the twenty first century. It continues to be a public health problem in several developing countries in which social, economical and cultural conditions favor the maintenance of this zoonosis.

This zoonosis is potentially eradicable if sanitary facilities are improved and pig farming is regulated. The disappearance of *T. solium* from most European countries was due to progress in environmental sanitation and adequate husbandry, and inspection of pig carcasses. Unfortunately, these measures have not yet been completely implemented in many developing countries. Therefore, alternative measures have to be undertaken. Creation of awareness about the disease through public health services and mass media would go a long way to curtail the disease. Diagnosis of human cysticercosis through scanning and serodiagnosis and proper treatment is another approach. The dosing of pigs with oxfendazole and introduction of the recombinant vaccine as is being extensively introduced in Latin American countries should be an enforced duty of veterinarians in this direction with institutional support.

References

Acha, P.N. and Aguilar, F.J. (1964). Studies on cysticercosis in Central America and Panama. *Am. J. Trop. Med.Hyg.*, 13: 48-53

Al-Shahrani, D., Frayha, H.H., Dabbagh, O. and Al-Shail, E. (2003). First case of neurocysticercosis in Saudi Arabia. *J. Trop.Pediat.*,49: 58-60

Allan, C.G., Martinez, N., Flisser, A., Aluja, A., Allan, J.C. and Craig, P.S. (1996). Immunocharacterization of *Taenia solium* oncosphere and metacestode antigens. *J. Helminthol.*, 70: 271-280

Allan, J.C., Avila, G., Garcia-Noval, J., Sarti, E. and Flisser, A. (1993). Dipstick dot ELISA for detection of *Taenia* coproantigens in humans. *Parasitol.*, 107: 79-85

Allan, J.C., Avila, G., Garcýa-Noval, J., Flisser, A. and Craig, P.S. (1990). Immunodiagnosis of taeniosis by coproantigen detection. *Parasitol.*, 101: 473-77

Antonio, A.H. (1982). *Economic impact of porcine cysticercosis*. In: Cysticercosis – Present state of knowledge and perspective (Flisser, A., Williums, K., Laclette, J.P.,Larrslde, C., Ridaura, C. and Beltran, F., eds), Academic press, New York, pp. 63-67

Blaton,R.E., Wachira,T.M., Zeyhle,E.M., Magambo,J.K. and Schantz,P.M. (1998). Oxfendazole treatment for cystic hydatid disease in naturally infected animals. *Antimicrob. Agents chemother.*, 42: 601-605

Boa,M.E.,Kassuku,A.A., Willingham,A.L.,Keyyu,J.D.,Phiri,I.K. and Namsen,P. (2002). Intensity, distribution and density of *Cysticercus cellulosae* by muscle groups and organs in naturally infected slaughter pigs in Mbulu district of Tanzania. *Vet. Parasitol.*,106: 155-164

Burger, A.J. (1984). In: Animal Parasitology, 3rdedn.(edited by J.D. Smyth), Cambridge University Press, pp. 327 and 345

Carbin,H., Budke,C.M., Cowan,L.D., Michael, L. and Willingham,A.L. and Torgerson,P.R. (2005). Methods for assessing the burden of parasitic zoonoses: echinococcosis and cysticercosis.*Trends Parasitol.*, 21: 327-333

Chandramuki, A. (2006). Neurocysticercosis.Compendium, IX National Training programme on New Insights in Parasite Disease- Epidemiology and Control. Feb. 6-26, conducted by the CAS, Department of Parasitology, Veterinary College, Bangalore, pp. 22-23

Colley, D. (2000). Parasitic Diseases: Opportunities and challenges in the 21stcentury. *Mem. Inst.Oswaldo. Cruz.*,95 (Suppl. 1): 79-87

Cruz, R.R, Vazquez, Z.G and Alanis, L.M. (1993). Retrospective study of the condemnation of pigs with cysticercosis from 1987-1991 in the municipal abattoir of Cuernavaca, Mexico. *Tecnica Pecuaria –en Mexico*,31: 102-111, *Helminthol. Abs.* 1994, 63:1244

De Aluja, A.S., Villalobos, N.M., Nava, G., Toledo, A.,Martinez,J.J., Plancarte,A.,Rodarte,L.F.,Fragoso,G. and Sciutto, E. (2005). Therapeutic capacity of the synthetic peptide based vaccine against *Taenia solium* cysticercosis in pigs. *Vaccine*, 23:4062-4069

Degiorgio,C., Pietsch-Esueta,S., Tsang,V., Corral-Leyva, G., N.L., Medina,M.T.,Astudillo,S.,Padilla,N.,Leyva,P., Martinez,L., Noh, J., Levine,M., del villasensor, R. and Sorvillo,F.(2005). SeroPrevalence of *Taenia solium* cysticercosis and *Taenia solium* taeniasis in California, USA. *Acta Neurol. Scand.*, 111: 84-88

Del Brutto, O.H., Rajshekhar, V., White, A.C., Jr. Tsang,V.C., Nash, T.E., Takayanagui, O.M., Schantz, P.M.,Evans, C.A., Flisser, A., Correa, D., Botero,

D., Allan,J.C., Sarti, E., Gonzalez, A.E., Gilman, R.H. and Garcia, H.H. (2001). Proposed diagnostic criteria for neurocysticercosis. *Neurol.*, 57: 177-183

Dhanalakshmi, H. (2003). Phenotypic and Genotypic characterization and immunodiagnosis of *Taenia solium* bladder worms of pigs. Ph.D. Thesis submitted to University of Agricultural Sciences, Bangalore

Dorny, P., Somers, R., Dang, T.C.T., Nguyen, V.K. and Vercruysse, J. (2004). Cysticercosis in Cambodia, Laos and Vietnam. *Southeast Asian. J. Trop. Med. Pub. Hlth.*,35: 223–226

Dorny, P., Brandt, J., Zoli, A. and Geerts, S. (2003). Immunodiagnostic tools for human porcine cysticercosis. *Acta Trop.*, 87: 79-86

Dorny, P., Geerts, S., Brandt, J. and Geerts, S. (2005). Detection and diagnosis. In: WHO/FAO/OIE Guidelines for the surveillance, prevention and control of Taeniosis/Cysticercosis (eds. Murrel, K.D.),pp. 44-52

D'Souza, P.E. (1996). Studies on porcine cysticercosis with special reference to serodiagnosis. PhD thesis submitted to Andhra Pradesh Agricultural University, Hyderabad

D'Souza, P.E. (2004). Cysticercosis in pigs- epidemiology, Immunodiagnosis, economic impact under Indian conditions and control. INV 27, presented at the 3rd global meet on parasitic diseases at Bangalore University, Jan. 12-16, pp.29

D'Souza, P.E. (2007). Cysticercosis: an old but persistent helminthosis in animals and man. Tropacon 2007- First National Conference of Indian Academy of Tropical Parasitology, Oct. 5-6, 2007, C.M.E. proc.

D'Souza, P.E. and Hafeez, M. (1999). Comparison of routine meat inspection, CIEP and ELISA to detect *Cysticercus cellulosae* infection in pigs. *Indian Vet. J.*, 76: 285-288

Dueger, E.L., Moro, P.L. and Gilman, R.H. (1999). Oxfendazole treatment of sheep with naturally acquired hydatid disease. *Antimicrob. Agents Chemoth.*, 42: 2263-67

Eom, K.S. and Rim, H.J. (1992). Natural infections of Asian *T. saginata*metacestods in the livers of Korean domestic pigs. *Korean J. Parasitol.*, 30: 15-20

Erhart, A., Dorny, P., Van De, N., Vien, H.V., Thach, D.C., Toan, N.D., Cong, L.D., Geerts, S., Speybroeck, N., Berkvens, D. and Brandt, J. (2002). *Taenia solium* cysticercosis in a village in northern Viet Nam: seroprevalence study using an ELISA for detecting circulating antigen. *Trans. R. Soc. Trop. Med.Hyg.*,96: 270-272

Erica, L.,Dueger, E.L., Pedro, L., Moro, P.L. and Gilman, R.H. (1999).Oxfendazole treatment of sheep with naturally acquired hydatid disease. *Antimicrob. Agents Chemoth.*, 43: 2263-2267

Fan, P.C., Chung, W.C., Lin, C.Y. and Wu, C. C. (1990b). The pig as an intermediate host for Taiwan *Taenia* infection. *J. Helminthol.*, 64: 223-231

Flisser, A. (1988). Neurocysticercosis in Mexico. *Parasitol. Today*, 4: 131-137.

Flisser, A., Gonzalez, D., Shkurovich, M., Madrazo, I., Correa, D., Rodriguez-Carbajal, J., Rodriguez del Rosal, E., Collado, M., Fernandez, B., Fernandez, F. and Aluja, A.S. (1990). Praziquantel treatment of porcine brain and muscle *Taenia solium* cysticercosis-I. Radiological, physiological and histo-pathological studies. *Parasitol. Res.*, 76: 263-269

Flisser, A., Guaci, C.G., Zoli, A., Martinez Ocana, J., Garza, A. Rodriguez, Dominguaz-Alpizar, J.L., Maravilla, P., Rodriguez-Canul, R., Avila, G., Aguilar-Vegas, L., Kyngdon, C., Geertz, S. and Lightowlers, M.W. (2004). Induction of protection against porcine cysticercosis by vaccination with recombinant oncosphere antigens. *Inf. Immun.*, 72: 5292-5297

Flisser, A., Perez-Montfort, R. and Laralde, C. (1979). The immunology of human and animal cysticercosis: a review. *Bull. WHO*, 57: 839-856

Gauci, C.G. and Lightowlers, M.W. (2001). Alternative splicing and sequence diversity of transcripts from the oncosphere stage of *Taenia solium* with homology to the 45W antigen of *Taenia ovis*. *Mol. Biochem. Parasitol.*, 112: 173-181

Gauci, C.G.P., Flisser, A. and Lightowlers, M.W. (1998). A *Taenia solium* oncosphere protein homologous to host-protective *Taenia ovis* and *T. saginata* 18kDa antigens. *Int. J. Parasitol.*, 28: 757–60

Gonzalez, A.E., Cama, V., Gilman, R.H., Tsang, V.C.W., Pilcher, J.B., Chavera, A., Castro, M., Montenegro, T., Verastegui, M., Miranda, E. and Bazalar, H. (1990). Prevalence and comparison of serologic assays, necropsy and tongue examination for the diagnosis of porcine cysticercosis in Peru. *Am. J. Trop. Med. Hyg.*, 43: 194-199

Gonzalez, A.E., Falcon, N., Gavidia, C., Garcia, H.H., Tsang, V.C.W., Bernal, T., Romero, M. and Gilman, R.H. (1998). Time-response curve of oxfendazole in the treatment of swine cysticercosis. *Am. J. Trop. Med. Hyg.*, 59: 832-836

Gonzalez, A.E., Garcia, H.H., Gilman, R.H. and Tsang, V.C.W. (2003). Control of *Taenia solium*. Cysticercosis working group in Peru. *Acta Trop.*, 87: 103-109

Gonzalez, A.E., Garcia, H.H., Gilman, R.H., Lopez, M.T., Gavidia, C., McDonald, J., Pilcher, J.B. and Tsang, V.C. (1995). Treatment of porcine cysticercosis with albendazole. *Am. J. Trop. Med. Hyg.*, 53: 571-574

Gonzalez, A.E., Verastegui, M., Noh, J.C., Gavidia, C., Falcon, N., Bernal, T., Garcia, H.H., Tsang, V.C., Gilman, R.H. and Wilkins, P.P. (1999). Persistence of passively transferred antibodies in porcine *Taenia solium* cysticercosis. The cysticercosis working group in Peru. *Vet. Parasitol.*, 86: 113-118

Gonzalez, A.E. (2002). Control of *Taenia solium* with porcine chemotherapy. In: *Taenia solium*cysticercosis. From Basic to Clinical Science (eds. Singh, G. and Prabhakar, S.),Wallingford,United Kingdok, CABI Publishing, pp. 431-435

Gonzalez,A.E., Gauci, C.G., Barber, D., Gilman, R.H., Tsang, V.C.W., Garcia, H.H., Verastegui, M. and Lightowlers, M.W. (2005). Short report: Vaccination of pigs to control human neurocysticercosis. *Am. J. Trop. Med. Hyg.*, 72: 837-839

Gonzalez,A.E., Gavida,C.,Falcon,N.,Bernal,T.,Verastegui,M., Garcia, H.H., Gilman,R.H. and Tsang, V.C. (2001). Protection of pigs with cysticercosis from further infections after treatment with oxfendalzole. Cysticercosis working group in Peru. *Am. J. Trop.Med.Hyg.*, 65: 15-18

Gonzalez, L.M., Montero, E., Sciutto, E., Harrison, L.J., Parkhouse, R.M. and Garate, T. (2002). Differential diagnosis of *T. saginata* and *T. solium* infections: from DNA probes to polymerase chain reaction. *Trans. Roy. Soc. Trop. Med. Hyg.*, 96: S243-250

Hall, A., Latham,M.C., Crompton, D.W.T. and Stephenson, L.S. (1981). *Taenia saginata* (Cestode) in western Kenya: the reliability of fecal examination in diagnosis. *Parasitol.*, 83:91-101

Hidalgo, R.R., Geysen, D., Ortiz, W.B., Geerts, S. and Brandt, J. (2002). Comparison of conventional techniques to differentiate between *Taenia solium* and *Taenia saginata* and an improved PCR-RFLP assay using a mitochondrial 12S rDNA fragment. *J. Parasitol.*, 88: 1007-1011

Hira, P.R., Francis, I., Abdella, N.A., Gupta, R., Al-Ali, F.M., Grover, S., Khalid, N., Abdeen, S., Iqbal, J., Wilson, M. and Tsang, V.C.W. (2004). Cysticercosis: imported and autochthonous infections in Kuwait. *Trans. Roy. Soc. Trop. Med.Hyg.*, 19: 172-175

Huerta, M., de Aluja, A.S., Fragoso, G., Toledo, A., Villalobos, N., Hernandez, M., Gevorkian, G., Acero, G., Diaz, A., Alvarez, I., Avila, R., Belrran,C., Garcia, G., Martinez, J.J., Sarralde, C. and Scitto, E. (2002). Synthetic peptide vaccine against *Taenia solium* pig cysticercosis: successful vaccination in a controlled field trial in rural Mexico. *Vaccine,* 20: 262-266

Huerta, M., Scitto, E., Garcia, G., Villalobos, N., Hernandez, M., Fragoso, G., Diaz, J., Diaz, A., de Aluja, A.S., Toledo, A., Gevorkian, G., Acero, G., Alvarez, I., Avila, R., Belrran,C., Martinez, J.J. and Sarralde, C. (2000). Vaccination against *Taenia solium* cysticercosis in underfed rustic pigs of Mexico: Roles of age, genetic background and antibody response.*Vet. Parasitol.*, 90: 209-219

Jeri, C., Gilman, R.H., Lescano, A.G., Mayta, H., Ramirez, M.E., Gonzalez, E., Nazerali, R. and Garcia, H.H. (2004). Species of identification after treatment for human taeniasis. *Lancet,* 363: 949-950

Julio, M., Martinez, J.J., Manoutcharian, K., Hernandez, M., Fleury, A., Gevorkian, G., Gonzalo, A.,Blancas, A., Toledo, A., Cervantes, J., Maza, V., Quet, F., Bonnabau, H., Aline, S., De Aluja, Fragoso, G., Carlos, L. and Sciutto, E. (2008). Inexpensive anti-cysticercosis vaccine: S3Pvac expressed in heat inactivated M13 filamentous phage proves effective against naturally acquired *Taenia solium* porcine cysticercosis. *Vaccine,* 26: 2899-2905

Kashi, N.P., Prasad, A., Gupta, R.K., Chandra, M.P. and Singh, U. (2007). Prevalence and associated risk factors of *Taenia solium* taeniasis in a rural pig farming community of north India. *Roy. Soc. Trop. Med. Hyg.,* 101: 1241-1247

Kaur, M., Joshi, K., Ganguly, N.K., Mahajan, R.C. and Malla, N. (1995). Evaluation of the efficacy of albendazole against the larvae of *Taenia solium* in experimentally infected pigs, and kinetics of the immune response. *Int. J. Parasitol.,* 25: 1443-1450

Krishnan, A., Saharaiah, S.U. and Kapoor, S.K. (2004). Cost of epilepsy in patients attending a secondary level hospital in India. *Epilesia,*45: 289-291

Lightowlers, M.W. (2003). Vaccines for prevention of cysticercosis. *Acta Trop.,* 87: 129-135

Lightowlers, M.W. (2004). Vaccines for prevention of cysticercosis. *Dev. Biol.,*119: 361-368

Lightowlers, M.W. (2006). Vaccines against cysticercosis and hydatidosis: Foundations in taeniid cestode immunology.*Parasitol. Int.,* 55: S39-S43

Manoutcharian, K., Diaz-orea, A., Gevorkian, G., Fragoso, G., Acero,G., Gonzalez, E., de Aluja, A., Villalobos, N., Gomez-Conde, E. and Sciutto, E. (2004). Recombinant bacteriophage based multiepitope vaccine against *Taenia solium* pig cysticercosis. *Vet. Immunol. Immunopathol.,* 99: 11-24

Marisela, H., Cabrera-Ponce, J.L., Gladis, F., Lopez-Casillas, F., Guevara-Garcia, A., Rosas, G., Leon-Ramirez, C., Juarez, P., Sanchez-Garcia, G., Cervantes, J., Gonzalo, A., Toledo, A., Cruz, C., Bojalil, R., Herrera-Estrella, L. and Sciutto, E. (2007). A new highly effective anti-cysticercosis vaccine expressed in transgenic papaya. *Vaccine,* 25: 4552-4260

Nakao, M., Okamoto, M., Sako,Y., Yamasaki, H., Nakaya, K. and Ito, A. (2002). A phylogenetic hypothesis for the distribution of two genotypes of the pork tapeworm *Taenia solium* worldwide. *Parasitol.,*124: 654-662

Nash, T.E. and Patronas, N.J. (1999). Edema associated with calcified lesions in neurocysticercosis. *Neurol.,* 53: 777-781

Nash, T.E., Del Bruttp, O.H., Butman, J.A., Corona, T., Delgado-Escueta, A., Duron, R.M., Evans, C.A., Gilman, R.H., Gonzalez, A.E., Loeb, J.A., Medena, M.T., Pietsch- Escueta, S., Pretell, E.J., Takayanagui, O.M., Theodore, W., Tsang,

V.C. and Garcia, H.H. (2004). Calcific neurocysticercosis and epileptogenesis. *Neurol.*, 62: 1934-1938

Nash, T.E., Pretell, J. and Garcia, H.H. (2001). Calcified cysticerci provoke perilesional edema and seizures. *Clin. Infect. Dis.*, 33: 1649-1653

Nguekam, Zoli, A.P., Vondou, L., Pouedet, S.M.R., Assana, E., Dorny, P., Brandt, J. and Geerts, S. (2003). Kinetics of circulating antigens in pigs experimentally infected with *Taenia solium* eggs. *Vet. Parasitol.*, 111: 323-332

Njoroge, E., Mbithi,P., Wachaira, T., Gathuma, J., Gathura, P., Maitho, T.E., Magambo,J. and Zeyhle, E. (2005). Comparative study of albendazole and oxfendazole in the treatment of cystic echinococcosis in sheep and goats. *Int. J. Appl. Res. Vet. Med.*, 3: 97-1001

Okamoto, M., Nakoo, M, Sako, Y. and Ito (2001). Molecular variation of *Taenia solium* in the world. *South-east Asian J. Trop. Med. Pub.Hlth.*, 32:S90-S93

Paranoli (1550). Cited by Nieto, D. (1982) in "Historical notes on cysticercosis". In: Cysticercosis- present state of knowledge and perspectives (Flisser, A., Willims, K., Laclette, J., Larralde, C., Ridaura, C. and Beltran, F., eds), Academic Press, New York, pp. 2

Pathak, K.M.L. and Gaur, S.N.S. (1989). Prevalence and economic implications of *T. solium* taeniasis and cysticercosis in Uttar Pradesh state of India. *ActaLeid.*, 57: 197-200

Pouedet, M.S., Zoli, A.P., NguekamVondou, L., Assana, E., Speybroeck, N., Berkvens, D., Dorny, P., Brandt, J. and Geerts, S. (2002). Epidemiological survey of swine cysticercosis in two rural communities of West Cameroon. *Vet. Parasitol.*, 106: 45-54

Priyadarshi, S.S., Subhash, C.P. and Pramod, K.S. (2008). Tear IgA-ELISA: A novel and sensitive method for diagnosis of ophthalmic cysticercosis. *Acta Trop.*, 106: 168-174

Rajshekhar, V., Joshi, D.D., Doanh, N.Q., De, N.V., Zhou, X.N. (2003). *Taenia solium* taeniosis/cysticercosis in Asia: epidemiology, impact and issues. *Acta Trop.*, 87: 53-60

Rickard, M.D. and Williams, J.F. (1982). Hydatidosis/Cysticercosis: immune mechanisms and immunization against infection. *Adv. Parasitol.*, 21: 229-296

Román, G., Sotelo, J., Del Brutto, O., Flisser, A., Dumas, M., Wadia, N., Botero, D., Cruz, M., Garcia, H., de Bittencourt, P.R.M., Trelles, L., Arriagada, C., Lorenzana, P., Nash, T.E. and Spina-França, A. (2000). A proposal to declare neurocysticercosis an international reportable disease. *Bull. WHO*, 78: 399-406

Sato, M.O., Yamasaki, H., Sako, Y., Nakao, M., Plancarte, A., Kassuku, A.A., Dorny, P., Geerts, S., Benitez-Ortis, W. and Hashiguchi, Y. (2003). Evaluation of tongue inspection and serology for diagnosis of *T. solium* cysticercosis in swine: usefulness of ELISA using purified glycoproteins and recombinant antigen. *Vet. Parasitol.*, 111: 309-322

Schantz, P.M., Moore, A.C., Munoz, J.L., Hartman, B.J., Schaefer, J.A., Aron, A.M., Persaud, D., Sarti, E., Wilson, M. and Flisser, A. (1992). Neurocysticercosis in an orthodox Jewish community in New York. *New. Eng. J. Med.*, 327: 692-695

Sciutto, E., G. Fragoso, K., Manoutcharian, G. Gevorkian, G. Rosas-Salgado, M., Hernandez-Gonzalez, L., Herrera-Estrella, J., Cabrera-Ponce, F., Lopez-Casillas, C., Gonzalez-Bonilla, A., Santiago-Machuca, F., Ruiz-Perez, J., Sanchez, F.,Goldbaum, A., de Aluja, A.S. and Larralde, C. (2002). New approaches to improve a peptide vaccine against porcine *Taenia solium* cysticercosis. *Arch. Med. Res.*, 33:371-378

Sciutto, E., Martinez, J.J., Villalobos, N.M., Hernandez, M., Jose, M.V., Beltran, C., Rodarte, F., Flores, I., Bobadilla, J.R., Fragoso, G., Parkhouse, M.E., Harrison, L.J. and de Aluja, A.S. (1998). Limitations of current diagnostic procedures for the diagnosis of *T. solium* cysticercosis in rural pigs. *Vet. Parasitol.*, 79: 299-313

Shey-Njila, O., Zoli, P.A., Awah-Ndukum, J., Nguekam, E. Assana, P., Byambas, P., Dorny, J., Brandt and Geerts, S. (2003). Porcine Cysticercosis In Village Pigs Of North-West Cameroon.*J. Helminthol.*, 77: 351-354

Sorvillo, F.J., Portigal, L., DeGiorgio, C., Smith, L., Waterman, S.H., Berlin, G.W. and Ash, L.R. (2004). Cysticercosis mortality in California. *Emerg. Infect. Dis.*,10:465-469

Torres, A., Plancarte, A., Villalobos, A.N., de Aluja, A.S., Navarro, R. and Flisser, A. (1992). Praziquantel treatment of porcine brain and muscle *Taenia solium* cysticercosis, three effects of one day treatment. *Parasitol.Res.*,7: 161-164

Varma, T.K. and Ahluwalia, S.S. (1985). Development of *Taenia solium* in cats and dogs. *Liv. Adv.*,10: 52-53

White, A.C. Jr., Robinson, P. and Kuhn, R. (1997). *Taenia solium* cysticercosis: host-parasite interactions and the immune response. In: Immunopathogenetic Aspects of Disease Induced by Helminth Parasites (eds. Freedman, D.O.),Basel,Karger, pp. 209–230

Wilkins, P.P., Allan, J.C., Verastegui, M., Acosta, M., Easom, A.G., Garcia, H.H., Gonzalez, A.H., Gilman, R.H. and Tsang, V.C.W. (1999). Development of a serologic assay to detect *T. solium*taeniasis. *Am.J.Trop.Med.Hyg.*, 60: 199-4

Willingham, A.L., De N.V., Doanh, N.Q., Cong, L.D., Dung, T.V., Dorny, P., Cam, P.D. and Dalsgaard, A. (2003). Current status of cysticercosis in Vietnam. *Southeast Asian J. Trop. Med. Pub. Hlth.*, 34: S35–S50

World Health Organization (2000). Bringing epilepsy out of the shadows of Africa (Press release, WHO 30, May 4, 2000)

World Health Organization (2001). Epilepsy: an historic over view. WHO Fact sheet 168, Geneva: World Health Organization

Yamasaki, H., Allan, J.C., Sato, M.O., Nakao, M., Sako, Y., Nakaya, K., Qui, D., Mamuti, W.,Craig, P.S. and Ito, A. (2004). DNA differential diagnosis of taeniasis/cysticercosis by multiplex PCR. *J. Clin. Microbiol.*,42: 548-553

Yamasaki, H., Nakao, M., Sako, Y.,Nakaya, K., Sato, M.O. and Ito, A. (2006). Mitochondrial DNA diagnosis for taeniasis and cysticercosis. *Parasitol. Int.*, 55:S81-85

Yamasaki, H., Nakao, M., Sako, Y. Nakaya, K., Sato, M.O., Qui, D., Mamuti, W., Okamoto, M. and Ito, A. (2002). DNA differential diagnosis of human taeniid cestodes by base excision sequence scanning thymine base reader analysis with mitochondrial genes. *J. Clin. Microbiol.*, 40: 3818-3821

Yasuhito, S., Minora, N., Kazuhiro, N., Hiroshi, Y. and Akira, I. (2006). Recombinant antigens for serodiagnosis of cysticercosis and echinococcosis. *Parasitol. Int.*, 55: S69-S73.

❑❑❑

Chapter 9

Theileriosis

Debdatta Ray
Division of Parasitology
IVRI, Izatnagar-245 122, India

Theileriosis is caused by the genus of the tick borne parasitic protozoa *Theileria,* which belongs to the phylum Apicomplexa and is closely related to *Plasmodium*. The two most important species infecting cattle and water buffalo (*Bubalus bubalis*) are *T. parva,* which causes East Coast fever (ECF), and *T. annulata,* which causes tropical theileriosis. *Theileria parva* can also infect African buffalo (*Syncerus caffer*), and waterbucks (*Kobus* spp.), whereas *T. annulata* may occur in yaks and camels. A number of other *Theileria* spp. including *T. mutans, T. buffeli, T. velifera, T. taurotragi* and *T. sergenti,* can also infect domesticated and wild ruminants. Many of these organisms are carried asymptomatically, but some can cause anemia, and concurrent infections may increase the severity of ECF or tropical theileriosis. *Theileria lestoquardi* (formerly *T. hirci*) is the most virulent spp. in sheep and goats. *Theileria separata* and the non-pathogenic spp., *T. ovis* also occur in small ruminants.

Theileriosis causes considerable losses for dairy farmers due to morbidity and mortality of their cattle. The disease is most severe in recently introduced animals and is a constraint on the selective improvement of the genotype of cattle in countries where the disease is endemic by importation of new breeds. In India, tropical theileriosis assumed noticeable importance only after the initiation of the national crossbreeding project in cattle in the beginning of 20th century when exotic breeds of *Bos taurus* or the cross-bred progeny (*Bos indicus* female x *Bos taurus* male) were introduced for improving productivity of Indian milch cattle. The general consensus is that the indigenous breeds of *Bos indicus* are not susceptible to *Theileria*. The Indian breed of cattle "Sahiwals" is inherently much more resistant to *T. annulata* infection than the European breed "Friesians" (Brown, 1996). The introduction of assorted breeds of *Bos taurus*, which came from *Theileria* free zones, upset the epidemiological balance and theileriosis became an emerging disease problem in India.

Epidemiology

Geographical distribution of Theileria spp. : T. parva is found in sub-Saharan Africa. *T. annulata* occurs from southern Europe and the Mediterranean coast through the Middle East and North Africa, and into parts of Asia. These two species are usually not found in the same region excepting probably southern Sudan (Morzaria *et al.*, 1981). *T. mutans* has been found in African and in some Caribbean islands, and is reported also from the U.S. *T. velifera* and *T. taurotragi* occur in Africa, while *T. sergenti* is reported from parts of Asia. *T. buffeli* is widespread, and has been reported from Europe, Asia, Australia, North America and parts of Africa. *T. lestoquardi* is documented in Asia, the Middle East and the parts of Africa and Europe. *T. ovis* and *T. separata* occur in Asia (Bishop *et al.*, 2004).

In India, existence of *T. annulata* has been verified based on tick vector specificity, pathogenicity in naive animals, the pattern of host responses including parasitological features, clinical symptoms and identification of postmortem lesions. The behaviour of field isolates of *T. annulata* from different parts of the country was studied extensively through experimental tick induced infections in naïve calves (Bhattacharyulu *et al.*, 1975; Gill *et al.*, 1976; Subramanium and Naithani, 1979). Earlier report of the existence of *T. mutans* in India, based on serological evidence of the disease (Dhar and Gautam, 1977) is not substantiated by tick vector specificity and other morphological features of the parasite. In many parts of the world the incidence of *T. mutans* is reported on the sole criteria of low pathogenicity and the percentage distribution of the pleomorphic forms (piroplasms) within the erythrocytes. However, it has been shown that *T. mutans* was essentially an African species, it was transmitted by the ticks of the genus *Amblyomma* and this parasite was not always of low pathogenicity in cattle (Uilenburg, 1981). The reported transmission of *T. mutans* by *Hyalomma anatolicum anatolicum* in Sudan (Morzaria *et al.*, 1981) is never confirmed in India.

Transmission and role of vectors : Theileria spp. are transmitted by ticks acting as biological vectors. Iatrogenic transmission can also occur via blood (eg. through reused needles). *Rhipicephalus appendiculatus* is the most important vector for *T. parva,* but *R. zembeziensis* and *R. duttoni* carry this organism in parts of Africa. *T. annulata* is transmitted by ticks in the genus *Hyalomma. Hyalomma* spp. also act as the vectors for *T. lestoquardi, T. ovis* and *T. separata,* while *T. buffeli* and *T. sergenti* are transmitted by *Haemaphysalis* spp. *T. mutans* and *T. velifera* are transmitted by *Amblyomma* spp. Ticks of the genus *Rhipicephalus* spread *T. taurotragi.*

The most common vector spp. in India for *T. annulata* is *Hyalomma anatolicum anatolicum* (Bhattacharyulu *et al.,* 1975). Gill *et al.* (1974) established that *H. detritum,* which is a two host tick and a barn-inhabitant (Pipano, 1974, 1976) also transmitted *T. annulata* and behaved as a three host tick. This would explain the frequent reports of very young calves getting infected with *Theileria,* even when they are tethered in well maintained sheds and not allowed to graze in the pasture.

Transmission of *Theileria* is trans-stadial with larva or nymph picking up the infection from sick or premune animals and the succeeding nymph or adult instars transmitting the sporozoites to animals present in the saliva .Ordinarily, the sporozoites only mature and enter the saliva after the tick attaches to a host for a few days during the blood sucking phase. However, if environmental temperatures are high, infective sporozoites of *T. parva* can develop in ticks on the ground, and may enter the host within hours of attachment. Transovarian transmission does not occur with *Theileria* spp. The accurate determination of *Theileria* infection in tick vectors in the field facilitates the quantitative approach to study the epidemiology of theileriosis. By this method the contact rates of vertebrate hosts with infected ticks and transmission coefficient between ticks and hosts can be estimated. In India, the overall prevalence of *T. annulata* (total number of infected ticks/total number of ticks examined x100) in *H. a. anatolicum* varies from 31 to 64% in different agro-climatic zones, however, the abundance of infection (total number of infected acini in the salivary glands /total number of ticks examined x100) is found to be only 0.9% (Sangwan *et al.,* 1986; Das and Ray, 2003). In contrast, the natural infection rates of *T. parva* in the vector ticks *R. appendiculatus* is generally low and varied from 1.5 to 2.3% in endemic areas of Africa (Leitch and Young, 1981). Both prevalence and abundance of infection are higher in females than male ticks irrespective of species of *Theileria.*

Strain variation of Theileria : The *in vivo* cross-protection test is originally the gold standard for evaluating the strain variations in different countries. In ECF-zones the strain variation is not very much pronounced as partial to complete cross-protection is observed among different strains of *T. parva* (Barnet, 1963, 1968). In contrast, the cross-immunity between different strains of *T. annulata* originating from Algeria, Iran and Israel is only partial or absent (Wilde, 1967; Pipano, 1974). The existence of 12 partially cross-protective strains of *T. annulata* is recorded from Iran (Rafyi *et al.,* 1965). In India, the commonly recognized *T. annulata* strains are named after their place of origin like Izatnagar, Hisar, Ludhiana, Anand, Chennai, Panagarh, Urlikanchan, Bangalore, Jaipur and considerable cross-protection between these strains is reported in limited *in vivo* studies (Gill *et al.,* 1980; Ray *et al.,*1987; Subramanian *et al.,*1987). The strain of *T. annulata* originated from Parbhani (Maharashtra) is found to be more virulent and antigenically distinct in compared to Izatnagar (UP) strain (Saravanan *et al.,* 2003a). MTT tetrazolium salt colorimetric assay is utilized as an *in vitro* marker system to establish a higher replication rate of *T. annulata* (Parbhani) strain in culture of bovine lymphocytes infected with macroschizonts. Higher virulence trait of the Parbhani strain is attributed to its higher rate of replication in compared to other (Saravanan *et al.,* 2003b).

Pathogenesis

Course of infection : At the site of injection by the vector ticks, the sporozoites of *T. annulata* preferentially infects macrophages *in vivo* in the lymph gland nearest to the tick bite. The incubation period for tropical theileriosis is thought to be approximately 1 to 3 weeks. The sporozoites undergo schizogonous replication to generate large number of merozoites which after lysing the host cell, invade erythrocytes and become piroplasms, the developmental stage infectious for ticks. The incubation period for ECF is 8 to 12 days in experimentally infected animals. It might be as long as three weeks in naturally infected animals. A similar series of events occur in *T. parva,* except that T and B cells (principally CD4+ T cells) rather than macrophages/monocytes are invaded by sporozoites (McKeever and

Morrison, 1998; Boulter and Hall, 2000). The severity of infection depends on virulence of the strain, host susceptibility and quantum of infection delivered by the vector ticks (Robinson, 1982). In general, the course of the acute disease may be of 10 to 28 days duration (Subramanian and Naithani, 1979). Cattle that recover from *Theileria* infections usually become carriers for months or years. The carrier animals may exhibit poor productivity and stunted growth.

Clinical symptoms : In ECF, the clinical signs include generalized lymphadenopathy, fever, anorexia and loss of condition with decreased milk yield. Petechiae and ecchymoses may be found on the conjunctiva and oral mucous membranes. Lacrimation, nasal discharge, corneal opacity and diarrhoea can also be seen. Terminally ill animals often develop pulmonary edema, severe dyspnea and a frothy nasal discharge. Some cattle have a fatal condition called "turning sickness". In this form of the disease, infected cells block capillaries in the central nervous system and cause neurological signs.

Tropical theileriosis generally resembles ECF, but these parasites also destroy red blood cells causing jaundice, anemia, and in some cases, haemoglobinuria. Haemorrhagic diarrhoea may be seen in the late stages. Petechiae are often found on the mucous membranes. Neurological signs have been documented in some terminally ill water buffalo, but "turning sickness" does not seem to be a feature of tropical theileriosis in cattle. Abortions can be seen.

Other species of *Theileria* including *T. mutans*, *T. sergenti* and *T. buffeli* can cause anemia in cattle or increase the severity of clinical signs in animals co-infected with *T. parva* or *T. annulata*. On their own, these organisms usually cause mild disease compared to ECF or tropical theileriosis. Some species such as *T. velifera* appear to be non-pathogenic.

T. lestoquardi is the most virulent species in small ruminants, and often causes fatal disease. The clinical signs may include fever, anorexia, weight loss, listlessness, lymphadenopathy, edema of the throat, dyspnea, anemia and icterus. Sub acute, chronic or mild cases can also be seen.

The course and the level of clinical symptoms in *T. annulata* infection have been studied in calves experimentally infected by "ground up tick sporozoite" (GUTS) (Gill *et al.*, 1978; Subramanian and Naithani, 1979; Samantray *et al.*, 1980; Ray and Subramanian, 1987). Generally, the time to onset of fever, swelling in the draining lymph node (when GUTS was given subcutaneously, close to the lymph gland), the maximum schizont index (MSI-number of intra-lymphocytic macroschizont per hundred cells), febrile response and level of maximum erythrocytic parasitaemia are dose dependent with higher doses of GUTS increasing the severity of host responses. The important clinical features of theileriosis are summarized in the Table 1.

Table1: Summary of clinical symptoms

Clinical symptoms	Healthy cattle	Theileriosis
Body condition	Good	Emaciated
Visible mucous membrane	Bright red, moistened	Congested with obvious lacrimation, corneal opacity, out ward visible protrusion of haemorrhagic conjunctiva
Rectal temperature	38.7 ^{0} C	40.6 ^{0} C
Pulse	57 beats /minute	76 beat /minute
Respiration	21 cycles /minute	36 cycle /minute
Lymph node	No swelling, movable, hotless, painless	Greatly swelled (prescapular>parotid> prefemoral), painful and hot during palpation
Urine	Light yellow	Straw yellow
Appetite	Normal	Slightly lost to total refusal to suckle /eat

Post-mortem lesions : Petechial and ecchymotic hemorrhages are often found on the serosal surfaces of internal organs, and the body cavities may contain serous fluid. In acutely infected animals, the lymph nodes are usually enlarged and may be oedematous and haemorrhagic. In chronic cases, they may be shrunken. The spleen is typically enlarged. The liver may also be larger than normal, and white foci of lymphoid infiltration (pseudoinfarcts) may be present in the liver and kidney. Gastrointestinal tract can have signs of hemorrhagic enteritis, particularly in the small intestine and abomasum. Prominent haemorrhagic ulcers and petechae in the abomasum are pathognomonic post-mortem lesions in theileriosis. Such lesions are, however, absent in the omasum, reticulum and rumen. Interlobular emphysema and severe pulmonary edema are common in animals that die of ECF. A frothy exudate may be found around the nostrils and in the trachea and bronchi. The lungs are hyperemic and full of fluid. Pulmonary edema also occurs in goats infected with *T. lestoquardi*.

Morbidity and mortality : Morbidity and mortality are variable and depend on the host's susceptibility, and the strain and dose of the parasite. The case fatality rate for untreated ECF can be as high as 100% in taurine, zebu or sanga cattle from non-endemic areas. In contrast, the morbidity rate approaches 100% among indigenous cattle, but the mortality rate is usually low. Similarly, tropical theileriosis is more severe in introduced breeds, with a mortality rate of 40-90%, while the mortality rate in indigenous cattle can be as low as 3%. The calves under three months old, belonging to either crossbred or pure Indian breeds, are most seriously affected by theileriosis. Thus, in cross-breeding programmes in endemic areas, the improved calves may be particularly valuable. Infections with *Theileria* spp. other than *T. parva* and *T. annulata* are rarely fatal in cattle. In sheep and goats, the morbidity rate from *T. lestoquardi* can approach 100%, with a mortality rate of 46-100%.

Diagnosis

The word "Diagnosis" will include detection, identification and characterization of *Theileria*. It will also include the use of biotechnological methods namely the use of PCR based techniques, monoclonal antibodies and genetically expressed antigens of *Theileria*. The conventional methods of diagnosis are as follows-

(i) *Clinical pathology* : Clinical pathology is comprised of clinical disease recognition, haematology, morbid anatomy and histopathology. Theileriosis should always be suspected in tick-infested animals with a fever and enlarged lymph nodes. Other cardinal symptoms of the disease are listlessness, inappetance, dyspnea, diarrhoea, mucosal discharge from eyes and nostrils. In severe cases death usually occurs in third week of infection.

In stained blood slides, lymphocytosis immediately followed by lymphopenia and signs of anemia like punctate basophilia in RBCs, poikilocytosis and anisocytosis are commonly recorded. The postmortem lesions are very important in diagnosis of the disease in dead animals.

(ii) Microscopic identification of the Parasite : The detection and identification of parasite in Giemsa (or other Romanowsky stain) stained lymph node biopsy smears and thin blood smears associated with evidence of clinical disease is of fundamental importance in diagnosis. Schizonts (Koch's blue bodies) may be found in the cytoplasm of lymphoblasts in lymph node biopsy smears in the acute stage of both ECF and tropical theileriosis (Fig 1). The schizonts also occur in blood leukocytes and in impression smears from a variety of tissues like the lungs, lymph nodes, spleen and kidney collected at necropsy. The macroschizont index (MSI) or percentage parasitosis in lymph node biopsy smears is considered as a guideline in assessment of the severity of the infection in early stage of the disease. The percentage of intra-erythrocytic piroplasms (parasitaemia) is always proportional to the degree of anemia and it dictates the prognosis of the disease to a great extent. The piroplasms are also most commonly sought in detection of the carrier stage. Morphologically the piroplasms of *T. parva* and *T. annulata* are predominantly comma and annular ring shaped, respectively. However, comma, rod and dot shaped structures are also detected for both the parasites (Fig. 1).

(iii) *Tick transmission :* The tick transmission of *Theileria* spp. is so vector specific that it offers the technique of "xenodiagnosis" to confirm the speciation of the pathogen. *T. annulata* can be visualized as pink to purple parasitic mass in hypertrophied acinar cells in the stained (Methyl-green and Pyronin stain) salivary glands of the infected *Hyalomma* spp. (Fig 2). The nucleus of the infected acinar cell also becomes hypertrophied (Das and Ray, 2003). The staining method cannot differentiate between *Theileria* spp. which co-exist in same tick vectors namely *T. parva* and *T. taurotragi* spread by *Rhipicephalus* spp. Similarly *T. lestoquardi*, infecting small ruminants in India, is also transmitted by *Hyalomma* spp. and looks alike *T. annulata* in stained salivary glands of vector ticks. Animal transmission studies may be of use in differentiation.

(iv) *Cross-immunity :*This is mainly important in discrimination of the strains of the species *Theileria.* Although isolates of the parasite from different places of India has been found to be immunologically indistinguishable, the isolate of the parasite originated from "Parbhani" (Maharashtra) is characterized as most virulent. A primary infection with this strain prevents re-infection with other less virulent strains but vice-versa does not occur.

(v) *Serology* : Many serological assays have been applied to detect the humoral anti-*Theileria* antibodies in cattle. Among these tests, the indirect fluorescent antibody test (IFAT) and Enzyme linked immunosorbent assay (ELISA) are widely accepted.

Indirect fluorescent antibody test (IFAT) : This is OIE recommended test for detection of antibodies to *T. annulata/T. parva* infection in cattle. The test is useful for monitoring the post vaccination seroconversion in cattle immunized with attenuated macroschizont of *T. annulata*, in assessing the disease transmission by infected ticks and in epidemiological survey of infections. IFAT can be done either with schizonts of *Theileria* grown in tissue culture or with erythrocytes of infected cattle (Burridge, 1971; Burridge and Kimber, 1972; Dhar and Gautam, 1977, Ray and Subramanian, 1986). For piroplasm antigens, infected erythrocytes are separated by centrifugation from blood of experimentally infected calves (free from plasma and buffy coat) at the height of parasitaemia (20% or more) and washed (x3) thoroughly in cold PBS. The packed infected RBC is diluted with PBS in doubling dilutions and spots of cells (5μl) are prepared on slide and stained with Giemsa. The dilution that gives a single layer of RBC spread uniformly on the spot is selected. Using this suspension, smears/spots of RBC are made on glass slides, air dried, fixed in cold acetone, wrapped in foils and stored in moisture free boxes at -200C.

Antigen can also be made in suspension which is suitable for transportation at 4°C and can be preserved indefinitely at -20°C. The washed cells (infected lymphoblasts/RBC) in final concentration as above are fixed for 24 hours at -20°C by adding two volumes of cold fixative (80% acetone, 0.25% formaline in PBS). The fixed cells are washed x3 times in cold saline and centrifuged at 200g for 20 minutes in cold. The fixed cells are distributed in 0.5 ml aliquots and stored/ transported (at 4°C) after adding 0.2% sodium azide. The cells can be used for making slides when required as above.

IFAT is performed by two step procedures in which the antigen spots on the glass slides are treated with test bovine sera, incubated at room temperature for 30 minutes in a humid chamber, washed and finally treated with anti-bovine rabbit antiserum conjugated with fluorescent dyes. The slides are incubated and washed as before, mounted with a coverslip in 50% glycerol in PBS, ph 8.0 and examined in a fluorescent microscope under ultra violet light. In positive cases, the schizonts/piroplasms are visualized as bodies with apple green fluorescence. Although a sensitive test, cross reaction between species of *Theileria* and *Babesia* occurs commonly in IFAT because being in the same phylum Apicomplexa, these two genera share many common antigens (Morzaria *et al.*, 1994).

Enzyme linked immunosorbent assay : The test was initially standardized with soluble piroplasm antigens when the antibodies to *T. annulata* and *T. parva* were detected on day 13 and day 16 post-infection, respectively (Gray *et al.*, 1980). The test has been successively refined for better sensitivity and specificity by using antigens which are conserved in a particular species of *Theileria* and capable of stimulating long lasting antibody response. The major conserved antigens of *T. parva* as identified by immune sera in immunoblots are 67 kDa (p67) and the polymorphic immunodominant molecule (PIM). The p67 molecule is a stage specific antigen which is expressed by the sporozoites, while the PIM occurs on the surface of sporozoites and schizonts (Toye *et al.*, 1991; Nene *et al.*, 1991). The major conserved antigens of *T. annulata* (Shiels *et al.*, 1989), which are detected in the sporozoites and schizonts are sporozoite surface antigen (SPAG) and surface antigen (TASP). The p67 and PIM have genetical similarities with SPAG and TASP, respectively. The third group of antigens of interest in *Theileria* spp. is the 30 kDa protein families representing moities of 30 to 33 kDa of the merozoite/piroplasm proteins. The 32 kDa merozoite surface protein (TAMS) of *T. annulata* (Shiels *et al.*, 1995) and *T. mutans* (Katende *et al.*, 1990) are characterized in this group. The DNA technology has been applied for preparation of large quantities of these antigens for development of diagnostic ELISA. The polymorphism in size exhibited by some of these antigens like PIM did not become a hindrance for serology. The purified recombinant antigens are used to coat the microtitre plates before introduction of test serum. This is followed by a second antibody, anti bovine immunoglobulins conjugated to horse radish peroxidase. The reaction is revealed by the addition of the substrate. The assay is simple to perform because negative sera can be discriminated from positive sera by the visual detection of the intensity of colour developed with the substrate. However, for the purpose of standardization, accurate diagnosis and interpretation of data an ELISA reader is required. For the future, development of more "field friendly" test like dot based ELISA with specific purified recombinant antigens is desirable.

(vi) *Biochemistry* : For biochemical differentiation, the piroplasms of *T. annulata* and *T. parva* is freed from blood of infected calves by suitable methods. Lysates of the purified piroplasms and control host cell material were examined electrophoretically for several enzymes. Zymograms stained for glucose phosphate isomerase showed distinct differences between the host cell enzyme pattern and parasite enzyme patterns. The isoenzyme pattern of *T. annulata* piroplasms differed from the isoenzyme pattern of *T. parva* piroplasms (Melrose *et al.*, 1980).

(vii) *Differential diagnosis* : In cattle, the differential diagnosis for theileriosis includes heart water disease, hemorrhagic septicemia, trypanosomosis, babesiosis, Rift Valley fever and malignant catarrhal fever. In sheep and goats, *T. lestoquardi* infections must be distinguished from babesiosis, Rift Valley Fever and malignant catarrhal fever.

(viii) *Biotechnological methods* : The recombinant DNA technology is mainly used to prepare purified antigens because the low abundance of the conserved antigens in the various parasite stages precludes biochemical purification. The DNA probe of *T. annulata* TaT17 and TaT21 are used to hybridize the DNA finger printings (RFLP) of different stocks of *T. annulata* to reveal genetic polymorphisms (Ben Miled *et al.*, 1994). However, the DNA hybridization technique has not been used as a routine diagnostic method.

The monoclonal antibodies to *T. annulata* have been raised against a number of life cycle stages of the parasite: schizont, piroplasm and sporozoites. Such antibodies are tried directly in antigen trapping ELISA to detect persistent circulating antigens in infected animals. They may also be used in affinity columns to purify native antigen, as a primary selective coat on the surface of wells in an ELISA plate in a competitive ELISA to identify specific antibodies within the test sera and as a reference positive serum in IFAT.

The technique of PCR is found to be sensitive in detecting very low levels of parasitosis/parasitaemia in lymph node biopsy samples and blood of carrier cattle. The PCR also provided an easier method to detect infection in the vector ticks for epidemiological studies as the staining of dissected salivary glands of the ticks is cumbersome, particularly when large sample sizes of ticks must be processed (Das and Ray, 2003). The genus and species specific oligonucleotide primers designed from genes encoding ribosomal RNA of *Theileria* have been used in PCR assays. The amplification of a 372 bp small subunit ribosomal DNA is used as a detection method of *T. annulata* infection in lymph gland biopsy (Ray *et al.*, 1999) and blood (Roy *et al.*, 2000) of cattle. The method is highly effective to detect and differentiate infection in lymph glands much earlier than the schizont specific antibodies are detected by serological tests. The early detection of the disease may be useful to impart chemotherapy prior to onset of severe schizont induced pathology. A combination of PCR and RFLP is implied to differentiate *B. bigemina* and *T. annulata* infection in which the restriction enzyme *kpn*1 yielded specific 466 and 98 bp DNA fragments in the PCR product indicative of *T. annulata* infection (Ravindran *et al.*, 2007).

Treatment

Tetracyclines : The tetracyclines has a suppressive effect on the schizogony of *Theileria,* if applied in multiple doses during the incubation period after an experimental infection, however, treatment after appearance of clinical symptoms is not useful.

Quinazolinones (Halofuginone) : The coccidiostat halofuginone lactate given orally at a dose of 1.2 mg/kg body weight as a single dose or two doses in 2-4 days intervals is found effective against schizonts of *Theileria.* But this drug is reported to have no effect on sporozoites and piroplasm stages of the parasite.

Nephthoquinones (Parvaquone, Buparvaquone) : "Menoctone", a hydroxynethoquinone is found to be effective against *T. parva* infection in a single injection at a dose rate of 10 mg/kg body weight. A cheaper analog with generic name "parvaquone" (Clexon, Coopers Animal Health Ltd., UK) is effective against theileriosis at a dose rate of 20 mg/kg body weight of cattle. Another analogue, "buparvaquone" (Butalex-Coopers Animal Health Ltd., UK) is more effective in the treatment of both experimental and natural infections of *T. annulata* and *T. parva* in cattle. In India, the drug is marketed by Sarabhai Zydus Animal Health product. Butalex is presented in 20 milliliter vials containing 50 mg buparvaquone per ml. The drug is recommended as 1ml intramuscularly per 20 kg body weight of cattle. In severe theileriosis, a repeat dose is required within 48-72 hours of initial injection. Milk and meat of the treated cattle are recommended as unfit for human consumption for 48 and 42 days, respectively following the treatment.

In addition to effective specific chemotherapy, supportive therapies for anaemia and secondary bacterial infections are necessary for successful treatment of theileriosis.

Control

The basic strategies for the control of theileriosis are control of vectors, vaccination of cattle with tissue culture schizont vaccine and effective chemotherapy. These methods are adopted in different endemic countries with variable success.

Control of vectors : The use of chemical acaricides belonging to the groups "organophosphates" and "synthetic pyrethroids" is the major tick control strategy in cattle. The chemicals are applied by spraying or dipping the animals in acaricide solution. However, the use of acaricides is often accompanied by serious drawbacks, including the selection of acaricide resistant ticks, environmental contaminations and contamination of milk and meat products with drug residues. The use of acaricides is also beset with limitations particularly in the three host ticks like *Hyalomma,* because of the availability of various alternative hosts other than cattle and greater length of time spent by these ticks off the hosts. At present, the development of environment friendly "herbal extracts" having proven acaricidal properties constitutes a major research thrust area in integrated control of pests. Efforts are also afoot to develop anti-tick vaccine in the line of vaccines used in Cuba (Gavac) and Australia (Tick guard).

Live vaccine against theileriosis : The live sporozoite derived vaccine along with subsequent treatment (infection and treatment method) has been widely used for controlling *T. parva* infection in Africa. In this method, cattle are deliberately infected with sporozoite stabilates containing pathogenic stocks of *T. parva* and subsequently treated with anti-*Theileria* drugs (Radly, 1981). Cocktail of different isolates of *T. parva* supplemented with *T. laurencei* stock engendered acceptable protection against field challenge (Mutugi *et al.*, 1988). The live sporozoite vaccine of *T. annulata* from infected ticks accompanied by chemoprophylactic treatment with tetracycline or buparvaquone is also formulated (Gill *et al.*, 1978; Dhar *et al.*, 1990). However, the method has not been applied in routine vaccination in the field.

The live attenuated vaccine of *T. annulata* is produced by prolonged *in vitro* cultivation of lymphoblasts of cattle infected with macroschizonts of *T. annulata* (Pipano and Tsur, 1966). The attenuated schizonts do not evoke parasitaemia or clinical symptoms but confer protection when inoculated in naive cattle. Complete attenuation of schizonts is reported after *in vitro* cultivation for 600-900 days depending on the nature of the isolates (Subramanian *et al.*, 1986,

1988; Singh, 1990). The attenuated cell line of bovine lymphoblasts infected with *T. annulata* (Tunisian isolate) is used at passage 100 (p100) of culturing in RPMI medium (Darghouth *et al.,* 1996). The time required for the attenuation of the macroschizonts appeared to be proportional to the virulence of the isolate of *T. annulata* as well as the rate of replication of the infected lymphoblastoid cells (Saravanan *et al.,* 2003b).

The protection engendered by the attenuated schizont vaccine is evaluated by laboratory challenge with live infected ticks or with ground up tick sporozoites (GUTS) inoculated through syringe passage. The results of such challenge ranged from no clinical response at all (Gill *et al.,* 1976; Subramanian *et al.,* 1988; Khatri *et al.,* 2001) through mild transient clinical reactions with low parasitaemia (Khdier and Latif, 1991), to death from acute theileriosis (Shukla and Sharma, 1991). In endemic areas, single vaccination appears to be adequate for protection when the animals receive continuous challenge from natural tick infestation (Ray and Bansal, 1997). The attenuated schizont vaccine of *T. annulata* was commercialized under the trade name of "Raksha Vac-T" and is produced and marketed by Indian Immunological at Hyderabad, India. The live schizont vaccine of *T. annulata* is a successful commercial endeavor in spite of the drawbacks like continuous requirement of liquid nitrogen for storage and transportation of this vaccine.

It is not possible to produce an attenuated vaccine to *T. parva,* as *T. parva* requires up to two orders of magnitude more schizonts in order to achieve transfer to the new host cells after inoculation. This transfer of the attenuated schizonts present in the vaccine to the host cells is considered as essential event for mounting immunity in the host. A suggested reason for this is that the macrophage targets of *T. annulata* are phagocytes and thus, the schizont has a natural, efficient route of entry, whilst the preferred host of *T. parva* is non-phagocytic T cell (Boulter and Hall, 2000).

Recombinant antigens as vaccine : Recombinant proteins of both *T. annulata* and *T. parva* are tried to immunize cattle to overcome the drawbacks associated with live vaccine. However, till now none of these proteins could be used for any commercial vaccine production. Immunization trial with full length sporozoite surface antigen (SPAG 1) of *T. annulata* mixed with either saponin based adjuvant (SBA) or immunostimulating complexes (ISCOMs) provided partial protections in naive calves against a challenge infection with sporozoites of *T. annulata* (Boulter *et al.,* 1988). The immune calves exhibit significant level of anti-SPAG antibodies and T-cell proliferative responses. There is a synergistic effect of vaccination of calves with both attenuated macroschizont vaccine and full length SPAG protein of *T. annulata* (Darghouth *et al.,* 2006). Immunization with recombinant p67 protein (surface protein of sporozoite of *T. parva*) rendered protection in two third of the experimental cattle against ECF. There is a lack of CMIR in hosts despite high specific antibody titre (Musoke *et al.,* 1995). A considerable sequence homology, serological cross reactivity and degree of cross-species protection between SPAG1 and p67 genes is found showing a prospect of developing a common vaccine for *T. annulata* and *T. parva* (Hall *et al.,* 2000). The allelic forms of Tams1 (Tams1-1 and Tams1-2) encoding 30 and 32 kDa major merozoite surface antigens of *T. annulata* are cloned and characterized. The recombinant proteins produced in *Escherichia coli* as well as in *Salmonella typhimurium* is recognized by monoclonal antibodies specific against 30 kDa protein and polyclonal serum of calf immunized with sporozoites of *T. annulata.* The calves immunized with adjuvanted recombinant proteins of Tams1-1 and Tams1-2, showed specific humoral antibody response and partial protection against challenge infection with homologous strain of *T. annulata* (d'Oliveira *et al.,* 1997).

Conclusions/future projections

One of the major constraints of the crossbreeding project in India was the emerging higher susceptibility of the exotic breeds and their F1 crossbred progenies to the tick-borne haemoparasite infections like *T. annulata* and the control was specifically problematic due to ubiquitous distribution of vector ticks. The interbreeding in crossbred cows although caused decline in the progress of milk production but it lowered the exotic inheritance and the susceptibility to diseases including bovine theileriosis. The presence of ubiquitous carrier status of *T. annulata,* particularly in nondescript indigenous cattle, contributes to development of an "endemic stability". Thus, the incidence of tropical theileriosis in India is gradually declined over the past decades although a high rate of seroprevalence is detected in the population of cross bred cattle (Bansal *et al.,* 1987). However, immunosuppression resulting from stress due to intercurrent diseases, malnutrition, pregnancy, parturition causes "endemic instability" and manifestation of clinical disease.

The most popular current control method for theileriosis is the live attenuated cell culture vaccine. However, due to declining incidence of the disease in successive generations of cross bred cattle, the live attenuated macroschizont vaccine of *T. annulata* has a low adoption rate through out the country excepting in some regions. The attempts to immunize cattle with genetically developed antigens have not been a commercial success till the present time. A future strategy of dual immunization of cattle with tick antigen and associated pathogens transmitted by the tick is also advocated with a view to achieve integrated protection in the host. Development of resistance in cattle against the vector ticks is shown to be effective in reducing the ability of the ticks to transmit *T. parva* (Fivaz *et al.,* 1989) or *T. annulata* (Rubaire- Akiki, 1990) infections. Reduction in the growth rate and viability of *T. annulata* infection in the salivary glands of ticks feeding on calves immunized with purified larval antigens of *H. a. anatolicum* is also reported (Das *et al.,* 2005). These studies indicated the prospect of blockade of transmission of theileriosis by immunization against vector ticks.

References

Bansal, G.C., Ray, D., Srivastava, R.V.N. and Subramanian, G. (1987). Seroprevalence of bovine theileriosis in some farms of India. *Indian J. Anim. Sci.,* 57: 366-368

Barnett, S.F. (1963). The biological races of bovine *Theileria* and their host-parasite relationship. In: "Immunity to Protozoa" (eds. Garnham, P.C.C, Pierce, A.E. and Roitt, I.), Blackwell Science Publication, Oxford, pp.180-195

Barnett, S.F. (1968). Theileriasis. In "Infectious Blood diseases of Man and Animals ", Vol. 2 (eds. Weinman, D. and Ristic, M.), Academic Press, pp. 269-329

Ben Miled, K. Dellagi, G. Bernardi, T. R., Melrose, M., Darghouth, A., Bouattour, J., Kinnaird, B., Shiels, A., Tait and Brown, C. G. D. (1994). Genomic and phenotypic diversity of Tunisian *Theileria annulata* isolates. *Parasitol.,* 108: 51-60

Bhattacharyulu,Y., Chaudhri, R.P. and Gill, B.S. (1975). Transtadial transmission of *Theileria annulata* through common ixodid ticks infesting Indian cattle. *Parasitol.,* 71: 1-7

Bishop, R., Musoke, A., Morzaria, S., Gardner, M. and Nene, V. (2004). *Theileria*: intracellular protozoan parasites of wild and domestic ruminants transmitted by ixodid ticks. *Parasitol.,* 129 Suppl.: S271-283

Boulter, N.R. and Hall, F.R. (2000). Immunity and vaccine development in the bovine theileriosis. *Adv. Parasitol.,* 44: 42–97

Boulter, N.R., Brown, C.G., Kirvar, E., Glass, E., Campbell, J., Morzaria, S., Nene, V., Musoke, A., d'Oliveira, C., Gubbels, M.J., Jongejan, F. and Hall, F.R. (1988). Different vaccine strategies used to protect against *Theileria annulata*. *Ann. NY Acad. Sci.*, 849: 234–246

Brown, C.G.D. (1996). DFAID Animal health Programme. R5569–The epidemiology and control of bovine theileriosis.

Burridge, M.J. (1971). Application of the indirect fluorescent antibody test in experimental East coast fever (*Theileria parva* infection in cattle). *Res. Vet. Sci.*, 12: 338-341

Burridge, M.J. and Kimber, C.D. (1972). The indirect fluorescent antibody test for experimental East coast fever (*Theileria parva* infection in cattle). Evaluation of a cell culture schizont antigen. *Res. Vet. Sci.*, 13: 451-455

Darghouth, M.A., Ben Miled, L., Bouattour, A., Melrose, T.R., Brown, C.G.D. and Kilani, M. (1996). A preliminary study on the attenuation of Tunisian schizont infected cell lines of *Theileria annulata*. *Parasitol. Res.*, 82: 647-655

Darghouth, M.A., Nicola, R., Boulter, N.R., Gharbi, M., Sassi, L., Tait, A. and Hall, R. (2006). Vaccination of calves with an attenuated cell line of *Theileria annulata* and the sporozoite antigen SPAG-1 produces a synergistic effect. *Vet. Parasitol.*, 142: 54-62

Das, G. and Ray, D.D. (2003). PCR- based detection of *Theileria annulata* infection in ticks collected from cattle of West Bengal, India. *J. Vet. Parasitol.*, 17: 11-14

Das, G., Ghosh, S. and Ray, D.D. (2005). Reduction of *Theileria annulata* infection in ticks fed on calves immunized with purified larval antigens of *Hyalomma anatolicum anatolicum*. *Trop. Anim. Hlth. Prod.*, 37: 345-361

Dhar, S. and Gautam, O.P. (1977). Indirect fluorescent antibody test for serodiagnosis in cattle infected with *Theileria annulata*. *Indian J. Anim. Sci.*, 47: 720-723

Dhar, S., Malhotra, D.V., Bhushan, C. and Gautam, O.P. (1990). Chemoimmunoprophylaxis against tropical theileriosis in young calves: a comparison between buparvaquone and long-acting oxytetracycline. *Res. Vet. Sci.*, 49:110-112

d'Oliveira, C., Feenstra, A., Vos, H., Osterhaus, A.D., Shiels, B.R., Cornelissen, A.W. and Jongejan, F. (1997). Induction of protective immunity to *Theileria annulata* using two major merozoite surface antigens presented by different delivery systems. *Vaccine*, 15: 1796–1804

Fivaz, B.H. (1989). Immune suppression induced by the brown ear tick *Rhipicephalus appendiculatus* Neumann, 1901. *J. Parasitol.*, 75: 946-952

Gill, B.S., Bhattacharyulu,Y., Kaur, D. and Sing, A. (1976). Vaccination against bovine tropical theileriasis (*Theileria annulata). Nature*, 264: 355-356

Gill, B.S., Bhattacharyulu, Y., Kaur, D. and Sing, A. (1978). Chemoprophylaxis with tetracycline drugs in the immunization of cattle against *T. annulata* infection. *Int. J. Parasitol.*, 8: 467-469

Gill, B.S., Bansal, G.C., Bhattacharyulu, Y., Kaur, D. and Singh, A. (1980). Immunological relation-ship between strains of *T. annulata* (Dschunkowsky and Luhs, 1904). *Res. Vet. Sci.*, 29: 93-97

Gill, B.S., Kaur, D. and Bhattacharyulu, Y. (1974). Transmission of *Theileria annulata* through the tick *Hyalomma detritum* (Schulze, 1919). *Bul. Int. Epizoot.*, 81: 805-811

Gray, M.A., Luckins, A.G., Rae, P.F. and Brown, C.G.D. (1980). Evaluation of an enzyme immune-assay for serodiagnosis of infection with *T. parva* and *T. annulata. Res. Vet. Sci.*, 29: 360-366

Hall, R., Boulter, N.R., Brown, C.G.D., Wilkie, G., Kirvar, E., Nene, V., Musoke, A.J., Glass, E.J. and Morzaria, S.P. (2000). Reciprocal cross-protection induced by sporozoite antigen SPAG1 from *Theileria annulata* and p67 from *Theileria parva*. *Parasite Immunol.*, 22: 223-230

Katende, J.M., Godderis, B.M., Morzaria, S.P., Nkonge, C.G. and Musoke, A.J. (1990). Identification of a *Theileria mutans* specific antigen for use in an antigen and antibody detection ELISA. *Parasite Immunol.*, 12: 419-433

Khatri, N., Nichani, A.K., Sharma, R.D., Khatri, M., Malhotra, D.V. (2001). Effect of vaccination in the field with *Theileria annulata* (Hissar) cell culture vaccine on young calves borne during winter season. *Vet. Res. Comm.*, 25: 179-188

Khdier, I.A., and Latif, B.M.A. (1991). Immunization of cattle against *Theileria annulata* infection using schizonts propagated in tissue culture. *Indian Vet. J.*, 68: 209-214

Leitch, B.L. and Young, A.S. (1981). In "Advances in the control of theileriosis. Proceedings of international conference Nairobi, Kenya, February 9-13, 1981 (eds. Irvin, A.D., Cunningham, M.P. and Young, A.S.), Martinus Nijhoff, The Hague, pp. 63-65

McKeever, D.J., Morrison, W.I. (1998). Novel vaccines against *Theileria parva*: prospects for sustainability. *Int. J. Parasitol.*, 28: 693–706

Melrose, T. R., Brown, C.G.D. and Sharma, R.D. (1980). Glucose phosphate isomerase isoenzyme patterns in bovine lymphoblastoid cell lines infected with *Theileria annulata* and *Theileria parva*, with an improved visualization method using meldola blue. *Res. Vet. Sci.*, 29: 298-304

Morzaria, S.P., Tatchell, R.J., Minor, R., Pederson, V., Julia, L., Rahim, A., Dyson, D. and Van, Aarle, F.A.M. (1981). Preliminary studies on the epidemiology of theileriosis in eastern eqatoria province of Sudan. In: "Advances in the control of theileriosis". Proceedings of international conference, Nairobi, Kenya, Feb. 9-13, 1981 (eds. Irvin, A.D., Cunningham, M.P. and Young, A.S.), Martinus Nijhoff, The Hague, p. 83-85

Morzaria, S., Nene, V., Musoke, A.J. and Bishop, R. (1994). Use of applicable biotechnological methods for diagnosing haemoparasites. Proceeding of the expert consultation FAO of United Nations, Merida, Mexico, October 4-6, 1993, pp.164-173

Musoke, A.J., Nene, V. and McKeever, D.J. (1995). Epitope specificity of bovine immune responses to the major surface antigen of *T. parva* sporozoites. In: chanock, R.M., Brown, F., Ginsberg, H.S., Norrby, E. (eds.). *Molecular approaches to the control of infectious diseases*. Cold Spring Harbor: Cold Spring Harbor laboratory Press, pp. 57-61

Mutugi, J.J., Young, A.S., Maritim, A.C., Ndungu, S.G., Linyonyi, A., Ngumi, P.N., Mining, S.K., Leitch, B.L., Stagg, D.A., Grootenhuis, J.G., Kariuki, D.P., Morzaria, S.P. and Dolan, T.T. (1988). Parasite stock used for East Coast Fever immunization in Kenya. In: T.T. Dolan (eds.), *Theileriosis in Eastern, Central and South Africa*. ILRAD, Nairobi, Kenya, pp. 39-45

Nene, V., Iams, K.P. and Musoke, A.J. (1991). Molecular characterization of a *Theileria parva* surface sporozoite antigen. *Vaccine*, 91: 369- 373

Pipano, E. (1974). Immunological aspect of *T. annulata* infection. *Bul. Int. Des. Epizoot.*, 81: 139-156

Pipano, E. (1976). Basic principals of *Theileria annulata* control. In: *Theileriosis, Report workshop, Nairobi, Kenya, December 7- 9, 1976* (eds. Hensen, J.B. and Campbel, M.), IDRC, Ottawa, Canada, pp.8-11

Pipano, E. and Tsur, I. (1966). Experimental immunization against *Theileria annulata* with a tissue culture vaccine. *Lab. Trials Refuah Vet.*, 23: 186-194

Radley, D.E. (1981). Infection and treatment method of immunization against theileriosis. Irvin A.D., Cunningham, M.P. and Young, A.S. (eds.), Martinus Njhoff, The Hague, pp. 227-237

Ravindran, R., Saravanan, B.C., Rao, J.R., Misra, A.K., Bansal, G.C. and Ray, D.D. (2007). A PCR-RFLP method for simultaneous detection of *Babesia bigemina* and *Theileria annulata* infection of cattle. *Cur. Sci.*, 93: 1840-1843

Ray, D.D. and Bansal, G.C. (1997). Duration of immunity in calves vaccinated with attenuated macroschizonts of *Theileria annulata*. *J. Vet. Parasitol.*, 11: 197-199

Ray, D.D. and Subramanian, G. (1986). Time course of antibody response to *Theileria annulata*. *Indian J. Exp. Biol.*, 24: 471-473

Ray, D.D. and Subramanian, G. (1987). *Theileria annulata*: Dose dependent virulence to bovines. *Indian J. Parasitol.*, 10: 181-183

Ray, D., Roy, K.C., Bansal, G.C. and Singh, R.K. (1999). Direct assessment of *Theileria annulata* infection in lymph gland of cattle by polymerase chain reaction. *Indian J. Anim. Sci.*, 69: 951-52

Ray, D.D., Bansal, G.C., Srivastava, R.V.N. and Subramanian, G. (1987). Characterisation of an isolate of *T. annulata* from Panagarh (West Bengal). *J. Vet. Parasitol.*, 1: 31-34

Rafyi, A., Maghami, G. and Hooshmand, P. (1965). The virulence of *Theileria annulata* and premonition against bovine theileriosis in Iran. *Bull. Off. Int. Epizoot.*, 64: 441-446

Robinson, P.M. (1982). *T. annulata* and its transmission- a review. *Trop. Anim. Hlth. Prod.*, 14: 3-12

Roy, K.C., Ray, D.D., Bansal, G.C. and Singh, R.K. (2000). Detection of *Theileria annulata* carrier cattle by PCR. *Indian J. Exp. Biol.*, 38: 283-284

Rubaire-Akiki, C.M. (1990). The effect of bovine tick resistance on the susceptibility of *H. a. anatolicum* to infection with *Theileria annulata* (Ankara). *Vet. Parasitol.*, 34: 273-288

Samantray, S.N., Bhattacharyulu, Y. and Gill, B.S. (1980). Immunization of calves against bovine theileriasis (*Theileria annulata*) with graded doses of sporozoites and irradiated sporozoites. *Int. J. Parasitol.*, 10: 355-358

Saravanan, B.C., Bansal, G.C. and Ray, D.D. (2003a). A comparative study on the clinico-parsitological responses of Izatnagar and Parbhani isolates of *Theileria annulata* in cattle. *J. Vet. Parasitol.*, 17: 161-162

Saravanan, B.C., Sreekumar, C., Bansal, G.C. (2003b). A rapid MTT colorimetric assay to assess the proliferative index of two Indian strains of *Theileria annulata*. *Vet. Parasitol.*, 113: 211-216

Sangwan, A.K., Chhabra, M.B. and Samantaray (1986). *Theileria* infectivity of *Hyalomma* ticks in Haryana, India. *Trop. Anim. Hlth. Prod.*, 18: 149-154

Shiels, B., Hall, R., Glascodine, J., Mcdougall, C., Harrison, C., Taracha, E., Brown, D. and Tait, A. (1989). Characterization of surface polypeptides on different life cycle stages of *T. annulata*. *Mol. Bioch. Parasitol.*, 34: 209-220

Shiels, B.., Oliveira, D., Christine, Mckeller, S., Ben-Miled, L., Kawazu, Shin-Lchiro, Hide, G. (1995). Selection of diversity at putative glycosylation sites in the immunodominant merozoite/piroplasm surface antigen of *Theileria* parasites. *Mol. Bioch. Parasitol.*, 34: 209-220

Shukla, P.C. and Sharma, R.D. (1991). Immunization of bovine calves with cell culture vaccine against *Theileria annulata*. *Acta Vet.*, BRNO, 60: 79-86

Singh, D.K. (1990). Method currently used for the control of *Theileria annulata*: their validity and proposal for future control strategies. *Parasitologia*, 32: 33-40

Subramanian, G. and Naithani, R.C. (1979). Studies on biology and control of theileriasis. Final ICAR scheme report, IVRI, Izatnagar

Subramanian, G., Ray, D. and Naithani, R.C. (1986). *In vitro* culture and attenuation of macro-schizonts of *T. annulata* (Dschunkowsky and Luhs, 1904). *Indian J. Anim. Sci.*, 56: 174-82

Subramanian, G., Naithani, R.C. and Ray, D.D. (1987). Cross- reactions among four isolates of *T. annulata* from India. *Vet. Parasitol.*, 25: 75-77

Subramanian, G., Srivastava , R.V.N., Bansal, G.C. and Ray, D.D. (1988). A field trial with live schizont vaccine for control of bovine theileriosis. *Indian J. Anim. Sci.*, 58: 635-639

Toye, P.G., Goddeeris, B.M., Iams, K. Musoke, A.J. and Morrison, W.I. (1991). Characterization of a polymorphic immunodominant molecule in sporozoites and schizonts of *Theileria parva. Parasite Immunol.*, 13:49-62

Uilenberg, G. (1981). Theilerial species of domestic livestock. In: *Advances in the control of theileriasis.* Proceedings of the international conference, *Nairobi, Kenya, February 9-13, 1981* (eds. Irving, A.D., Cunningham, M.P. and Young, A.S.), Martinus Nijhoff, The Hague, pp. 4-37

Wilde, J.K.H. (1967). East Coast Fever. In: Advances in Veterinary Science, Vol. II (eds. Brandly, C.A. and Charles, C.), AP, New York, pp. 207-253

□□□

Chapter 10

Tropical Fasciolosis in Ruminants: Epidemiology, Pathophysiology, Diagnosis and Control

R. Godara, R. Katoch and Anish Yadav
Division of Veterinary Parasitology, Faculty of Veterinary Sciences and Animal Husbandry, Sher-e-Kashmir University of Agricultural Sciences and Technology-Jammu, R.S. Pura-181 102

Introduction

Fasciolosis is an important digenetic trematode infection of ruminants. Since decades, the disease has been recognized as an incessant major constraint on ruminant productivity and a recognized impediment to global food production of animal origin (Kendall, 1954; Schillhorn VanVeen, 1980; Kumar *et al.*, 1982; Okao, 1984; Swarup and Pachauri, 1987a; Bhatia *et al.*, 1989; Roy and Tandon, 1992; Gupta and Singh, 2002; Garg *et al.*, 2009; Sharma and Godara, 2010; Sharma *et al.*, 2011). In India, the disease is primarily caused by three species of *Fasciola* (*F. gigantica, F. hepatica* and *F. jacksoni*). Of these, *F. gigantica* has been a fluke of major pathogenic and economic consequence to ruminant industry. The parasite survives in the bile ducts of primarily ruminants and causes high mortality in growing stock and morbidity incidental to loss of metabolisable energy, anaemia, poor live weight gain and feed conversion efficiency, stress and reduced productivity in adults (Mehra *et al.*, 1999; Yadav *et al.*, 1999b; Ganga *et al.*, 2007; Edith *et al.*, 2010a, b). In recent past, global losses incidental to fasciolosis were estimated over US $3,200 million per annum. The disease is widely prevalent in the country. The establishment of new irrigation systems (irrigation channels and dams) has further increased the distribution, creating more water bodies suitable habitats for propagation of Lymnaeid snails that act as intermediate hosts. Thus, the semi-arid and arid regions of western India, where the parasite was hitherto non-existing, the disease has been started emerging.

Herein, the varied epizootiological factors that offers possible explanation to pathophysiological clinical signs, deleterious effects of the tropical liver fluke involving hepato-biliary system, haemopoitic system, endocrine glands and their secretions, oxidative stress, altered metabolism, and significant fall in food conversion efficiency with unaffected digestibility of nutrients have been described. Besides, the developments and significance of successful immunodiagnostic approaches for detecting the disease during early prepatency and feasibility of developing a cost effective immunoprotection strategies against tropical fasciolosis have been discussed.

Life cycle and epizootiology

The epizootiological determinants and prevalence of the disease mainly influenced by agro-climate of the region, exposure of ruminant population to *F. gigantica* contaminated biomass on grazing lands and in cultivated crop residue used as fodder, quantum and periodic intake of *F. gigantica* metacercariae and their release by the infected snail host in the surroundings, above all scientific healthcare and management of the host. Recent epizootiological studies have shown that *F. gigantica* is better adapted to buffaloes than cattle and/or small ruminants.

The parasite matures in the bile ducts of the definitive host, produces oval, operculated, pale yellow eggs. The incubation period for hatching of eggs varies from 7-20 days depending upon the temperature which ranges from 13-37°C (Thapar and Tandon, 1952). In winter months, the period may prolong, with lower hatching rate (Sarwar, 1950; Khajuria, 1981). Khajuria (1981) demonstrated that the hatching did not occur at freezing temperature, the eggs survived at different stages of development (4-16 cell stage) up to 18 months at 4°C and they hatched when kept at room temperatures (29-35°C). The development of *F. gigantica* eggs is not affected by the depth of the water. After hatching of eggs, miracidia are released in the water and could survive for 18-26 hours prior to invading and penetrating into the body of susceptible snail intermediate host. Temperatures between 25-26°C is necessary for the purpose. The penetration is maximal after few hours of their emergence till 4-5 hours before their death.

In Indian subcontinent, fresh water snail *Lymnaea auricularia* var *rufescens* (Kendall, 1954; Dutt and Bali, 1977; Khajuria, 1981) or *L. acuminata* (Bhalerao, 1933; Thapar and Tandon, 1952), belonging to family Lymnaeidae, act as intermediate host for *F. gigantica*. These snails breed throughout the year in favourable environmental conditions. In India, these snail species do not appear as the sole intermediate host. In Kashmir, *L. auricularia sensu stricto* (Dhar and Sharma, 1986) and in Sikkim, *L. andersoniana* (Katiyar *et al.*, 1983) have also been recorded as intermediate hosts for *F. gigantica*. These snail species are phytophagous and true aquatics, adapted well to a slight alkaline condition and are found in low lying swampy areas with slow moving water, small water bodies, streams and/or spring discharging luke warm underground water and ponds, with high oxygen content and abundant aquatic vegetation, beside in irrigated rice fields in lowland tropical areas (Kendall, 1954; Gupta and Singh, 2002; Sharma *et al.*, 2011). Sluggish putrid streams, swift current, turbid water with suspended organic matter and deep water without much aquatic vegetation appear unfavourable for the development of snail vector of *F. gigantica* (Khajuria, 1981). Patnaik and Ray (1968) from Orissa reported that the distribution of snail vector of *F. gigantica* is limited to permanent bodies of water and are seldom found in stagnant water. Agricultural crops frequently irrigated with contaminated water, constituted the most preferred and suitable sites for shelter, propagation, breeding and burrowing of the snail population. In dry conditions, *L. auricularia* survives periods of desiccation (about one month) and plays an important role in the epidemiology of tropical fasciolosis.

Snails once infected with *F. gigantica*, normally do not accept other trematode infections, life-long remain positive for the infection, and have a shorter life span of 5-85 days than non-infected snails of 50-150 days (Dhar and Sharma, 1986). In an experimental infection, Prasad (1989) observed that ten to fourteen mm long *L. auricularia* snails, aged less than 14 weeks were most susceptible to *F. gigantica* miracidial infection. These snails had smaller prepatent but longer period of patency discharging *F. gigantica* cercariae. The survival of the infected snail in nature depends upon optimum temperature, snail density, altered aquatic pH and the depth of the water table.

A detailed geographical distribution and ecology of *L. auricularia* var *rufescens* was studied by Patnaik and Ray (1968) in Orissa and they reported that only 0.14% snails were harboured developmental stages of *F. gigantica*. In an another study at Bareilly, 9% snails shed cercariae of *F. gigantica* (Gupta and Yadav, 1994), while Garg *et al.* (2009) demonstrated that 5.48% snails were positive for larval stages of *F. gigantica* in different geo-climatic regions of North India. In a detailed study, Yadav *et al.* (2007) documented two annual peaks of infection in snails on the basis of meteorological data and an analysis of snail population *vis-à-vis* prevalence of the disease in cattle and buffaloes in Uttaranchal, revealed 18.06% and 17.84% snails, respectively were harbouring the larval stages of *F. gigantica* in May and September.

In the snail host, miracidia develop into sporocysts, rediae and cercariae which emerge about 10-12 weeks later depending on the temperature (Khajuria, 1981; Soulsby, 1982). The incubation period in snails increases as temperature decreases. The optimal temperature for the development of miracidia and cercarial production is 25±0.5°C (range 12-33°C) (Dhar and Sharma, 1986). However, Sharma *et al.* (1989) demonstrated that at 25-27°C, cercarial shedding commenced as early as 20 days after the infection of snails. An infected snail continues to shed cercariae for a period of 10-20 days. The emergence of cercariae from the snail host is fairly a regular process with only minor changes depending on climatic variations. Cercariae are shed in up to 15 waves (usually three) and at each wave of shedding, 50-70 cercariae are released (Da Costa *et al.*, 1994). The number of cercariae develop from a miracidium vary from 15-600 (Khajuria, 1981). Yadav *et al.* (1997) demonstrated that the escaping sites of *F. gigantica* cercariae from *in situ* developing rediae are not confined to birth pore(s) unlike that of *F. hepatica*. The freely floating cercariae could emerge out from any site of the redial elastic, acellular but sticky tegument, leaving behind a self-healing indentation. Cercarial shedding by the infected snail mainly (80-95%) occurs during night between 6pm-6am next day (Gurlap *et al.*, 1964; Gupta and Yadav, 1994).

Most of cercariae after releasing from the snail host settles on aquatic grass blades or plants just below the water level, cast off tail and get encysted into metacercarial cyst. Cercariae that fail to encyst on an aquatic object, transform into floating cysts. It is influenced by the size of the snail at miracidial infection (Dreyfuss and Rondelaud, 1994; Vareille *et al.*, 1994). The percentage of floating cysts is high in the first few waves of cercerial shedding but it declines in subsequent waves (Da Costa *et al.*, 1994). The floating cysts float and move with water to far off distances and serve as potent source of infection in snail population free areas where climate is not condusive for development of snails (Spithill *et al.*, 1999). In laboratory, under optimum temperature (14-21°C) and humidity (>70%) metacercariae can survive for a period of 6-10 months, but under natural conditions, on herbage, a large population may die within 6-8 weeks. The survival of metacercariae in water is also affected by the host of origin (al-Kubaisee and Altaif, 1989). Contaminated biomass harvested in moist conditions and not properly sun cured may remain infective up to 35 days. Fermentation process during preparation of silage from the contaminated paddy straw kills the metacercariae (Gupta and Kamra, 1987).

The rate of *F. gigantica* infection is not consistent throughout the year. It depends more upon epizootiological determinants favourable to snail population, survival of metacercariae on the pastures and grazing management of livestock. In late summer (May-June) there is a close contact between infected animals or their faeces and snails, as there is shrinkage of water bodies during summer with concentration of snails in the bottom of the water bodies, where ruminant host frequently go for drinking water, as well as for grazing the lush green pastures. The cercarial shedding by the infected snails starts about two and half months later and result in the high prevalence of fasciolosis during rainy season (July-August), particularly in sheep and goats that closely graze or browse the infected biomass throughout the year, including the summer (Garg *et al.*, 2009). However, high prevalence in cattle and buffaloes was recorded in December-January (Chaudhri *et al.*, 1993; Velusamy *et al.*, 2004; Singh *et al.*, 2005; Yadav *et al.*, 2007; Garg *et al.*, 2009). Cattle and buffaloes are stall fed during summer due to the lack of sufficient green pastures available. With the onset of rainy season, they are let loose for grazing and pick up freshly discharged metacercariae, resulting in concurrent *in situ* building-up of fluke burden. Thus, it is responsible for higher prevalence of fasciolosis in cattle and buffaloes during December-January.

The metacercariae are not fully infective just after encystation. At room temperatures, they require at least 2-3 days to become fully infective to definitive host. In definitive host, the metacercariae after excystation become infective in 24 hours. Adolescercariae migrate and develop in the liver parenchyma (9-12 weeks), and finally reach to the bile ducts. *F. gigantica* requires a longer incubation period for its *in situ* growth, development and maturation than *F. hepatica*. The prepatent period of *F. gigantica* in riverine buffaloes is 92-97 days (Yadav *et al.*,

1999b). Faecal egg counts increases during patency from 13 to 21 weeks then start declining, suggestive of the end of the patent stage and animal become immune carrier.

Pathogenesis and clinical signs

The pathogenesis of tropical fasciolosis in ruminants has been remarkably complex, involving *in situ* migratory and an aerobic phase of active adolescercariae causing traumatic hepatitis and the anaerobic ductal phase of maturation and the establishment of the adult distome, causing hyperplastic obstructive cholangitis (Radostits *et al.*, 1994; Aiello and Mays, 1998; Edith *et al.*, 2010a). The pathological manifestations and the severity and the course of the disease vary with the dose of metacercariae ingested, in a primary single massive dose or perpetual and recurrent lower doses, over a shorter or a prolonged period that accumulate and persistently damage hepatic parenchyma, but much depends on the nutritional and immunological status of the host.

The parasite does not cause much damage during its migration through the intestinal wall or the peritoneal cavity. The pathogonomic lesions are seen in the liver parenchyma or in the major bile ducts. Damage caused by spiny tegument and the prehensile action of the suckers are responsible for severe haemorrhage in hepatocytes, beside during massive feeding of the hepatic tissues by the extended oral sucker. Macerated hepatic cells have been observed inside the sucker and pharynx (Dawes and Hughes, 1964). It is believed that the fluke secretes a huge quantity of amino acid proline which is essential for collagen synthesis by fibroblasts. The increased concentration of proline causes hyperplasia of epithelial and sub epithelial cells of the duct walls, resulting in enlargement of the bile duct walls and lumen much before the fluke reach the bile ducts (Isseroff *et al.*, 1979). The flukes have a great affinity for the hepatic tissues, capable of crossing the placental membranes and get access to foetal tissues and cause prenatal infections in pregnant ewes and cows (Sinclair, 1962). Usually the lobe situated nearest to the small intestine (left or ventral lobe) is more prone and get heavily infested. Consequently, the unaffected hepatic lobes become hypertrophied to compensate the liver functions of damaged tissues. During their migration through liver parenchyma, many flukes become trapped and only few reach the bile ducts. In an infected liver, both fresh as well as lesions undergoing resolution may occur simultaneously in the same section of the tissue. The adult flukes in the bile ducts exhibit prolonged longevity extending into several years.

Fasciolosis in sheep and goats mainly occurs as acute or sub-acute and devastating, and is often fatal. It is mainly seen in late summer and during post rainy season when a large number of adolescercariae migrate through the liver parenchyma. Sudden deaths after two to three months of the start of grazing on swampy pasture in fluke prone areas is a typical scenario and it can be predicted by a study of bio-climatograph. The much damage in the liver parenchyma is caused during early prepatency (1-6 weeks postinfection). The disease is evidenced by distended painful abdomen, severe anaemia associated with sub capsular haemorrhages and death during prepatency, prior to discharge of the fluke eggs in faeces. The diseased animals tend to lag behind, assume sternal recumbency and die within few hours. The acute fasciolosis, at times, get associated with "Black disease" caused by *Clostridium novyi*. However, due to widespread vaccination against clostridial diseases, the incidence of "Black disease" has been reduced dramatically.

The sub-acute disease occurs when a large number of metacercariae are ingested over a longer period of time. Some flukes have reached bile ducts causing cholangitis, while others are still migrating through liver parenchyma, causing lesions less severe than the acute disease. The affected sheep survive longer duration until coproscopically positive for fluke eggs, with greater damage to the liver. The affected animals show clinical signs for 1-2 weeks prior to death which include loss of appetite, appear dull and depressed, with pale mucous membranes, dyspnoeic and have palpable enlarged livers associated with abdominal pain. On necropsy, the liver parenchyma shows numerous haemorrhagic tracks undergoing different stages of resolution.

The chronic disease is more common and occurs when a moderate number of metacercariae are ingested over a prolonged period causing cholangitis, biliary obstruction, hypertrophy and hyperplasia of bile duct epithelium coupled with periductal fibrosis, thickening of hepatic arterioles and egg granulomas in the hepatic parenchyma (Arora and Iyer, 1974). The ductal walls yet remain pliable and accommodate the adult fluke population (Dow *et al.*, 1967). The chronic infection in sheep is characterized by reduced feed intake, anaemia, submandibular oedema, weight loss, wool break, reduced fertility and a fall in production. In the bile ducts, nearly 0.5 ml of blood per fluke can be lost each day, beside additional loss of plasma proteins by leakage through the hyperplastic biliary mucosa. Animal may die with obvious signs discharging fluke eggs in faeces. Sometimes, the flukes may *in situ* migrate to unusual sites/organs such as lungs, kidney and duodenum (Srivastava, 1939; Sahoo and Mohanti, 1966; Alibasoglu and Gurlap, 1969; Pandit *et al.*, 1991).

In cattle and buffaloes, the course of the disease ranges from acute (young animals below one year of age) to an asymptomatic course in immune carrier adults, and is rarely fatal (Radostits *et al.*, 1994; Sharma, 2003; Sharma and Godara, 2010). The pathogenesis of fasciolosis in large ruminants is similar to that in sheep but has added features of calcification of bile ducts and distended gall bladder. Calcium deposits in the bile ducts start after 16-20 weeks of infection, resulting in enlargement of the ducts (up to 3 cm in diameter) which become prominent on the surface of the liver. In cattle, the flukes may show aberrant migration and encapsulated parasites are often seen in the lungs (Urquhart *et al.*, 2003).

In experimental infection in Murrah buffalo yearlings, with a primary infection dose of 1000 *F. gigantica* metacercariae caused acute clinical disease, chronologically exhibiting pathognomonic clinical manifestations viz. apyrexic inappetance, anaemia, poor live weight gain, diarrhoea, and sub-mandibular and facial oedema, respectively from 5, 6, 8, 16 and 17 weeks post infection (Yadav *et al.*, 1999b). These signs were synchronous with *in situ* growth and maturation of the infection dose and associated hepato-biliary lesions. They reported that a hepatic load of 368±110 adult flukes could cause death in buffalo calves, aged above six months by day 140 postinfection. They also concluded that a coprological egg counts >300 per gram was suggestive of acute fasciolosis, while its subsequent fall to 100-200 per gram was symbolic to onset of chronic phase of the disease and/or immune carrier status of the affected host. On necropsy, the carcasses were emaciated and icteric in appearance. Characteristic necropsy lesions included extensive gelatinization of subcutaneous fat, thickened, mineralized and prominent bile ducts beneath the liver capsule, distended gall bladder, hepatomegaly (1.5 times) and the liver had rounded margins with grey coloured necrotic foci on the surface. The histopathological sections revealed intense vascular congestion of hepatic parenchyma, widened portal areas, with massive fibrosis, pseudolobulations and network of developing collateral bile ductules (Yadav *et al.*, 1999b, Edith *et al.*, 2010a, b).

Pathophysiology

The liver being an important vital organ, it plays a major role in biochemical alterations, affecting normal functioning of various vital systems. The tissue damage inflicted to the hepatic tissues by *in situ* invading fluke population brings about varied systemic alterations that ultimately result into decreased productivity of the affected animals. Deleterious effects of *Fasciola* spp. do not confine to liver alone. It is a sort of syndrome, influences normal functioning of hepato-biliary and haemopoitic systems, normal function of hypothalamus-pituitary axis and secretions of hormones from the target endocrine glands. Precise understanding of the overall impact of *in situ* fluke population on the health, growth and development during the course of disease seems quite interesting.

Apyrexic inappetance, weight gain and production losses : Sewell (1966) observed a linear relationship between adult *F. gigantica* worm counts and weight gain in zebu cattle, with each fluke reducing 200 g weight annually. Nour *et al.* (1979) demonstrated that the sheep fed poorer/basal diets affected more severely by infection with *F. gigantica* than those fed a high protein diet. They concluded that the extent to which weight gain is affected, depends more upon the level of nutrition, *in situ* worm burden, age and breed of the animal. It is also documented that delayed onset of puberty; longer inter calving intervals and/or infertility in *F. gigantica* infected cows in the endemic hilly areas were incidental to the fluke infestation. It was finally inferred that the anaemia caused by fluke might be one of the contributing factors to this effect (Spithill *et al.*, 1999, Kumar and Sharma, 1991).

Investigations on impact of the adverse effects of *F. gigantica* on milk yield in dairy animals revealed that there was increase in milk yield of 5.5 liters per animal per week in *F. gigantica* infected buffaloes after treatment with albendazole (Kumar and Pachauri, 1989). Recently, a reduction of 30.55% in milk production was documented in *F. gigantica* infected cows. Further, the milk yield increased up to 18.18% following treatment with triclabendazole (Kumar *et al.*, 2006). Significant fall in intake of nutrients appears to be contribute towards conspicuous fall in milk production in the lactating animals

Anaemia is the persistant feature of fasciolosis that ultimately results into a sharp fall in metabolizable energy. It causes an impaired appetite and nitrogen utilization, adversely affecting the feed conversion efficiency of the deceased host. Consequently, there is decreased body weight gain (Hope Cawdery and Conway, 1971; Hope Cawdery *et al.*, 1977; Sharma *et al.*, 2011). Mehra *et al.* (1999) observed apyrexic anorexia in *F. gigantica* infected buffaloes from the five weeks after infection with mean *in situ* adult fluke counts of 368±110. The inappetance was more marked during the biliary stage of fluke development. Marked reduction (30%) in dry matter intake was observed in the first twelve weeks of infection. Thereafter, there was a moderate increase in dry matter intake but it continued to be approximately 16% lower during the 165 days of the experiment. They recorded a sharp decline in feed conversion efficiency (unit intake per unit gain) from 9.6 to 33.4 was evidenced in the diseased buffaloes. The digestibility of the nutrients, however, remained unaffected. It was finally inferred that the fall in feed conversion efficiency was due to fall in intake of feed. There was 75% reduction in daily body weight gain in the diseased buffaloes which was mainly ascribed to the adverse pathophysiological impact of *in situ* sexually mature and adult *F. gigantica* and/or their metabolites discharged in the host circulation.

Anaemia : In ruminants, anaemia and hypoalbuminaemia are the most common and glaring manifestations of the fasciolosis. These are more marked in sheep than cattle and buffaloes (Berry and Dargie, 1978; Kumar *et al.*, 1982; Ganga *et al.*, 2007; Edith *et al.*, 2012). The developing *Fasciola* spp. juveniles and the adults have been considered non-haematophagous and tissue feeding parasites yet the fluke causes severe anaemia in animal suffering from acute, sub acute and chronic course of the disease (Ganga *et al.*, 2004b). Obviously, the pathogenesis of anaemia in fasciolosis has been debatable. Haematophagia (Spengler and Isseroff, 1981), haemodilution (Dargie and Berry, 1979), haemorrhages during migratory phase (Yadav *et al.*, 1999b; Edith *et al.*, 2012), intrabiliary haemorrhages by the adult flukes (Holmes *et al.*, 1968) and injurious nature of the fluke metabolites discharged into the host circulation significantly contribute to the development of anaemia. In the diseased host, a significant fall in erythrocytic indices started from the six to eight weeks after infection and therefore increased in severity and it is more pronounced during late prepatency. The ultimate degree of anaemia is related to the erythropoitic ability of the host adversely affected by the sharp reduction in protein and iron intake. Recent work evidenced that intra-peritoneal inoculation of the fluke metabolites for a period of seven days in the fluke free rats was progressively associated with significantly declined erythrocytic indices and caused normochromic and normocytic anaemia (Ganga *et al.*, 2004b). It has been postulated that *in situ* flukes, at times, accidentally feed blood oozed out from traumatic lesions in the liver and immuno-suppressive metabolites discharged by the fluke into the host circulation possibly contain proline, injurious to the host circulating erythrocytes (Isseroff *et al.*, 1979). In the chronic phase, hypoalbumineamia is more marked than anaemia yet an immune carrier host, on partial recovery from the acute course of the disease, continues to suffer from hypochromic and normocytic anaemia.

Endocrine gland dysfunction : It is believed that the fluke metabolites discharged into the host circulation coupled with generalized oxygen starvation at tissue level, incidental to the severe and prolonged anaemia could influence normal functioning of the hypothalamus-pituitary axis, consequently, the altered physiological plasma levels of the tropic hormones leading to dysfunctioning of the target endocrine gland(s), especially thyroid and adrenals that in turn influence and shift the entire metabolism to enhance catabolism in the fluke affecting animals.

(a) Thyroid gland : Although *Fasciola* infected animals do not show classical clinical signs (obesity and myxoedema, etc.) of hypothyroidism but lower concentrations of tri-iodothyronine (T_3) and thyroxine (T_4) in the host circulation indicate a clear picture of non-clinical hypothyroidism resulting in poor appetite and the onset of loss in body weight from the six weeks postinfection onwards (Mehra *et al.*, 1999; Ganga *et al.*, 2003). Ganga *et al.* (2007) in an experimental infection observed that the physiological levels of T_3 and T_4 were depressed by 54.7% and 16.21%, respectively during the thirteen weeks after the infection in riverine buffaloes. The histopathological evidences of hypothyroidism in the diseased host include appearance of peripheral vacuoles and atrophy of the thyroid follicles and lymphocytic thyroiditis with diffuse mononuclear cell infiltration (lymphocytes, plasma cells and macrophages) in inter and intracellular spaces causing progressive destruction of thyroid hormone secretory cells and follicles. Some of the follicles evidenced complete loss of colloidal mass due to excessive infiltration and invasion of the thyroid tissues by the inflammatory cells.

Obviously, in *Fasciola* infected animal, entire metabolism and mitochondrial oxygen consumption at cellular levels got affected due to hypothyroidism. Anabolic activities of the hormones in conjunction with the growth hormone and insulin to synthesize proteins and excretion of nitrogen in urine got altered. At mitochondrial level, the events had direct negative and/or depressing impact on oxygen consumption and release of energy in the form of adenosine tri-phosphate and onset of catabolism, thereby adversely affecting nutrient utilization, the growth and differentiation, lipid, carbohydrate and protein metabolism. Hence, it is strongly speculated that the thyroiditis in fasciolosis affected animals could be incidental to circulating anti-thyroglobulin antibodies, follicular atrophy and/or pituitary insufficiency (Kaneko *et al.*, 1997; Pineda and Dooley, 2003; Ganga *et al.*, 2007).

(b) *Adrenal glands :* The adrenals are the most sensitive and versatile steroid hormone producing endocrine glands. These glands spontaneously interact with the altered *in situ* environment/stimuli from a stressor, refluxed gluco-corticosteroids, especially cortisol into the circulation from the activated zona fasciculata, seemingly under the influence of adrenocorticotrophic hormone (ACTH) from the hypothalamus-anterior pituitary-adrenal axis. The long-term effect of such stressors on the growth, development, production and reproduction was monitored and quantified in different situations and was correlated with *in situ* elevated blood levels of cortisol (Johnson *et al.*, 1976; Stephens, 1980; Schoental, 1986; Ganga *et al.*, 2007; Edith *et al.*, 2010b).

Recent *in vivo* investigations on adrenocortical response in *F. gigantica* infected Murrah buffaloes during the course of the disease revealed that the response was variable in severity, depending much upon the clinical phase of the disease, *in situ* activities and location of the *F. gigantica* adolescercariae or adult fluke population in the hepatic tissues. A marked increase in concentration of the hormone occurred during the first six weeks of experimental infection in buffaloes (Edith *et al.*, 2010b), when the highest degree of disease stress is suffered by infected animals. It was synchronous with severity of hepato-cellular traumatic injury inflicted by the flukes during early prepatency. Subsequent progressive fall in the levels of hormone in circulation synchronised well with the arrival and establishment of the adult flukes in the hepato-biliary network, caessation of traumatic activities of the flukes and partial resolution of the lesions in the hepatocytes and/or recovery of the animals from the disease stress. The histopathological evidences to this effect comprised of hypertrophy of cellular elements in zona fasciculata, with a remarkable increase in its width occupying major portion of the cortex and altered cellular architecture in the cortex. The long-term secretion of cortisol (>112 days post infection) influenced the on going *in situ* metabolic activities, suppressed immune response, consequently, results in hepatomegaly, loss of collagen and elastin in the dermis, skeletal muscle weakness of the extremities and abdomen, lipolysis, etc. often evidenced on necropsy in an animal died of fasciolosis (Aiello and Mays, 1998; Pineda and Dooley, 2003; Ganga *et al.*, 2007; Edith *et al.*, 2010b).

Oxidative stress : Experimentally *per os* infected riverine buffaloes with 1000 *F. gigantica* metacercariae exhibited an increasing lipid peroxide profile from the fourth weeks post-infection onwards and it was much marked during late prepatency and patency stage of the disease (Ganga *et al.*, 2004a). The disease stress was further confirmed by synchronous hyperplastic changes in the adrenal cortex and higher levels of cortisol in the host circulation (Ganga *et al.*, 2007). It is speculated that the increased levels of lipid peroxide in fasciolosis could be a synergistic effect of one or more factors operative in the infected host, such as activation of CN-insensitive respiratory burst of the phagocytic cells due to *F. gigantica* invasion in the hepatic parenchyma (Facino *et al.*, 1990), hypothyroidism and/or hypoalbuminaemia in an animal suffering from fasciolosis (Ganga, 2001).

Altered serum enzyme levels : The elevated serum enzyme concentrations refluxed into the host circulation by the traumatized, inflamed and/or damaged hepatic tissues in fasciolosis are being exploited for early and semi quantitative diagnosis of the disease before the animal is coproscopically positive for fluke eggs. Activities of serum enzymes glutamate dehydrogenase (GLDH), glutamate-oxaloacetate aminotransferase, aspartate transaminase (AST) and alanine transaminase (ALT) increase during early prepatency, following a progressive fall during late prepatency and patency stage of the disease. These events are suggestive of hepatic tissue injury, whereas the elevated levels of alkaline phosphatase (AP) and gamma-glutamyl transpeptidase (GGT) are suggestive of patency or biliary phase of the infection (Anderson *et al.*, 1977; Kumar *et al.*, 1982; Wyckoff and Bradley, 1985; Swarup and Pachauri, 1987b; Reichling and Kaplan, 1988; Pachauri, 1995; Edith *et al.*, 2010a, 2011).

Recently, *in vivo* investigation revealed that an increasing pattern of the serum enzyme concentrations in *F. gigantica* infected buffalo yearlings had two clearly demarcated stages (Edith *et al.*, 2010a). The first stage was of massive invasion of parenchymal tissue by the fluke juveniles during early prepatency. The stage coincides with the onset and significant increase in the hepatic enzymes (AST and ALT) in the host circulation from the second weeks of the infection. A remarkable increase (3.4 times) of serum ALT (140.0%) and AST concentration (40.8%) was evidenced during prepatency, suggesting severe parenchymal tissue damage, whereas moderate but persistently higher levels of these enzymes in the serum indicated parasitic hepatopathy/ cirrhosis, onset of the regenerative process and/or partly resolution of traumatic lesions in the liver tissues during patency stage of the disease.

The second phase (patency) in the infected buffaloes was synchronous with overall 107.9% increase in the serum AP concentrations. In contrast to AST and ALT, the elevated levels of AP were ascribed to decreased biliary excretion of the enzyme or obstruction of bile flow stimulate *de novo* synthesis of the hepatic AP and synthesized enzyme is refluxed into the host circulation. Over 28% increase in AP concentration indicates obstructive hepato-biliary lesions and less than 8% increase in AP concentration is suggestive of chronic form of the disease or post-patency immune carrier status of the host (Edith *et al.*, 2010a, 2011).

The periodical monitoring of serum concentrations of the hepatic enzymes and exploiting them as marker enzymes in the animals would not only reveal the factual status of fasciolosis but would also elucidate the extent of traumatic hepatitis and obstructive/hyperplastic cholangitis suffered by the host. These can also be exploited for the purpose of disease forecasting and in time application of control strategies in the endemic areas.

Diagnosis

In the endemic areas, diagnosis of fasciolosis is of prime importance for timely chemotherapeutic intervention and to prevent further contamination of water bodies. Following methods are in practice to diagnose fasciolosis in ruminants.

Conventional methods : An animal infected with *F. gigantica*, in tropics and subtropics, essentially suffers from the deleterious pathophysiological effects during its prolonged prepatency period of 12-13 weeks. The onset of the adverse effects is much before (5th week PI onwards) coprological detection of the fluke eggs (during the 13th week PI) and confirmatory diagnosis of acute/subacute fasciolosis at necropsy. Evidently, coprological examination for fluke eggs is of little consequence in animals suffering from the acute course of the disease. However, its application even in patent phase of the disease and/or in subclinical and chronic infections although cannot be under estimated yet it is of limited value on account of marked fluctuations in day to day copro egg counts and, at times, it is very difficult to demonstrate low grade infections in immune carrier host. Therefore, repeated faecal examination seems mandatory before declaring an animal free from disease or forecasting disease in the endemic areas. Egg floatation technique using potassium mercury iodine solution is more sensitive method for ante-mortem diagnosis of fasciolosis in ruminants, as compared to direct smear examination and/or sedimentation technique. Technique has its own limitations as it causes morphological distortion of fluke eggs (Morel, 1987; Braun *et al.*, 1995; Aguirre *et al.*, 1998; Kumar *et al.*, 2002). However, examination of bile is more sensitive than faecal examination but it cannot be used for ante-mortem diagnosis. Garg *et al.* (2009) in a study compared faecal, bile and necropsy examination and found that the examination of liver at necropsy was the most specific and sensitive method than faecal or bile examination, because these methods failed to detect the presence of *in situ* immature flukes in the hepatic tissues.

Care should be taken to ascertain as to infection with flukes could be the main cause of disease or it has occurred with other debilitating factors (copper or cobalt deficiencies, John's disease or other internal parasitism). Clinical signs must be analyzed in relation with copro egg counts. In fasciolosis and ostertagiosis concurrent infections, particularly in cattle, preponderance of diarrhoea is suggestive of ostertagiosis, whereas preponderance of anaemia is suggestive of fasciolosis. In sheep, the disease is differentiated with "Black disease", as acute fasciolosis mainly occurs in young animals, and the "Black disease" affects animals in the 2-4 years age group. At necropsy, acute fasciolosis can be differentiated from other causes of acute, heavy mortality (haemonchosis, anthrax, enterotoxaemia) by heavily damaged liver and the presence of immature flukes in liver tissues (Soulsby, 1982; Radostits *et al.*, 1994; Taylor *et al.*, 2007).

Meteorological forecasting : It is applicable in endemic areas. It facilitates early warning of disease occurrence so that control measures are timely applied, prior to shedding of cercariae by the infected snails and intake of metacercariae infection by the host. Two computer based systems (Ground surface wet index and Wet days index) are practiced in advanced countries and the disease is being kept under control (Soulsby, 1982).

Biochemical methods : It is possible to predict/suspect fasciolosis as early as Day-40 post-infection onwards, using non-invasive methods of diagnosis in the endemic areas. The migration of juvenile flukes inflicts hepatic tissue damage. Elevated levels of marker enzymes in circulation, especially GLDH, AST and ALT are suggestive of acute disease, whereas elevated levels of AP and GGT during late prepatency and patency stages are suggestive of cholestasis and the presence of sexually mature flukes in the hepatic bile duct network.

Immunological methods : Immunodiagnosis has advantage over coproscopic examination, as it successfully predict prepatent infections. In the past few decades, a remarkable progress has been made in this direction. The disease is diagnosed during early prepatency by detection/demonstration of anti-fluke specific antibodies, fluke antigen(s) and immune complexes in serum of infected host, with significant success to diagnose acute/sub-acute fasciolosis as early as second week post-infection. Details reviews on the subject are available (Gupta and Singh, 2002; Dixit *et al.*, 2008; Sharma and Godara, 2010).

Amongst various immunodiagnostic techniques used (Immuno-diffusion, IHA, IFAT, ELISA, Immuno-blot, RIA and CFT), ELISA is the most sensitive and acceptable technique but, at times, suffers from false positive reactions due to concurrent *in situ* metazoan infections (Radostits *et al.*, 1994; Edith, 2004; Dixit *et al.*, 2008). Sincere and intensive efforts were made to isolate, characterize and identify the *F. gigantica* specific immunodominant moieties in complex somatic and excretory antigens (Yadav *et al.*, 1999a). Role of metabolites released during the development of adolescercariae in conferring acquired immunity in the host, immune evasion and diagnosis of the disease was thoroughly investigated. Ultimately, glutathione-S-transferase (GST) and cathepsin L cysteine proteinase (CS) have been identified as antigens of diagnostic importance. Cathepsin L cysteine proteinase was further purified, characterized and designated as FgCL-3 antigens. Using this antigen in ELISA revealed 100 and 97% sensitivity, respectively in experimental and natural *F. gigantica* infection in small as well as large ruminants (Dixit *et al.*, 2004; Raina *et al.*, 2006; Sriveny *et al.*, 2006).

Demonstration of *Fasciola* specific antibodies in circulation fails to indicate *in situ* parasite status of the host, as anti-fluke antibodies can persist for a longer time after elimination of the parasite. Therefore, seropositivity is considered a complementary tool to diagnosis.

Improved and specific techniques are in offing to demonstrate anti-fluke specific antibody or fluke antigens in the circulation of infected host, as during prepatency, demonstration of anti-fluke specific antibody /fluke antigens corresponds well with the presence of *in situ* flukes rather than faecal egg counts.

Control

The control of fasciolosis has been a challenging task since decades. It mainly comprised of guarded husbandry practices, proper disposal of animal excreta, drainage of water logged areas, breeding disease resistant livestock and the effectively harnessing measures to control the intermediate hosts coupled with the specific integrated therapeutic management in herd/flock. *L. auricularia* can be successfully controlled by fresh water fishes *Heteropneustus fossilis* and *Mystus vitatus*, which are potent malacophagous (Khajuria, 1981). However, the elimination of snails, using molluscicides or predators like ducks, fishes and frogs seems not feasible because of being costly, labour intensive and ecological reservations (Rai *et al.*, 1996). Since decades, strategic anthelmintic prophylaxis of animals exposed to the infection in endemic areas has been the most preferred option to control fasciolosis. Benzimidazoles (triclabendazole), Salicylanilides (rafoxanide, closantel, oxyclozanide) groups of drugs and substituted phenol (nitroxynil) are considered drugs of choice and are in use against *F. gigantica* (Khajuria, 1981; Gupta *et al.*, 1989; Sanyal and Gupta, 1996; Pal *et al.*, 2003). The efficacy of the drug used depends upon the drug, dosage and administration modalities. Although triclabendazole has shown high efficacy against immature and mature flukes in cattle but it has lowered efficacy against bubaline fasciolosis due to its poor intake (Gupta *et al.*, 1989). In order to overcome this limitation, intraruminal administration of the drug at higher dose (24 mg/ kg) improved the efficacy of the drug in buffaloes (Sanyal and Gupta, 1996). Use of Triclabendazole in feed pellets and strategic application of the anthelmintic delivery device claimed to reduce fluke burden in dairy animals (Sanyal, 1998). Silage preparation of agro waste successfully killed the *F. gigantica* metacercariae in 20 days. For control of the disease and its use as feed supplement to susceptible animals is recommended (Gupta and Kamra, 1987). It is advised that rice fields near to snail infested bodies in the villages should not be grazed for at least six weeks after harvest. In the endemic areas, epizootiology based specific therapeutic management of the disease in mid-summer (April-May), in autumn (September-October), and in late winter (January) when the animals are usually confined to indoor housing and are stall fed, have been practiced. In rice cultivated areas, it is advised to deworm animals at least three months prior to planting the rice crop. Such strategies may be effective, but are not practiced, because of poor awareness and costly proposition. Above all, in the endemic areas, meteorological forecasting facilitates early warning of the disease occurrence, so that control measures are timely applied, prior to shedding of cercariae by the infected snails and intake of metacercariae by the susceptible hosts.

Immunoprophylaxis

Of late, an alternative approach aiming at early diagnosis of the disease and development of acquired resistance in the susceptible host, using different viable or non-viable antigens of the fluke has been quite interesting, on account of being an efficient, cost effective, environmentally friendly and reliable long-term solution to control and/or possible eradication of the disease, so much so to ensure optimum health and productivity of the animals in the endemic areas and minimum losses to their owners. Global approaches adopted by different workers in this direction are being briefly presented in Table I. Further protection conferred by live attenuated *F. gigantica* metacercariae in the different experiments is summarized in Table II.

The immunoprotection strategies against fasciolosis, using non-viable soluble purified parasite defined protein molecules as antigens, including fatty acid binding proteins, glutathione-S-transferase, leucine aminopeptidase, paramyosin and cathepsin L cysteine proteinases which having the potency of inducing acquired protective response against the fluke in laboratory and large animal models is presented in Table III. Amongst these, the parasite enzymes belonging to cysteine proteinase family, secreted by the fluke to help it burrow deeper through various host tissues, nutrient acquisition, egg production and cleavage the immunoglobulins of the host (Dalton *et al.*, 1996; Dixit *et al.*, 2008), were most intensively investigated. Ultimately, cathepsin L secreted by Mehlis gland was resolved as the target of the immune response in vaccinated animals. Its *in vivo* use resulted in interference of egg shell synthesis, reduced egg production and hence reducing available metacercariae on pasture for subsequent infection to ruminants. However, immunization of Brahman-cross cattle against tropical liver fluke with cathepsin L was claimed to be discouraging. It conferred poor protection against the fluke and caused no reduction in faecal egg count despite stimulating high total antibody titres (Estuningsih *et al.*, 1997). It was concluded that the protection level depends more on the use of different adjuvants, and better results can achieved if cathepsin L proteases are used in conjunction with other liver fluke antigens (Dalton *et al.*, 1996). Wijffels *et al.* (1994) demonstrated that sheep vaccinated with purified cysteine proteinases of *F. hepatica,* had shown decreased worm fecundity, recovered flukes were morphologically normal, suggesting that their development was not retarded by vaccination. Contrary to these biometric observations of the flukes, Dalton *et al.* (1996) and Edith (2004) did observe a longer prepatent period, low mean copro egg counts, significantly lesser mean wet fluke weight, and lesser mean length and width of the flukes recovered from experimentally immunized and infected cattle and riverine buffaloes, respectively. A reduction in size of adult flukes recovered from vaccinated cattle and buffaloes suggested that immune responses to cathepsin L fluke antigen in cattle and buffaloes *vis-à-vis* sheep could be different. It needs further critical analysis.

Table1: Various immunoprotective approaches against fasciolosis

Period	Immunogen	Host	Protection(%), Max (Range)
1. 1973-89	Live attenuated mc	Goat, cattle, sheep	86 (29 -86)
2. 1972-85	Crude antigen		
	* Sonicat ed cultures	Sheep	79
	* Freez dried SAg	Rats	41-55
	* Immature fluke ESAg	Rabbits	Significant
3. 1973-81	Passive immunization (Immune Sera)	Rats Rabbits	25-48
4. 1990-96	Defined antigens		
	* GST	Cattle	18-69
	* FABP	Cattle	55
	* Cathepsin L	Sheep	69
		Cattle	42-69
	* Cathepsin L + Fluke Haemoglobin	Cattle	52 -72

Table2: Immunoprotection against tropical fasciolosis using live attenuated metacercariae

Parasite	Host	Immunogen	Radiation Dose (GY)*	% Protection/ Findings	References
F. gigantica	Cattle	1000 irradiated MC	300	100	Bitakaramire (1973)
		200/2000 MC	200	83	Haroun *et al.* (1988)
	Sheep	6 doses of 100 MC	30	64	Dargie *et al.* (1974)
		Single dose of 100 MC	40	100	Khajuria (1981)
				Significant protection	Haroun *et al.* (1988)
	Goat	Double or triple dose of 400 MC at 15 days	35	83-86	Yadav and Gupta (1989)

*GY- Absorbed dose of radiation, 10 GY =1 sm k rads, MC- metacercariae

Table 3: Immunoprotection against fasciolosis using purified immunogens

Parasite	Host	Protein	Vaccine Protection (%)	References
F. hepatica	Cattle	FABP	55	Hillyer *et al*. (1987)
F. hepatica	Sheep	GST	57	Sexton *et al*. (1990)
F. gigantica	Cattle	FABP	31	Estuningsih *et al*. (1997)
F. gigantica	Cattle	GST	18 (ns)	Estuningsih *et al*. (1997)
F. gigantica (1997)	Cattle	Cathepsin L	0	Estuningsih *et al*.
F. gigantica (1997)	Cattle	Paramyosin	0	Estuningsih *et al*.
F. hepatica	Sheep	Cathepsin L	69	Wijiffels *et al*. (1994)
F. hepatica	Cattle	Haemoglobin	44	Dalton *et al*. (1996)
F. hepatica	Cattle	Cathepsin L + Haemoglobin	52-78	Dalton *et al.* (1996)
F. gigantica	Rats	32 kDa NEJ protein	90 protection	Florine *et al*. (2000)

NEJ- Newly excysted juvenile fluke, ns- non-significant

Despite persistent efforts, a vaccine with adequate protection against fasciolosis has not yet been developed to the point of commercialization. This can largely be attributed to the fact that immune responses to immunogens are influenced by the route of administration, nature of antigens, delivery system and the adjuvants used in the trial. Native cathepsin L could be purified from liver fluke excretory-secretory products in sufficient quantities, detailed analysis of their biochemical and physio-chemical properties, and their evaluation as protective immunogen under defined experimental conditions may find solution for application in the field. Ultimately, for field trials, recombinant cathepsin L cysteine proteinase could be cloned and produced in large quantities (Dixit *et al.*, 2008). Immunoprotection properties of both native and recombinant cathepsin L can be intensively studied, standardized and tested in the endemic areas for their effectiveness, before release of vaccine for field use.

Conclusions

- A majority of metazoan parasite species exert pathogenic lesions and directly influence the functioning of the target organ that explains pathogenesis and characteristic clinical signs of the disease caused. However, fasciolosis has been an exception; it is a sort of syndrome, synchronously involving and collectively influencing normal functioning of hepato-biliary system, haemopoitic system, hypothalamus-pituitary axis, and secretions of hormones from the target endocrine glands, thereby affecting tissue level carbohydrate, protein and lipid metabolism and consequential feed conversion and live body weight gain efficiency of the infected animal(s).
- More planned *in vivo* investigations are therefore needed to elucidate pathophysiological impact of *F. gigantica* on erythrocytic membrane, bone marrow so as to precisely define the genesis of the deleterious effect of the fluke and its metabolites in circulation discussed above, such as anaemia and hypoxemia, oxidative stress, delayed onset of puberty and/or infertility in growing female hosts, poor growth and development, etc. in growing hosts incidental to *in situ F. gigantica* population.
- As early as 1883, it was believed that fasciolosis is preventable and its control ought to be integrated. In the endemic areas,

control of fasciolosis requires strategic, integrated and well planned programmes, including (a) generating epizootiological and demographic data on the disease from different agro-climatic zones, (b) identification of endemic areas and forecasting of the disease, (c) immunoprophylaxis in susceptible livestock, and (d) timely diagnosis of the disease during early prepatency and cost effective chemotherapy.

- The containment of economic losses due to *F. gigantica* in ruminants by immunological intervention seems to be an achievable objective. However, before entering into the developmental phase of liver fluke diagnostics/vaccine, the best and cheapest options will have to be evolved and considered.
- In this context, large scale production of recombinant infection specific immunodiagnostic/protective proteins, using the most suitable and acceptable vector(s) that mimic the required optimum level of specificity and sensitivity for diagnosing the disease during early prepatency and confer required level of acquired immunity in the susceptible host against *F. gigantica*, could facilitate achieving the ultimate objective and prove beneficial in longer run.
- The vaccination programme may not completely eradicate *in situ* fluke population. Innovative immunization strategies are expected to confer adequate level of immunity and should reduce *in situ* fluke population to a tolerable levels (<100 flukes), without a compromise with any sort of production losses.
- The effectiveness of the immunogen can be improved by searching a commercially viable and efficient adjuvant(s) and selecting the most appropriate route of delivery system such as oral route or the immunogen adapted and administered with live viral vector(s) for immunoprotection purpose, development of disease specific antigen delivery system into the host for effective immunization.

References

Aguirre, D.H., Vinabal, A.E. and Gaido, A.B. (1998). Comparative study of three coprological techniques for *Fasciola hepatica* diagnosis in ruminants. *Veterinaria Argentina*, 15: 421-427.

Aiello, S.E. and Mays, A. (1998). *Merck Veterinary Manual*, 8th ed., Merck & Co Inc., New Jursey, USA, pp. 1196-98.

Alibasoglu, M. and Gurlap, N. (1969). Pathological changes in sheep experimentally infected with *Fasciola gigantica. Vet. Fak. Derg. Ankara. Uni.,* 16: 110-121.

Anderson, P.H., Berrett, S., Brush, P.J., Hebert, C.N., Parfitt, J.W. and Patterson, D.S. (1977). Biochemical indicators of liver injury in calves with experimental fascioliasis. *Vet. Rec.,* 100: 43-45.

Arora, R.G. and Iyer, P.K.R. (1974). Studies on the pathology of fascioliasis (*Fasciola gigantica*) in sheep and goats. *Indian J. Anim. Sci.,* 43: 720-723.

Berry, C.I. and Dargie, J.D. (1978). Pathophysiology of ovine fascioliasis : the influence of dietary protein and iron on the erythrokinetics of sheep experimentally infected with *Fasciola hepatica. Vet. Parasitol.,* 4: 327-339.

Bhalerao, G.D. (1933). Preliminary note on the life history of the common liver fluke in India, *Fasciola gigantica. Indian J. Vet. Sci.,* 3: 120-121.

Bhatia, B.B., Upadhyaya, D.S. and Juyal, P.D. (1989). Epidemiology of *Fasciola gigantica* in buffaloes, goats and sheep in tarai region of Uttar Pradesh. *J. Vet. Parasitol.,* 3: 25-30.

Bitakaramire, P. (1973). Preliminary studies on the immunization of cattle against fasciolosis using gamma irradiated metacercariae of *Fasciola gigantica.* Isotopes and radiation in Parasitology-III pp. 23-32.

Braun, U., Walfensberger, R. and Hertzberg, H. (1995). Diagnosis of liver fluke in cows- a comparison of the findings in the liver, in the faeces and in the bile. *Schweizer-Archiv-fur-Tierheilkunde,* 137: 438-444.

Chaudhri, S.S., Gupta, R.P., Kumar, S., Singh, J. and Sangwan, A.K. (1993). Epidemiology and control of *F. gigantica* infection of cattle and buffalo in Haryana, India. *Indian J. Anim. Sci.,* 63: 600-605.

Da Coata, C., Dreyfuss, G., Rakotondravao, C., Rondelaud, D. and Da Costa, C. (1994). Several observations concerning cercarial shedding of *F. gigantica* from *Lymnaea natalensis. Parasite,* 1: 39-44

Dalton, J.P., McGonigle, S., Rolph, T.P. and Andrews, S.J. (1996). Induction of protective immunity in cattle against infection with *Fasciola hepatica* by vaccination with Cathepsin L proteinase and with haemoglobin. *Infect. Immun.,* 64: 5066-5074

Dargie, J.D. and Berry, C.I. (1979). The hypoalbuminaemia of ovine fascioliasis : the influence of protein intake on the albumin metabolism of infected and of pair-fed control sheep. *Int. J. Parasitol.,* 9: 17-25.

Dargie, J.D., Armour, J., Rushton, B. and Murray, M. (1974). Immune mechanisms and hepatic fibrosis in fasciolosis. In: E.J.L. Soulsby (Editor), Proc. Sixth Intl. Conf. World Assoc. Adv. Vet. Parasitol., Academic Press, NY, pp. 119-122.

Dawes, B. and Hughes, D.L. (1964). Fascioliasis: The invasive stages of *Fasciola hepatica* in mammalian hosts. In: Advances in Parasitology, edited by B. Dawes, Academic Press, London and New York, 2: 97-168.

Dhar, D.N. and Sharma, R.L. (1986). Laboratory studies on the life cycle of *Lymnaea auricularia sensu stricto. Indian Vet. J.*, 63: 621-623.

Dixit, A.K, Yadav, S.C. and Sharma, R.L. (2004). Kinetics of antibody response using 28 kDa *Fasciola gigantica* cysteine proteinase as antigen. *Trop. Anim. Hlth Prod.*, 36: 49-54

Dixit, A.K, Dixit, Pooja and Sharma, R.L. (2008). Immunodiagnostic/protective role of Cathepsin L cysteine proteinases secreted by *Fasciola* spp.-a review. *Vet. Parasitol.*, 154: 177-184.

Dreyfuss, G. and Rondelaud, D. (1994). Comparative study of cercarial shedding by *Lymnaea tomentosa* infected with either *Fasciola gigantica* or *F. hepatica. Bull. de la Soc. Francaise de Parasitologie*, 12: 43-54.

Dow, C., Ross, J.G. and Todd, J.R. (1967). The pathology of experimental fascioliasis in calves. *J. Comp. Pathol.*, 77: 377-386.

Dutt, S.C. and Bali, H.S. (1977). Snails of Punjab and their trematode infections. Proc. All India Symposium on Helminthology, Srinagar, pp. 31-32.

Edith, R. (2004). Comparative immunoprotection profile of infection specific and excretory- secretary protein of *Fasciola gigantica* against tropical fasciolosis in buffaloes. M.V.Sc thesis submitted to IVRI Deemed University, pp. 1-96.

Edith, R., Godara, R., Sharma, R.L. and Thilagar, M.B. (2010a). Serum enzyme and haematological profile of *Fasciola gigantica* immunized and experimentally infected riverine buffaloes. *Parasitol. Res.*, 106: 947-956.

Edith, R., Godara, R., Thilagar, M.B. and Sharma, R.L. (2011). Alterations in serum enzyme profile of riverine buffaloes (*Bubalus bubalis*) experimentally infected with *Fasciola gigantica. J. Vet. Parasitol.*, 25: 50-55.

Edith, R., Sharma, R.L. Godara, R., and Thilagar, M.B. (2012). Experimental studies on anaemia in riverine buffaloes (*Bubalus bubalis*) infected with *Fasciola gigantica. Com. Clin. Pathol.*, 21: 415-419.

Edith, R., Thilagar, M.B., Godara, R. and Sharma, R.L. (2010b). Tropical liver fluke induced stress in the experimentally infected and immunized buffaloes. *Vet. Rec.*, 167: 571-575.

Estuningsih, E., Smooker, P.M., Wiedosar, E., Widjante, S. Vaiano, S., Partoutoms, S. and Spithill, T.W. (1997). Evaluation of antigens of *Fasciola gigantica* as vaccines against tropical fasciolosis in cattle. *Int. J. Parasitol.*, 11: 1419-1428.

Facino, R.M., Carini, M., Ganchi, C., Tofanetti, O., Casciarri, I. and Bedohu. D. (1990). Antihepatotoxic properties of uridine-diphosphoglucose in liver fluke infection in rat. *Agz-For-Schung*, 40: 490-498.

Florine, J., Van Milligen, Jan, B.W.J., Cornelisen Ben and Bokhout, A. (2000). *Fasciola hepatica*: An antigen fraction derived from newly excysted juveniles, containing an immunoreactive 32 kDa proteins, induces strong protective immunity in rats. *Exp. Parasitol.*, 94: 163-171.

Ganga, G. (2001). Experimental studies on bubaline fasciolosis. Ph.D Thesis submitted to IVRI Deemed University, Izatnagar, India.

Ganga, G., Varshney, J.P., Sharma, R.L., Varshney, V.P. and Kalicharan (2003). Hypothyroidism associated with bubaline fasciolosis. *Indian J. Anim. Sci.*, 73: 640-651

Ganga, G., Varshney, J.P. and Sharma, R.L. (2004). Oxidative stress in *F. gigantica* infected buffaloes. *J. Vet. Parasitol.*, 18: 71-71.

Ganga, G., Varshney, J.P. and Sharma, R.L. (2004a). Effect of *F. gigantica* excretory-secretary antigen on rat hematological indices. *J. Vet. Sci.*, 7: 123-125.

Ganga, G., Varshney, J.P., Sharma, R.L., Varshney, V.P. and Kalicharan (2007). Effect of *F. gigantica* infection on adrenal and thyroid glands of buffaloes. *Res. Vet. Sci.*, 82: 61-67.

Garg, R., Yadav, C.L., Kumar, R.R., Banerjee, P.S., Vatsya, S. and Godara, R. (2009). The epidemiology of fasciolosis in ruminants in different geo-climatic regions of north India. *Trop. Anim. Hlth. Prod.* 41: 1695-1700.

Gupta, S.C. and Kamra, D.N. (1987). Influence of wastelage fermentation on viability of *F. gigantica* metacercariae. *Biological Wastes*, 22: 311-313.

Gupta, S.C. and Singh, B.P. (2002). Fasciolosis in cattle and buffaloes in India. *J. Vet. Parasitol.*, 16: 139-145.

Gupta, S.C. and Yadav, S.C. (1994). Emergence of *F. gigantica* cercariae from naturally infected *L. auricularia*. *Indian J. Parasitol.*, 18: 53-56.

Gupta, S.C., Chandra, R. and Yadav, S.C. (1989). Efficacy of triclabendazole against experimental *F. gigantica* infection in sheep, goats, buffaloes and rabbit: a comparative study. *Indian Vet. J.*, 66: 680-682.

Gurlap, N., Ozcan, C. and Simms, B.T. (1964). *Fasciola gigantica* and fascioliasis in Turkey. *Am. J. Vet. Res.*, 25: 196-210.

Haroun, E.M., Yagi, A.I., Yogi, A.I., Yunis, S.A., Sanhouri, A./A., Gadir, H.A., Gameel, A.A., Bushara, E.I. and Taylor, M.G. (1988). Use of ionizing radiation in the development of vaccine against *Fasciola gigantica* and *Schistosoma bovis* in Sudanese cattle, sheep and goats. In: Nuclear techniques in the study and control of parasitic diseases of livestock, International Atomia Energy Agency Vietnam, pp. 1-21.

Hillyer, G.V., Haroun, E.M., Hernandez, A. and De Galanes, M.S. (1987). Acquired resistance to *Fasciola hepatica* in cattle using a purified adult worm antigen. *Am. J. Trop. Med. Hyg.*, 37: 363-369.

Holmes, P.H., Dargie, J.D., MacLean, J.M. and Mulligan, W. (1968). The anaemia of fascioliasis : studies with "Cr-labelled red cells". *J. Comp. Pathol.*, 78: 415-420.

Hope Cawdery, M.J. and Conway, A. (1971). Production effects of the liver fluke *Fasciola hepatica* on beef cattle. *Vet. Rec.*, 89: 641-643.

Hope Cawdery, M.J., Strickland, K.I., Conway, A. and Crowe, P.I. (1977). Production effects of the liver fluke in cattle. 1. The effects of infection on live weight gain, feed intake and feed conversion efficiency in beef cattle. *Br. Vet. J.*, 133: 145-159.

Isseroff, H., Spengler, R.N. and Charnock, D.R. (1979). Fascioliasis: similarities of anaemia in rats to that produced by infused proline. *J. Parasitol.*, 65: 705-714.

Johnson, H.D. and Vajonack, W.J. (1976). Effect of environmental and other stressors on blood hormone patterns in lactating animals. *J. Dairy Sci.*, 59: 1603-1607.

Kaneko, J.J., Harvey, J.W. and Bruss, M.L. (1997). Clinical Biochemistry of Domestic Animals, 5th edn., Singapore Academic Press, Harcourt Brace and Company Asia PTE Ltd., pp. 327-349.

Katiyar, R.D., Srivastava, V.K., Khera, R.C. and Lepcha, N.T. (1983). Occurrence of fasciolosis in livestock in Sikkim. *Livestock Advisor*, 8: 37-39.

Kendall, S.B. (1954). Fascioliasis in Pakistan. *Ann. Trop. Med. Parasitol.*, 48: 307-313.

Khajuria, J.K. (1981). Studies on some aspects of life history and control of *Fasciola gigantica*. M.V.Sc thesis submitted to Punjab Agricultural University, Ludhiana, pp. 1-114.

Al-Kubaisee, R.Y. and Altaif, K.Y. (1989). Comparative study of sheep and buffalo isolates of *F. gigantica* in the intermediate host *Lymnaea auricularia*. *Res. Vet. Sci.*, 47: 273-274.

Kumar, M., Pathak, K.M.L. and Pachauri, S.P. (1982). Clinico-pathological studies on naturally occurring bovine Fascioliasis in India. *Br. Vet. J.*, 138: 241-246.

Kumar, P. and Pachauri, S.P. (1989). Efficacy of albendazole against *Fasciola gigantica* infection in buffaloes with particular reference to milk production. *J. Vet. Parasitol.*, 3: 35-39.

Kumar, R.R., Vatsya, S. Yadav, C.L. and Singh, V.S. (2006). Economic impact of helminths infestation control on milk production in cattle. *J. Vet. Parasitol.*, 20: 133-136.

Kumar, S. and Sharma, M.C. (1991). Infertility in rural cows in relation to fascioliasis. *Indian J. Anim. Sci.*, 61: 838-840.

Kumar, V., Banerjee, P.S., Ram, H., Garg, R. and Yadav, C.L. (2002). Faecal examination *vis-à-vis* bile examination for the diagnosis of bubaline fasciolosis. *J. Vet. Parasitol.*, 16: 185-186.

Mehra, U.R., Verma, A.K., Dass, R.S., Sharma, R.L. and Yadav, S.C. (1999). Effect of *Fasciola gigantica* on growth and nutrient utilization by buffalo calves. *Vet. Rec.*, 145: 699-702.

Morel, A.M. (1987). Detection of *Fasciola gigantica* eggs in faeces. A comparison of methods. *Vet. Rec.*, 120: 90-91.

Nour, A.M., Abou, A.A.K., Badr, M.F. and El, S.K. (1979). The effect of type of ration on some blood components and daily gain of sheep infected with *Fasciola gigantica*. *Alexandria J. Agri. Sci.*, 27: 523-530.

Okao, E.T. (1984). An appraisal of the incidence and economic losses due to *F. gigantica* infection in Zebu cattle (*Bos indicus*) in Uganda. *Bull. Anim. Hlth. Prod. Africa*. 23: 423-429.

Pachauri, S.P. (1995). Clinico-biochemical profile in fasciolosis of buffaloes. *Buff. Bull.*, 14: 7-10.

Pal, D., Kumar, V., Yadav, C.L. and Banerjee, P.S. (2003). Efficacy of certain drugs against naturally acquired bubaline fasciolosis and amphistomosis. *Indian Vet. J.*, 80: 3-5.

Pandit, B.A., Mir, A.S. and Banday, M.A. (1991). An unusual recovery of *Fasciola gigantica* in the lungs and duodenum of sheep. *Indian Vet. J.*, 68: 193-194.

Patnaik, M.M. and Ray, S.K. (1968). Studies on geographical distribution and ecology of *Lymnaea auricularia* var *rufescens*, the intermediate host of *Fasciola gigantica* in Orissa. *Indian J. Vet. Sci.*, 38: 264-268.

Pineda, M.H. and Dooley, M.P. (2003). *Veterinary Endocrinology and Reproduction*, 5th ed., Iowa, Blackwell Publishing Company, pp. 35-70; 165-200.

Prasad, A. (1989). Experimental infection of *L. auricularia* var. *rufescens* for mass harvesting of metacercariae of *F. gigantica*. *J. Vet. Parasitol.*, 3: 31-34

Radostits, O.M., Blood, D.C. and Gay, C.C. (1994). *Veterinary Medicine- A text book of the diseases of Cattle, Sheep, Pigs, Goats and Horses*, 8th ed., London, Bailliere Tindall, UK, pp. 1230-1236.

Rai, R.B., Sevai, S., Ahlawat, S.P.S and Kumar, B.V. (1996). Studies on control of fasciolosis in Andaman and Nicobar Islands. *Indian Vet. J.*, 73: 822-825

Raina, O.K., Yadav, S.C., Sriveny, D. and Gupta, S.C. (2006). Immunodiagnosis of bubaline fasciolosis with *Fasciola gigantica* Cathepsin L and recombinant Cathepsin L 1-D proteases. *Acta Trop.*, 98: 145-151.

Reichling, J.J. and Kaplan, M.M. (1988). Clinical use of serum enzymes in liver disease. *Dig. Dis. Sci.*, 33: 1601-1614.

Roy, V. and Tandon, V. (1992). Seasonal prevalence of some zoonotic trematode infection in cattle and pigs in the north-east mountain zone in India. *Vet. Parasitol.*, 41: 69-76.

Sahoo, B.N. and Mohanti, G.C. (1966). Histopathological studies of lesions in lungs of sheep and goats encountered in the abattoir. 1. Study of lesions due to *Fasciola*. *Indian Vet. J.*, 43: 585-588.

Sanyal, P.K. (1998). Pharmacokinetics and efficacy of triclabendazole incorporated urea molasses block against experimental immature fasciolosis in cattle and buffaloes. *J. Vet. Parasitol.*, 12: 25-29.

Sanyal, P.K. and Gupta, S.C. (1996). Efficacy and pharmacokinetics of triclabendazole in buffalo with induced fasciolosis. *Vet. Parasitol.*, 63: 75-82.

Sarwar, M.M. (1950). Observations on the bionomics of ova of *Fasciola gigantica* in West Pakistan plains. *Proc. Pakistan Sci. Conf.*, 3(2): 74.

Schillhorn van Veen, T.W. (1980). Fasciolosis (*Fasciola gigantica*) in West Africa: a review. *Vet. Bull.*, 50: 529-533.

Schoental, R. (1986). Endogenous opioids and slaughter induced stress. *Vet. Rec.*, 119: 223.

Sewell, M.M.H. (1966). The pathogenesis of fasciolosis. *Vet. Rec.*, 78: 98-105.

Sexton, J.L., Milner, A.R., Panaccio, M., Waddington, L., Wijffels, G., Chandler, D., Thompson, C., Wilson, L., Spithill, T.W., Mitchell, G.F. and Campbell, N.J. (1990). Glutathione-S-Transferase: Novel vaccine against *Fasciola hepatica*, infection in sheep. *J. Immunol.*, 145: 3905-3910.

Sharma, R.L. (2003). Helminthic diseases of livestock in Jammu and Kashmir. In: Helminthology in India (ed. M.L. Sood), International Book House, Dehradun, pp. 231-245.

Sharma, R.L., Dhar, D.N. and Raina, O.K. (1989). Studies on the prevalence and laboratory transmission of fasciolosis in animals in Kashmir. *Br. Vet. J.*, 145: 57-61.

Sharma, R.L. and Godara, R. (2010). Metazoan diseases of livestock in the Greater Himalayan region of India and their diagnosis- an overview. *J. Vet. Parasitol.*, 24: 1-16.

Sharma, R.L., Godara, R. and Thilagar, M.B. (2011). Epizootiology, pathogenesis and immunoprophylactic trends to control tropical bubaline fasciolosis: an overview. *J. Parasit. Dis.*, 35: 1-9.

Sinclair, K.B. (1962). Observations on the clinical pathology of ovine fascioliasis. *Br. Vet. J.*, 118: 37-53.

Singh, B.P., Jayrao, A.K., Gupta, S.C., Raina, O.K. and Ghosh, S. (2005). Prevalence of *Fasciola gigantica* infection amongst *Lymnaea auricularia* population in surrounding regions of Bareilly, India. In proceedings of 16th National Congress of Veterinary Parasitology, Durg, Dec. 6-8, 2005, pp. 19-20.

Soulsby, E.J.L. (1982). Helminths, arthropods and protozoa of domesticated animals, 7th ed, Bailliere and Tindal, London, UK.

Spengler, R.N. and Isseroff, H. (1981). Fascioliasis: Is anaemia caused by haematophagia? *J. Parasitol.*, 67: 886-892.

Spithill, T.W., Smooker, P.M. and Copeman, D.B. (1999). *Fasciola gigantica*: epidemiology, control, immunology and molecular biology. In: Fasciolosis (Dalton, J.P., ed.), CAB International, pp. 465-525.

Srivastava, H.D. (1939). Occurrence of liver fluke *Fasciola gigantica* on the lung of goats. *Indian J. Vet. Sci.*, 9: 225-227.

Sriveny, D., Raina, O.K., Yadav, S.C., Chandra, D., Jayaraw, A.K., Singh, M., Velusamy, R. and Singh, B.P. (2006). Cathepsin L cysteine proteinase in diagnosis of bovine *Fasciola gigantica* infection. *Vet. Parasitol.*, 135: 25-31.

Stephens, D.B. (1980). Stress and its management in domestic animals: A review of behavioural changes and physiological studies under field and laboratory conditions. In: Advances in Veterinary Science and Comparative Medicine (Brandy, C.A., Cornelius, C.F., eds), 24: 179-208.

Swarup, D. and Pachauri, S.P. (1987a). Epidemiological studies on fasciolosis due to *Fasciola gigantica* in buffaloes in India. *Buff. Bull.*, 6: 4-9.

Swarup, D. and Pachauri, S.P. (1987b). Pathophysiology of fasciolosis in buffaloes: some biochemical indices. *Indian J. Anim. Sci.*, 57: 1083-1085.

Taylor, M.A., Coop, R.L. and Wall, R.L. (2007). Veterinary Parasitology, 3rd ed., Blackwell Publishing LTD, UK, pp. 85–89.

Thapar, G.S. and Tandon, R.S. (1952). On the life history of liver fluke, *Fasciola gigantica* Cobbold, 1885, in India. *Indian J. Helminthol.*, 4: 1-36.

Urquhart, G.M., Armour, J., Duncan, J.L., Dunn, A.M. and Jennings, F.W. (2003). Veterinary Parasitology, Blackwell Science LTD, UK pp. 1-307.

Vareille, M.C., Dreyfuss, G. and Rondelaud, D. (1994). *Fasciola gigantica* and *F. hepatica*: the numerical variations of floating cysts in relation to the snail species and its size at miracidial exposure. *Bull. de la Soc. Francaise de Parasitologie*, 12:161-166.

Velusami, R., Singh, B.P., Gupta, S.C. and Chandra, D. (2004). Prevalence of *Fasciola gigantica* infection in buffaloes and its snail intermediate host at Bareilly. *J. Vet. Parasitol.*, 18: 171-173.

Wijffles, G.L., Panaccio, M., Salvatore, R., Wilson, L., Walker, I.D. and Spithill, T.W. (1994). The secreted Cathepsin L-like proteinases of the trematode *Fasciola hepatica*, contain 3-hydroxy preoline residue. *Biochem. J.*, 299: 781-790.

Wyckoff, J.H. 3rd and Bradley, R.E. (1985). Diagnosis of *Fasciola hepatica* infection in beef calves by plasma enzyme analysis. *Am. J. Vet. Res.*, 46: 1015-1019.

Yadav, C.L., Garg, R., Kumar, R.R., Banerjee, P.S. and Godara, R. (2007). Seasonal dynamics of *Fasciola gigantica* infection in cattle and buffaloes in Uttaranchal, India. *Indian J. Anim. Sci.*, 77: 133-135.

Yadav, S.C. and Gupta, S.C. (1989). Immune response of goats against *Fasciola gigantica* induced by irradiated metacercariae. *J. Vet. Parasitol.*, 3: 121-123.

Yadav, S.C., Kumar, S., Sharma, R.L. and Gupta, S.C. (1997). Observation on escaping sites of cercariae from redia of *F. gigantica* in *L. auricularia*. *J. Parasitic Dis.*, 21: 189-191.

Yadav, S.C., Mandal, S. and Sharma, R.L. (1999a). A comparative evaluation of *Fasciola gigantica* antigens in immunodiagnosis of bubaline fasciolosis. *Rivista Di Parassitologia.*, 16: 73-81.

Yadav, S.C., Sharma, R.L., Kalicharan, Mehra, U.R., Dass, R.S. and Verma, A.K. (1999b). Primary experimental infection of riverine buffaloes with *Fasciola gigantica*. *Vet. Parasitol.*, 82: 285-296.

□□□

Chapter 11

Trypanosomosis (Surra) in Livestock

Veer Singh[1] and L.D. Singla[2]
[1]Department of Parasitology, College of Veterinary Sciences and Animal Husbandry, S.D. Agricultural University, Sardarkrushinagar-385 506, Gujarat
[2]Department of Veterinary Parasitology, College of Veterinary Science, Guru Angad Dev Veterinary and Animal Sciences University, Ludhiana-141004, Punjab

Introduction

Trypanosomosis (Surra) caused by haemoprotozoan parasite *Trypanosoma evansi* constitutes one of the major veterinary problems worldwide as it leads to progressive emaciation, anaemia, oedema, pyrexia, reduced weight gains, lowered milk and meat yields, abortion and mortality in animals. It is widely prevalent serious disease of considerable economic importance widely affecting a wide variety of domestic, wild and zoo animals. The disease has devastating effect on livestock health and leads to incalculable economic loses (Soulsby, 1982; Singh and Chhabra, 2008). It is endemic in most parts of the Indian sub-continent, and epizootics have occurred particularly in cattle and buffaloes with mortality rate ranging from 20 to 90% (Gill, 1991). Humans are refractory except in a very few instances of mutation of Apo L-1 protein where atypical trypanosomosis is seen (Lun *et al.*, 2009). Recently, a case of surra has been reported from human beings (Joshi *et al.*, 2005). This chronic disease caused by the first pathogenic trypanosome *T. evansi* which was identified by Griffith Evans, a British Veterinary Physician at Dera Ismail Khan in erstwhile Punjab (now in Pakistan) in 1880 from the blood of Indian horses and camels. India has the distinction of being the country where the first two mammalian trypanosomes i.e. *T. lewisi* and *T. evansi* were discovered. After the discovery of this protozoan parasite enormous literature has published on all aspects of diseases. In India, *T. evansi* being the mostly commonly occurring species of trypanosomes while *T. theileri* has been occasionally encountered (Sood *et al.*, 2011). The third important species, *T. equiperdum* causes dourine in horses has been eradicated from the country and there is no report of its occurrence since 1921. Strict application of preventive measures against 'Dourine' so called Venereal disease of horses became a noticeable disease under the Dourine Act V of 1910 of Indian Penal code.

Parasite morphology

Trypanosoma evansi is a monomorphic leaf like parasite measuring about 18–34 μ in length and 1.5–2.5μ in width. The kinetoplast is subterminal, undulating membrane is well developed and has a long free flagellum (5-6 μ) situated anteriorly. The nucleus is vesicular type situated centrally (Killick Kendrick 1968; Raisinghani and Lodha, 1982). Dyskinetoplastic forms also appear after treatment of *T. evansi* with a variety of trypanocidal drugs including berenil and prothidium.

Local names

A variety of local names, descriptive of the clinical signs of the disease are used by the livestock owners e.g., many Hindi names as "Surra" meaning rotten or emaciation is the name used almost universally to describe the disease caused by *T. evansi* in all species of livestock in many countries (Gill, 1991). Similarly other names are there as "Dubla" (emaciated), "Purana" (chronic or old) and "Tibursa" (three years diseases). Some Gujrati names based on Gujarat province (State) in India have also been coined as "Dance makhi no rog" (*Tabanus* biting fly diseases) and "Chakri no rog" (circling movement in acute stage).

Classification

The disease in Equines has been placed and listed by Office International Epizootics (OIE) under list 'B' diseases.

Susceptible hosts

Trypanosoma evansi has a wide host range. It principally infects horses and camels. Other species that develop severe disease include donkeys, mules, deer, llamas, dogs, cats, cattle and buffalo. Sheep, goats, pigs and elephants may occasional develop mild or chronic disease. The buffaloes act as reservoir of infection.

Distribution

The geographical area affected by enzootic trypanosomosis caused by non tsetse-borne *T. evansi* is about three times greater than that caused by tsetse-borne trypanosomes (Woo, 1977). Surra is present in North Africa, the Middle East, Asia and South America. It has never been reported in the Pacific Region. The disease is endemic in India, China, Southeast Asia, northern Africa, the Middle East, South America, Philippines, Bulgaria, parts of former USSR and Indonesia. The incidence of surra is comparatively higher in north and northwestern parts than the eastern and southern parts of India. Significant incidences have been reported from Haryana, Punjab, Rajasthan, M.P., U.P., Gujarat, Maharashtra, Tamilnadu, Kerala, Assam, Andhra Pradesh and Karnataka states. India seems to the major source from where surra has spread within livestock throughout the continent of Asia and Islands of Indian Ocean. There was introduction of *T. evansi* from India to Australia when camels were exported from India to Port Hedland in 1907. This invasion was eradicated by the rapid identification and slaughter of infected animals.

Transmission

Trypanosoma evansi is the member of subgenus Trypanozoon, which also include *T. brucei* and *T. equiperdum*. *T. evansi* differs from these species by the absence of kDNA maxicircle, which renders it unable to develop cyclically in insect vectors. Thus *T. evansi* is transmitted mechanically from the infected carrier animal to healthy animals through the haematophagous Dipteran flies belonging the genera *Tabanus, Stomoxys, Haematopota, Lypersia* and *Hippobosca*. No development takes place inside the vector. Efficiency of transmission is dependent on the interval between two successive feedings and intensity of fly challenge. The increase in fly activity of *Tabanus* and related flies is expected to increase the likelihood of *T. evansi* transmission and hence contribute towards disease outbreaks during monsoon and post monsoon seasons. Transmission with tabanid flies is achieved mostly by interrupted feeding habit and structure of their mouth parts which are highly adapted for transmission and wide spread distribution in monsoon season associated with increased prevalence. Tabanids are pool feeders. After cutting the skin with their mouth parts, they lap pooled blood along with connective tissue fluid. As a result the parasitaemia in jugular blood may not be a good indicator of infectivity for *Tabanus* spp. transmission. Rather, the trypanosome density in capillary blood, lymph or connective tissue in the skin could be more important. The trypanosomes remained alive in the food canal of tabanid flies for varying periods, up to four hour in *T. nemocallous*, up to eight hours in *T. rubidus*. Earlier the time for interrupted feeding on healthy animals after taking infection from diseased animals better are the chances of transmission.

It has been reported that during an acute stage of infection the trypanosomes were transported via the placenta to the foetus of camel. There is also possibility of sexual transmission of *T. evansi* as smears from the cauda epididymal fluid of *T. evansi* infected rodents revealed equivalent number of *T. evansi* and spermatozoa (Singla *et al*., 2003). Another probable route of transmission could be iatrogenic transmission such as during herd vaccination. Dogs and other wild carnivores may get the infection through the ingestion of the infected meat. In American trypanosomosis vampire bats also play significant role in transmission.

Incidence

The outbreaks of surra occur during the rainy and post monsoon seasons because high density of the vector. Sporadic cases are reported through out the year. Infectivity depends upon the strain, heterogeneity of susceptibilities of the host, number of organisms and host parasite contact. The predisposing factors include age of the host, inter-current infection, starvation, physical exertion/fatigue/stress, debility, weakness, introduction of animal into surra infected area or infected animal into a healthy herd. The vaccination against bacterial and viral infections is also flair up infection.

Risk of introduction

Surra could be introduced by importation of infected live animals or by introduction of infective vectors. Importation of semen does not present a risk of introducing surra.

Economic losses

The disease has a major economic impact in India, but it is difficult to assess the economic losses because of incomplete information of the exact epidemiological data. About 500 million cattle, 100 million buffaloes and 12 million camels are at risk all over the world due to the disease. It is responsible for 30 per cent morbidly and 3 per cent mortality. However, economic losses caused by surra in Asia may be higher than those caused by the African trypanosomes, which are estimated to be US$ 1.3 billion in relation to cost of meat and milk (Kristjanson *et al.*, 1999). Most of the direct losses in the animals are due to mortality and cost of chemotherapeutic interventions. The indirect losses due to infection have not been adequately defined, but remained an important factor in the field due to failure of vaccination against bacterial and viral infections, due to severe immunosuppression produced by the disease. Further losses are occurring through reduced yield of milk, reduced weight-gain in animals grown for meat and reduced ability shown by the draught animals.

Pathogenesis

Usually there are three stages in the disease process. Initially there is pyrexial stage during which intermittent fever occurs followed by anaemic stage in which erythrocyte count is reduced by 25% or even more. The end stage is the nervous stage during which trypanosomes enter into the brain by crossing the blood brain barrier.

Pathology

Basic mechanism involves in the pathology include utilization of host's nutrients and excretion of metabolites, excretion of toxic substances, mechanical disruption of host's tissue and immunologically mediated injury. Though different hosts show variable pathogenicity to *T. evansi*, the most common clinical feature is progressive anaemia due mainly to haemolysis of red blood cells as well as erythrophagocytosis (Bhatia *et al.*, 2006). Apart from progressive anaemia and intravascular coagulation, toxins and proteolytic enzymes liberated by the parasite, hypoglycaemia is considered to be the cause of death.

Haemolytic anaemia is macrocytic which may be associated with leucopenia or leucocytosis and thrombocytopenia. Predominant lesion is found in the connective tissue of various organs, blood and lymphoid system. Trypanosomes usually localize in connective tissue with mononuclear cell aggregation and exudation in body cavities. Wide spread distribution of parasites leads to subcutaneous oedema of head, limbs, genitalia, urticarial plaques, keratitis, opthalmitis, enlargement of lymph nodes, spleen and accumulation of fluid in the body cavities. Destruction of R.B.C. and platelets is regarded to be due to cytotoxic reaction associated with immune complexes formation ultimately causing disturbances in clotting mechanism and acute glomerulonephritis. Utilization of tryptophan by tryps in the brain has been proposed as basis for functional disturbances of CNS. CNS malfunction is due to generation of phenyl pyruvate and indole–3– ethanol by the trypanosomes in the brain. Mechanism of immunological injury is by delayed hyper-sensitivity reaction also generate substances causing direct inflammatory changes.

Immune exhaustion due to antigenic variation result into polyclonal B cell activation and IgM hypergamma globinaemia. This results into immunosuppression at both cellular and humoral levels. Immuno-suppression due to *T. evansi* results in failure of vaccination against bacterial and viral diseases (Sarmah *et al.*, 1997; Singla *et al.*, 2010) and secondary/concurrent infection with other pathogens (Gupta *et al.*, 2009).

The changes in blood chemistry and cellular component include increased serum enzyme levels of sorbitol dehydrogenase, alanine aminotransferase aspartate amino transferase and decrease in Serum alkaline phosphatase which is responsible for tissue damage. Hypoglycemia results in the breakdown of the liver function and fatal intoxication. Impairment of blood brain barrier and increased intra-cerebral immunoglobulin biosynthesis are other observations reported (Singla *et al.*, 1998).

The lysosomal secretory proteinases, phospholipases and other hydrolytic enzymes of trypanosomes are considered potentially important factors in the development of disease caused by trypanosomes. The E/S proteases released into blood stream may degrade the host tissue proteins and contribute to the pathogenesis. Immune targeting of such proteinases may protect the infected host. Death may occur due to endotoxin that may be set free by the lysis of parasites and hypoglycaemia which results from the consumption of large amount of blood sugar by trypanosomes. The other reason may be asphyxia due to increased blood lactic acid thus interfering with the normal absorption of oxygen by the haemoglobin. Asphyxiation may also occur due to mechanical blocking of the lung capillaries by agglutinated trypanosomes, which may cause pulmonary oedema result fatal termination. Erythrocyte production is inhibited by toxins. Trypanosomes may liberate proteolytic ferments, which digests proteins and may liberate toxic products.

Pathogenic effects of infection

i. *Pyrexia* : In trypanosomosis, pyrexia may or may not reflect the degree of parasitaemia and it is due to: (a) Direct contact of monocytes and macrophages with *Trypanosoma* antigen producing pyrogen, and (b) Antigen: Antibody complex stimulate for pyrogen release.

ii. *Thrombocytopenia* : Thrombocytopenia is caused due to immunological alterations; Decreased platelet count is related to number of trypanosomes per unit of blood.

iii. *Disseminated intravascular coagulation (DIC)* : In *Trypanosoma* infection, intravascular activation of clotting system leading to deposition of fibrin thrombi in small organs causing ischaemia and functional loss of the organ.

iv. *Anemia* : Anaemia in *Trypanosoma* infection is due to (a) erythrop hagocytosis (b) haemolysis (factors from *Trypanosoma* damage the erythrocytes).

In acute cases, the anemia is normally macrocytic normochromic and in chronic cases, it is microcytic hypochromic.

General Clinical Manifestations

These are observed during acute/sub-acute/chronic forms. Commonly observed signs are pyrexia which is intermittent type may be seen during paroxysms as well as during intermission phase and ranges from 102°F to 106°F, with rigors and sweating, appetite is usually normal. The fever relapses. Sometimes no fever is seen at all but parasites persists in peripheral circulation as observed by authors. Congested mucous membranes are seen in acute/sub-acute phase only. Conjunctivitis (sometimes haemorrhagic), opthalmitis, dullness (sleepy look), lethargy, weakness/loss of body weight /emaciation and anemia are commonly observed. But jaundice is very rare, ascites in few cases only. Pica can be seen in young calves and camels. Oedema is observed first around the genitalia, and lower part of the body including sub-orbital fossa. Oedema of tongue is there in some cases in buffaloes. Urticarial plaques are recurrent. Keratitis and corneal opacity are observed in dogs. Slight enlarged superficial lymph nodes, knuckling of fetlock joints, Loss of milk production especially in buffaloes and abortion in pregnant animals are other manifestations seen. Nervous signs include ataxia, aimless walking, circling movement, blindness, frenzy, hyperaesthesia (mild degree only), convulsions are seen in terminal cases. Muscular weakness of hind quarters is observed leading to paralysis.

Clinical Signs

Species wise clinical signs normally observed are as under:

Camel : In acute cases signs include: intermittent fever/no fever, dullness/tiredness/lethargy, petechial haemorrhage of the mucosa, discharge from eyes, subcutaneous oedematous swelling and progressive anaemia. In chronic form, the course of disease is 1-3 years (Tibersa). Signs include anaemia, emaciation, weakness, development of skin abscess and pica in young camel

Equines : In horses, mules and donkeys the incubation period is 5-60 days, the severity of disease varies from mild to per acute. Per-acute disease results in sudden death. In acute form the course is 2 weeks to 4 months. Typical clinical signs include intermittent pyrexia, weakness, lethargy, sweating, weight loss, lacrimation and nasal discharge. Hyperaesthesia is observed during pyrexial stage. Petechial haemorrhages on mucous membrane and extravasations of blood at muco-cutaneous junctions of the eyelids, nostrils and anus, urticarial plaques on the skin of neck, back and oedematous swelling on legs, lower abdomen, and scrotum are the other signs observed during acute phase. In chronic form, weakness and emaciation are seen. Mucous membrane becomes pale and icteric and superficial lymph nodes are enlarged. The outcome of infection is fatal.

Cattle and Buffaloes : In cattle and buffaloes infection is mostly chronic (cryptic) and asymptomatic. Sometimes, the animals suffer from per-acute form of disease showing nervous signs and animal die all a sudden after showing nervous signs (convulsions, ataxia, apparent blindness, frenzy and circling movement). In per acute form neural signs can be confused with anthrax, neural form of ketosis and tumor or cyst or abscess in brain. The cause of death in such animals may be occlusion of minute cerebral blood vessels leading to anoxia and fatality.

In acute form animal is dull, show staggering gait, staring wide open eyes, encircling movement, pyrexia and death in 6 to 12 hrs. In sub-acute form there is initial rise of temperature with intermittent fever, dullness and depression, circling movement, sudden drop in milk production in milking animals, slight enlargement of pre-scapular lymph nodes, conjunctivitis and white mucoid discharge from eyes.

Anaemia, loss of body weight, weakness, emaciation, knuckling of fetlock joints and abortion in pregnant animal are also reported during sub acute phase. In most of the cases there is no correlation of pyrexia with parasitaemia (Singh and Raisinghani, 1990; Singla *et al.,* 1996a). Sometimes, they may be correlated. In chronic form weakness, emaciation, anaemia, corneal opacity and lowered efficiency/ production losses are there due to surra.

Dogs and Cats : In dogs and cats, surra is often acute and fatal. In dogs, oedema of larynx and change of voice can be seen, hence can be confused with rabies; bilateral corneal opacity and corneal ulcers may be observed.

Immunity

The trypanosome's ability to escape the host immune response is through antigenic variation. Trypanosomes are known for evading host immune system and producing pathological effect. Trypanosomes possess mixtures of antigen which are released in different sets. Major types of antigen released in the first set elicit antibody production where as no antibody production for minor type of antigen hence these keep the infection going on, Moreover, antibody produced against major type also may become waste. This is because the trypanosomes release second or subsequent set of antigens, soon after releasing the first set of antigens. Thus, despite an effective host immune response mediated through IgM and IgG antibodies directed against their surface coat antigens, trypanosomes are able to evade it by altering the antigenic composition of their surface glycoprotein coat.

With the aim of reducing the pathological consequences of trypanosome infection, immunomodulation has been used in surra. Impairment of Blood Brain Barrier (BBB) and increased intra-cerebral immunoglobulin (Ig) biosynthesis occurred in *T. evansi* infected cow calves and marked improvement was observed after levamisole treatment (Singla *et al.*, 1998). Immunostimulatory effect of levamisole is also observed by hypergammaglobulinaemia (Singla *et al.*, 1992) and increased Ig production (Singla *et al.*, 2000). Levamisole also produced leucocytosis and lymphocytosis in *T. evansi* infected calves to combat the disease but dexamethasone flared up the infection.

Immunosuppression

The trypanosomes are also held responsible for producing a state of severe immunosuppression, which renders the infected host more susceptible to secondary infections and to produce poor immune response to bacterial and viral vaccines. Substantial immunosuppressive effect to haemorrhagic septicaemia (HS) vaccination was recorded in experimental *T. evansi* infection in buffalo calves (Singla *et al.*, 2010).

Post-mortem findings

The lesions are not very specific. The post mortem findings include pale mucous membranes with emaciated body, anaemia and petechiae on some internal organs. Oedema of lungs with accumulation of sero-sanguineous fluid in peritoneal, pericardial and thoracic cavities is sometimes seen. Yellow gelatinous exudates are seen under skin. Sub endocardial haemorrhages with enlarged lymph node, splenomegaly and hepatomegaly, and some times ulceration and patechial haemorrhages of GIT, serosa and mucosa are commonly observed post mortem findings. The parasites can be detected in brain, lung, spleen and liver.

Specimens required for diagnosis

Identification of the parasite can be attempted from blood smear. It is the prescribed test by the OIE. Sampling from deep vessels will increase the chances of having a positive result. The trypanosomes can be concentrated to increase the sensitivity of the test. An antigen ELISA and latex agglutination antigen tests are recent developments.

Serological tests are available, including complement Fixation, indirect haemagglutination, indirect fluorescent antibody test and enzyme linked immunosorbent assay (ELISA) or card agglutination tests (CATT). For declaring disease-free status, ELISA followed by re-testing of suspect samples by CATT is recommended.

Diagnosis

Generally, diagnosis of the disease is based on (a) the history on which the prevalence of *Trypanosoma* infection and of biting flies which acts as vectors responsible for transmission of the disease (b) clinical symptoms (c) laboratory examination of the blood and body fluids by direct examination, chemical tests, animal inoculation and immuno diagnostic test. Although trypanosomes have been studied for more than 125 years, there definite diagnosis still suffers from low sensitivity and specificity. The diagnosis is mainly based on conventional parasitological techniques. Additionally, new approaches are being developed from all the corners of the globe. This needs laboratory and field validation so that a suitable effective diagnostic technique is followed for early detection of surra.

Clinical signs of progressive emaciation, anaemia and oedema are indicative but not pathognomonic enough for making more than a provisional diagnosis. Accurate diagnosis of disease is extremely important both for identifying the animal for treatment as well as for tracking the prevalence of disease. The varied and non-specific clinical signs of surra as well as chronic non parasitiaemic form of the disease manifestation make it difficult to diagnose it under field condition. Traditional parasitological methods are less sensitive. As for as the animal inoculation method is concerned its sensitivity and specificity is higher but takes more time. Serological methods are more sensitive and based on the detection of antibodies, antigens and Ag-Ab complexes. Molecular diagnosis is highly sensitive and specific (Singh *et al.*, 1994, 1995).

Demonstration and identification of trypanosomes from the body fluids remains the basis of exact diagnosis. The limitations in terms of low sensitivity of parasitological diagnostic methods are a driving force for research into alternative techniques including immunodiagnostic, antigen detection assays and DNA-based methods. FAO and OIE are working to develop simple, sensitive, reliable and easily applicable method in field conditions. Various tests include parasite detection techniques, antibody detection test, antigen detection test, immune complex detection techniques and nucleic acid detection techniques.

(A) Parasite detection techniques

It is actual demonstration of trypanosomes in blood which is a Gold standard test. It is important that blood from the major or deep blood vessels is more likely to yield a positive test result than blood obtained from peripheral sites. Demonstration of trypanosomes in fresh blood smears from infected animals is the surest way of establishing the acute infection since the organisms are readily demonstrable in freshly stained blood smears. However, the diagnosis of chronic infections may be difficult because parasitaemia is usually low. In such cases, thick and thin blood smears or lymph node puncture smears should be attempted. Blood smears taken at height of temperature may be positive for the parasites. The number of parasite in blood between two paroxysms is less.

- *Wet blood examination (WBE) : T. evansi* is an active motile organism which is easily detected under x40 objective of a microscope. In cattle, the other species of trypanosome, *T. theileri,* is larger than *T. evansi* and can be easily differentiated from the later.

- *Stained blood film examination :* Stained thin blood smear by light microscopy is still the most readily applied method for diagnosis of surra in field. For diagnosis of acute cases, it is very useful, but this method is not suitable for diagnosis of subacute or chronic cases or for detection of carrier animals. The Giemsa stained thin blood smears have a low sensitivity equivalent to 10^5 trypanosomes/ml. So in subclinical infection it is often difficult or impossible to demonstrate parasites in the blood mainly because of the periodically cryptic nature of the parasitaemia. This results in the long periods during which the host has no detectable parasites in the blood.

  Thin blood smears, prepared in humid climate, should immediately be fixed after drying or should be kept in desiccator. Giemsa, Leishman or Wright stains are commonly used for staining the blood smears. Red blood cells in the thick blood films should be lysed before fixation with methanol and stained with Giemsa at a dilution of 2 drops of stain to 1 ml of water, buffered at pH 7.2. Dry thick films are also stained aqueous methylene blue for 1 second, then lysed in distilled water, fixed in methanol and stained with Giemsa stain.

  For the diagnosis of *T. equinum,* the blood is mixed with 20% sodium citrate, centrifuged, and suspension fluid is examined for trypanosomes. Arecoline hydro bromide can be tried to flush out trypanosomes from the aqueous humour of eyes in blindness and opacity.

- *Lymph/CSF/Aqueous humor examination :* The lymph node smears are prepared by injecting small quantity of normal saline into the lymph gland with the help of a tuberculin syringe and subsequently messaged and fluid aspirated.

- *Mouse sub-inoculation (MSI)/ Animal sub-inoculation :* Albino mice and rats are most suitable hosts for detecting sub-patent infection. Guinea pig and rabbit are less suitable because of their greater innate resistance to *T. evansi.* In white mice, 0.5 ml of suspected blood with an Alseverse solution is inoculated intra-peritoneally.

The 2-4 ml of blood is inoculated in other experimental animals. In mice, trypanosomes appear in its blood 2-3 days after inoculation while in other animals, 7-8 days are required for parasitaemia. The animals are observed for appearance of trypanosomes for up to 4 weeks. The blood smears from the infected experimental animals are stained and examined for the organism.

This sub-inoculation test is more reliable than the direct microscopic examination. It can detect microscopically sub-patent infection in blood following chemotherapy or infections breaking through chemoprophylaxis. It is useful in the detection of latent infection of bovines and cryptic infection of goats. By inoculating the mice with buffy coat, the sensitivity is further increased to one trypanosome per four ml of the blood. This test is time consuming and not very useful under field situations.

- *Cultivation :* Cultivation of *T. evansi* is not usually attempted as it is easy to maintain in the experimental animals. *T. evansi* can be cultivated in developing chick embryo. A window is cut in hens' egg after the embryo is 10-day-old. An injection of 0.5 ml of inoculum containing the trypanosomes is injected into the allantoic cavity. The chick blood becomes heavily infected with trypanosomes and the embryo dies within 4-5 days of infection.

- *Micro hematocrit technique (MHCT)/Woo technique :* This concentration technique is devised to overcome the problem of scanty/low grade parasitaemia and is considered the most efficient parasitological test. In subclinical infection it is often difficult or impossible to demonstrate the parasite in thin blood film mainly because of periodically cryptic nature of the parasitaemia. More that 50 to 80% infection may remain undiagnosed by direct microscopy. The diagnostic capability could be significantly increased by adopting single low cost alternative, the MHCT that has sensitivity equivalent to 85 trypanosomes/ ml (Reid *et al.*, 2001). Further, it was suggested that the sensitivity of MHCT was improved 10-fold through the use of buffy coat in place of whole blood.

- *Miniature anion-exchange centrifugation technique (MAECT) :* This technique is very much useful for detection of low level of parasitaemia. The technique is considered more sensitive method for detecting trypanosomes in the blood and is able to detect one trypanosome per two ml of blood (Reid *et al.*, 2001). Although preparation of separate column for diagnosis of separate animal is the disadvantage of this technique, but in absence of other facilities diagnosis of the disease, this technique could be used.

- *Quantitative buffy coat method (QBC)* : This assay has been found sensitive for detection of *T. evansi* infection in blood of asymptomatic carriers and found better than conventional light microscopy technique. For detection of *T. evansi* in the field, the test could be used as a rapid method diagnosis.

(B) Chemical tests

The following tests have been used for detecting changes in chemical composition of the blood produced by *T. evansi* organisms. Such disease-induced alteration of serum gamma globulins can occur in other infections as well. The tests, therefore, are non-specific and far less reliable, but may find place in the field for immediate tentative diagnosis.

Mercuric chloride test : A drop of serum from suspected camel is added to 1 ml of 1:25,000 solution of mercuric chloride in a tube, which is gently shaken to mix the two. Appearance of white precipitate after 15 min denotes a positive reaction. The utility of the test is limited to camels having 1 month or more old infection.

Formal-gel test : The test is reliable in camels. Commercial formalin (2 drops); 40% formaldehyde are added to 1 ml of serum of suspected case in a test-tube. The tube is shaken and allowed to stand. A gel starts forming in positive cases after 1 hr. Final reading may be taken after 24 hr after keeping at 4°C. Distinct opalescence, with or without gelatin indicate positive reaction for surra.

Thymol turbidity test : The test is similar to mercuric chloride test as it detects excess serum globulin fraction in infected animals. The test is indicated for cryptic cases of Surra in camel and is proved to superior to mercuric chloride test. Alkaline thymol buffer (3ml) is mixed with 1 drop of suspected serum inactivated at 56°C for 30 min. Immediate white turbidity, increasing maximum up to 1 hr, appears in positive cases.

Jone's nitric acid test: Its application is similar to mercuric chloride test and is done for the diagnosis of African trypanosomosis of chronic or latent status. The test is performed by adding 1 drop of clear serum to 1 ml of 1.8%w/v nitric acid. Positive reaction is indicated by the appearance of yellow colour/turbidity in 1 hr.

Stilbamidine test: This test is used in the diagnosis of latent trypanosomosis in bovines in India. Utility of this test is limited to surra in cattle. About 0.5-2.5 ml of freshly prepared 10% aqueous solution of stilbamidine is taken in a small tube. One drop of inactivated suspected serum is added on the surfaces of the above solution. A positive case shows coagulation which begins to sink down in half a minute and dissolves in 5-10 min.

(C) Immunodiagnostic techniques

Although direct demonstration of trypanosomes in the infected animal gives conclusive proof of infection, the limitations of parasitological diagnosis has been the driving force for a great deal of research into alternative techniques that provide indirect evidence of infection, namely immunodiagnostic techniques.

Problems in the control and standardization of another sensitive test, the indirect haemagglutination (IHA) test, have precluded its general use although it was used in the diagnosis of *T. evansi* in camels (Jatkar and Singh, 1971) and in a control programme for buffalo and cattle. In tests with *T. vivax,* it was considered too unreliable.

(i) *Antibody detection test* : The breakthrough in immunological diagnosis came with the introduction of primary binding assays for the detection of trypanosomal antibodies. These tests directly measure the interaction between antigen and antibody rather than relying on a secondary reaction consequent upon the initial binding. There are several methods for detection of specific humoral antibodies of *T. evansi* antigens.

- *Immunodiffusion test :* This testis not useful for detection of antibodies in suspected animals because it is a time consuming test. More over during the course of the infection Abs could not be detected by this test or the test found negative when IFAT was found positive.
- *Complement Fixation test :* The CF test was used successfully in the control and eradication of dourine in North America (Watson, 1920) and was also used in the diagnosis of surra in buffalo in the Philippines. This test is based on reactions of

1gM Abs, which are mainly produced early in primary infections. Due to chronic nature of the disease in most test animals, low sensitivity of the test noticed.

- *IFAT :* The indirect fluorescent antibody test (IFAT) has been used extensively in the detection of trypanosomal antibodies in animals and humans. Antigens are usually prepared from blood smears which are fixed in acetone and then stored at a low temperature. The IFAT has proven to be both specific and sensitive in detecting trypanosomal antibodies in infected cattle and camels (Luckins *et al.*, 1979).

  However, cross-reactions between different trypanosome species do occur. Ashkar and Ochilo (1972) found that more than 85 percent of cattle infected with *T. vivax* or *T. congolense* reacted with *T. brucei* antigen in the IFAT. When sera were tested against all three pathogenic trypanosome species, between 45 and 66 percent of sera reacted in the assay, and only by combining all the results did the test detect 94 percent of infected animals. Hence, although there is considerable cross-reactivity, these results indicate a degree of species specificity that requires the use of all three antigens in order to obtain maximum efficiency. Modifications in the preparation of antigens involving fixation of the parasites in acetone and formalin have provided antigens which are stable even at 4°C, can be kept in suspension until required and are capable of discriminating between different trypanosome species.

  The major drawback of the IFAT - apart from its requiring sophisticated microscopy - is its subjectivity, which can make comparison of results quite difficult.

- *Card agglutination test :* CATT has been recommended by OIE for serodiagnosis of *T. evansi* (Songa and Hamers, 1998). RoTat 1.2 VSG is a predominant variant antigen type and it is the diagnostic Ag in CATT/*T. evansi* experimentally and naturally infected animals, this test was done with encouraging result for detection of Abs. Immunodiagnostic test relies on the presence of a widely distributed variable surface antigen. The card agglutination test (CATT) uses the formalin fixed variable antigen types of *T. evansi* that are used in the agglutination test. The test, which is simple to perform, has been used for diagnosis of *T. evansi* but is unlikely to be of use for *T. vivax* or *T. congolense* because of the difficulty of identifying suitable variable antigens of these species. Test is useful for sero-epidemiology of *T. evansi* (Dhami *et al.*, 1999).

- *Antibody detection ELISA :* ELISA is a sensitive and efficient test, large number of samples could be handled at a time and the data could be analysed by computer. Undoubtedly, the introduction of enzyme-linked immunosorbent assays (ELISA) for use as diagnostic tests for animal trypanosomosis has increased interest in the possibility of a universally applied immunodiagnostic assay. In addition, species-specific monoclonal antibodies developed against *T. brucei, T. vivax* and *T. congolense* (Nantulya *et al.*, 1989) and *T. evansi* will allow isolation and purification of defined specific antigens for use in indirect ELISA.

  For detection of Abs raised in the host system during *T. evansi* infection, Ab detection ELISA is used. Ag prepared from crude sonicated trypanosomal extracts showed that sensitivity and specificity of the test is almost similar to the IFAT. The test has been used epidemiological survey and for detection of Ab in camel, horse, cattle and buffalo and found to have higher sensitivity than parasitological method of diagnosis. Advancement in research on characterization of trypanosome Ags have been done to the immunodominant proteins in order to obtain the highest diagnostic sensitivity by purification of defined specific Ags for use in Ab-ELISA (Singh *et al.*, 1995, 1997).

  Antibody detection EL1SA can not differentiate between active infection and past infection as Abs persists also after the treatment of the affected animals, but it is useful for epidemiological tools rather than diagnosis of clinical cases (Pathak and Singh, 2005). Although it is clear that detection of Abs does not mean active infection, but together with knowledge of trypanocidal use, conclusion of current infection can often be drawn from positive results. In the absence of facilities of Ag-ELISA or PCR technique, Ab-detection ELISA can be used extensively for epidemiological study of surra to know the seroprevalence.

- *Dot-ELISA :* It is the modification of antibody ELISA, where nitrocellulose membrane is used as a carrier of protein. Dot

ELISA-detection of Abs against *T. evansi* infection has been used in sheep, in immunized rabbits (Singla *et al.*, 1996b) and in camel (Shahardar *et al.*, 2002).

(ii) *Antigen detection test* : Detection of *T. evansi* released Ags in the blood and tissue fluids of the infected animals is a useful tool for diagnosis of current infection.

- *Counter immune-electrophoresis (CIEP)* : The test has been used for diagnosis of experimental as well as natural *T. evansi* infection. The test has been found simple reproducible.
- *Antigen Detection ELISA* : A modification of the ELISA, currently of great interest, is based on an antigen capture assay which enables detection of circulating trypanosomal antigen in the blood of infected animals. Antibody against trypanosomal antigen is used to coat ELISA plates and any antigen present in test sera binds. The complex so formed is then incubated with the same antibody, conjugated with enzyme and visualized with a suitable substrate. Early assays using polyclonal antibodies raised against crude trypanosomal antigen preparations were found to detect antigen in animals infected with *T. evansi* and *T. congolense* within ten to 14 days of infection, and after trypanocidal drug treatment they disappeared within 21 days (Rae and Luckins, 1984). Later, the species specificity of the assay was improved following the development of monoclonal antibodies as capture antibodies that recognized antigens present in *T. brucei*, *T. vivax* and *T. congolense*. Specific circulating antigens could be detected in cattle from eight to 14 days after infection, but within 14 days of treatment they were no longer detectable (Nantulya and Lindqvist, 1989).

Detection of *T. evansi* Ags using polyclonal or monoclonal Abs by ELISA have been used successfully for diagnosis of the disease. Ag ELISA was found to be more sensitive and specific compared with Ab-ELISA and wet blood examination and could be used for epidemiological studies of latent trypanosomosis in livestock. Although Ag-ELISA is very much useful for diagnosis of surra particularly for detection of active infection, but the test gives some false negative results in the early stage of infection, still this technique should be disseminated in the field for detection of active infection.

- *Latex Agglutination* : Surratex detects circulating trypanosome antigens (Nantulya, 1994). The Surratex reagent is a suspension of latex particles that have been sensitized with a monoclonal antibody against *T. evansi* internal antigen. The test kit is marketed by Brentec diagnostics, Nairobi.
- *Immune complex detection* : For detection of circulatory immune complex of cattle and buffaloes, sandwich ELISA has been done and compared with wet blood film examination and microhaematocrit centrifugation techniques and the test detected 37.8% aparasitaemic animals (Jeyabal *et al.*, 2003).

(D) Nucleic acid detection

Latest molecular diagnostic techniques have been developed to overcome the problems related to parasitological and serological methods of diagnosis of surra.

- *DNA Probes* : In this technique nucleic acid probes are used for the detection of parasite DNA. DNA probes constructed from *T. evansi* genomic DNA and kinetoplast DNA has been used for sensitive detection of the parasite in infected blood. Hybridization of total genomic DNA with a DNA probe has been found useful for detection of bubaline, cameline and equine strains of *T. evansi.* Highly sensitive PCR technique has superseded the technique of diagnosis by DNA probes. The application of DNA probes for identification and characterization of *T. evansi* strains has opened up the use of this technology for strain differences and antigenic variation.
- *PCR* : Amplification of a specific DNA sequence of the genome of *T. evansi* is done to produce an easily detectable product. PCR has been found more sensitive in detecting *T. evansi* infection than parasitological and serological tests.
- *PCR-ELISA* : For products are subsequently examined by ELISA in this method. The technique of PCR-ELISA is not only beneficial for diagnosis of the parasite but also useful for epidemiological study and control programme.

Treatment, control and prevention

Trypanosoma evansi control programme should be selected taking into account the complex epidemiology involving many hosts, vectors, predisposing diseases and possible stress factors. Control can be based on control of the causal agent, control of the vector and use of innate resistance of the host to the effect of the infection

Chemotherapy and chemoprophylaxis : Control of the disease mainly depends on chemotherapy and chemoprophylaxis, but this approach has not been without problems. The major problems are high price of drugs, difficulties in diagnosis, availability of few drugs and the development of drug resistance.

The first successful attempts at the treatment of cattle suffering from "nagana" were made with tartar. The emetic (= antimony potassium tartrate) early in the twentieth century. The drug is extremely irritant at the site of injection and has to be given intravenously. Another disadvantage was that several injections were needed to achieve a cure. The drug suramin is also one of the earliest, but is only active against trypanosomes of the *brucei* group (subgenus *Trypanozoon*). For a long period, few other drugs were available and it was only after the 2nd World War that a few new compounds reached the market stage that were both effective and practical, able to effect a cure by a single injection.

In the past, pharmaceutical companies routinely screened a great numbers of chemical compounds for their antitrypanosomal activity. Few of the promising ones, however, were developed up to the market stage, either due to their too toxic nature in domestic animals, or because they did not show the expected efficacy in practical field situations. Sometimes, the trypanosomes quickly developed resistance to the drug and disappeared from the market due to this reason. However, the fact that at present there are only very few commercially available effective products against trypanosomosis because of economic reasons. It should be realized that the chemical industry is not actively seeking to develop new compounds, because the market is rather uncertain and not very profitable.

Curative drugs : Curative drugs are mainly used where disease incidence is low and only a limited number of animals in a herd contract the disease during the course of a year. This is often the case when the threat mainly occurs seasonally. This is true in the case of *T. evansi* in which the higher risk situations occur during the rainy or post rainy season. Curative drugs are meant to cure individual infected animals, not to protect the whole herd or group for a longer period.

Curative treatment is most effective in herds that are inspected and treated at regular intervals. The more frequently the visits are carried out, the more effective the treatment regimen. Block treatment of all animals in a herd should not be carried out with curative drugs, at least not with one that possesses a residual effect, because of the high risk of drug resistance developing during the period that the drug reaches a subcurative level. All curative drugs also possess some residual effect, but in the case of diminazene aceturate, this is practically negligible.

Prophylactic drugs : These are used where the risk is so high that the health of the herds cannot be maintained by individual application of curative compounds. In such a situation many animals contract the disease too frequently. Although curative treatments may prevent a high death rate, the overall health of the affected herds is not satisfactory, with loss of condition, poor (re)productive performance, many clinical cases and some deaths, despite a relatively large number of treatments at each regular visit. The other condition in which there may be requirement of prophylactic drugs when the infected animals cannot be reached e.g. inaccessibility during the rainy season, transhumant herds and trade cattle moving to distant markets.

Available drugs in India include diminazene aceturate, quinapyramine sulphate and chloride combination and quinapyramine sulphate alone as curative for treatment and prophylactic use against trypanosomosis in domestic animals.

- Quinapyramines (Antrycide prosalt, Tevansi, Triquin, Tribexin, Trypnil, etc.) is normally available as 2.5 gm with Quinapyramines prosalt available in mixture of quinapyramine methyle sulphate (1.5 gm) and quinapyramine methyle chloride (1.0 gm). This drug is given by subcutaneous route at 3.0 mg to 5.0 mg/kg body weight. (Singh *et al.*, 1987).
- Diminazine aceturate (Berenil) is administered as 3.5 mg to 5.0 mg/kg deep intramuscular injection.
- Isometamedium (Samorin) is used @ 0.5– 2.0 mg/kg body weight intramuscular injection.
- Cymalarsan can cross the blood brain barrier and can be used in nervous form of surra. This is not available in India. It can be used @ 0.75 mg/kg body weight intramuscular injection.

- Suramines (Antrypol, Nagapol, Gilpol) are used @12mg/kg body weight 10% solution intravenous injection.
- Experimentally human sera were found to be trypanolytic. However, this activity was transient in nature (Juyal *et al.*, 1998).

Drug resistance : Drug resistance may be defined as a loss of sensitivity by a strain of an organism to a compound to which it had previously been susceptible. The discovery of the first compound active against *T. brucei rhodesiense* was rapidly followed by reports of resistance to that drug. Sooner or later, newly developed trypanocidal drugs have failed to cure some cases of human or animal trypanosomosis after a period of use. Every time that new drugs are released by the manufacturers and used in the field, drug resistance has appeared. It is especially by misuse of trypanocides, by their mistaken and inefficient application, that resistance develops.

Vaccination : All attempts for developing a vaccine against trypanosomosis have failed. With the rapid advances in molecular biology the situation may change at some point in the future, but so far this approach has been cut off by the almost unlimited ability of trypanosomes in the host to change their surface antigens frequently. With the new antigens appearing, antibodies elicited against previous types of antigens are no longer effective and the immune system has to start all over again to produce new antibodies, until it becomes exhausted. Also, the antigen repertoire is different between different strains, types and subspecies of the same trypanosome species.

Control of flies : Vector control or control of flies for prevention of disease has traditionally been used since long and should be based on specialized large-scale operations as insects recognize no boundaries between farms, districts, or even countries.

Tabanid flies are susceptible to the action of insecticides, and different products, starting with DDT and dieldrin up to the more recently introduced and less harmful pyrethroids, have been used over the past 50 years to control. Today, with DDT banned in most countries and the general shift towards a more sophisticated use of insecticide and ground spraying has practically been abolished. A different way of using insecticides is to apply these on domestic animals, so that flies settling on such animals are killed. Synthetic pyrethroid formulations are applied by spraying, dipping or used as a "pour-on" formulation, which is more expensive but does not need any pump, spray-race or dip. Depending on the particular insecticide used, ticks (and other ectoparasites) may also be reduced. Although the frequency of application needed for the effective control of ticks is greater. This method of insecticide application is much less polluting than spraying the environment. In brief, organochlorine insecticides, organophosphates or other pesticides such as synthetic pyrethroids for controlling the flies should be done. Another approach is the use of traps or insecticide-impregnated targets (screens).

Following adaptive measures can also be followed for the control of disease:

1. To protect the susceptible animals during the high risk period use chemoprophylactic drugs before the onset of rainy season.
2. To avoid spreading of disease and reducing the risk of infection sick animals must be given immediate attention and proper treatment.
3. Trypanocides must be selected keeping in mind the problem of drug resistance in the area.
4. As immunosuppression caused by trypanosomes can interference with vaccination programme, the animals must be treated for surra, before adopting any vaccination programme.
5. Mass campaign should be implemented for eradication of *Tabanus* and other biting flies by spraying insecticides. It has limited value under Indian conditions.
6. Need for diagnostic centers all over the country.
7. Search for new chemotherapeutic agents.
8. Herbal medicines must be investigated for the treatment of surra.
9. Regular disease surveillance and monitoring in apparently healthy animals.
10. Treatment and control against other diseases, deworming and vitamin supplements.
11. Sporadic cases of *T. evansi* infection should also be taken as seriously as the outbreaks and the treated with proper doses of suitable curative drugs/ proper administration.
12. For repeating the prophylactic injection one should not wait for the end of the protective period of the previous injection i.e. if

the protective period is three months the next injection should be made at 75 days.

References

Ashkar, T. and Ochilo, M. (1972). The application of the indirect fluorescent antibody test to samples of dried sera and blood from cattle in the Lambwe Valley, South Nyanza, Kenya. *Bull. World Hlth Organ.*, 47: 769-772

Bhatia, B.B., Pathak, K.M..L and Banerjee, D.P. (2006). *Text Book of Veterinary Parasitology.* 2nd ed., Kalyani Publishers, Ludhiana, pp. 304–315

Dhami, D.S., Juyal, P.D. and Singla, L.D. (1999). Sero-epidemiology of *Trypanosoma evansi* using CATT. *Indian Vet. J.*, 76: 842-44

Gill, B. S. (1991). *Trypanosomes and trypanosomiases in Indian livestock.* Indian Council of Agricultural Research, New Delhi, pp. 191

Gupta, M. P., Kumar, H. and Singla, L.D. (2009). Trypanosomosis concurrent to tuberculosis in black bucks. *Indian Vet. J.*, 86: 727–28

Jatkar, P.R. and Singh, M. (1971). Diagnosis camels by the passive of surra in haem-agglutination test. *Br. Vet. J.*, 127: 283-288

Jayabal, L., Chaudhri, S.S., Singh, A. and Kumar, D. (2003). Detection of circulating antigens in immune complexes of *Trypanosoma evansi* infected cattle and buffaloes by ELISA. *J. Vet. Parasitol.*, 17: 85-88.

Joshi, D.P., Shegokar, V.R., Powar, R.M., Herder, S., Katti, R., Salkar, H.R., Dani, V.S., Bhargava, A., Jannin, J. and Truc, P. (2005). Human trypanosomiasis caused by *Trypanosoma evansi* in India: the first case report. *Am. J. Trop. Med. Hyg.*, 73: 491–495

Juyal, P.D., Singla, L.D. and Saxena, H.M. (1998). In vivo activity of human serum against *Trypanosoma evansi* in Swiss albino mice. *J. Parasit. Dis.*, 22: 67-68

Killick-Kendrick, R. (1968). The diagnosis of trypanosomiasis of livestock– a review of current technique. *Vet. Bull.*, 33: 77-191

Kristjanson, P., Swallow, D., Rowlands, G.J., Kruska, R. and Leeuw, P. (1999). Measuring the cost of African animal trypanosomosis, the potential benefits of control and return to research. *Agri. Systems*, 59: 79-98

Luckins, A.G., Boid, R., Rae, P., Mahmoud, M.M., El-Malik, K.H. and Gray, A.R. (1979). Serodiagnosis of infection with *Trypanosoma evansi* in camels in the Sudan. *Trop. Anim. Hlth Prod.*, 11: 1-12

Lun, Z.R., Reid, S.A., Lai, D.H. and Li, F.J. (2009). Atypical human trypanosomiasis: a neglected disease or just an unlucky accident? *Trends in Parasitol.*, 25: 107–08

Nantulya, V.M. (1994). Surratex a simple latex agglutination antigen test for diagnosis of *Trypanosoma evansi* infection (Surra). *Trop. Med. Parasitol.* 45: 9-12

Nantulya, V.M. and Lindqvist, K.J. (1989). Antigen detection enzyme immunoassays for the diagnosis of *Trypanosoma vivax, T. congolense* and *T. brucei* infections in cattle. *Trop. Med. Parasitol.*, 40: 267-272.

Pathak, K.L.M. and Singh, N. (2005). Animal trypanosomosis. *Intas Polivet*, 9: 194-98

Rae, P.F. and Luckins, A.G. (1984). Detection of circulating trypanosomal antigens by enzyme immunoassay. *Ann. Trop. Med. Parasitol.*, 78: 587-596

Raisinghani, P.M. and Lodha, K.R. (1982). Note on biometrical observations of *Trypanosoma evansi* in camel. *Indian J. Anim. Sci.*, 52: 1003-1005

Reid, S.A., Husein, A. and Copeman, D.B. (2001). Evaluation and improvement of parasitological tests for *Trypanosoma evansi* infection. *Vet. Parasitol.*, 102: 291-297

Sarmah, P.C., Bhattacharyulu, Y. and Joshi, V.B. (1997). Effect of *Trypanosoma evansi* infection on the antibody response in guinea pigs vaccinated with haemorrhagic septicaemia oil adjuvant vaccine. *J. Vet. Parasitol.*, 11:161-164

Shahardar, R.A., Mishra, A.K. and Rao, J.R. (2002). Dot-ELISA for detection of antibodies against *Trypanosoma evansi* dromedary camel. *J. Vet. Parasitol.*, 16: 163-64

Singh, Veer, Chaudhri, S.S., Kumar, S. and Chhabra, M.B. (1995). Polyclonal antibody-based antigen-detection immunoassay for diagnosis of *Trypanosoma evansi* in buffaloes and horses. *Vet. Parasitol.*, 56: 261-267

Singh, Veer and Chhabra, M.B. (2008). Trypanosomosis (surra) in India: an update. *J. Parasit. Dis.*, 32: 104-110

Singh, Veer, Gahlot, A.K. and Chhabra, M.B. (1994). Evaluation of some serodiagnostic tests for *Trypanosoma evansi* infection in camels. *J. Camel Pract. Res.*, 1: 30-33

Singh, Veer and Raisinghani, P.M. (1990). Clinical observation in experimental surra in buffalo calves. *Indian J. Anim. Res.*, 24: 72-74

Singh, Veer, Raisinghani, P.M., Lodha, K.R. and Manohar, G.S. (1987). Trypanocidal value of a drug in experimental *Trypanosoma evansi* infection in camels. *Indian Vet. J.*, 64: 467-470

Singh, Veer, Singh, A. and Chhabra, M.B. (1997). Antigenic specificities of several Indian stocks of *Trypanosoma evansi* by western blot analysis. *Indian J. Anim. Sci.*, B67: 369-372

Singla, L.D. and Juyal, P.D. (1992). Immunomodulatory effects of levamisole against *Trypanosoma evansi* infection in cow-calves: serum gamma globulins. *J. Vet. Parasitol.*, 6: 9-14

Singla, L.D., Juyal, P.D. and Ahuja, S.P. (1998). Blood brain barrier status in experimental *Trypanosoma evansi* infected and levamisole treated cow-calves. *Indian Vet. J.*, 75: 109–12

Singla, L.D., Juyal, P.D. and Ahuja, S.P. (2000). Serum protein changes of cross bred calves experimentally infected with *Trypanosoma evansi* and immuno modulated with levamisole. *Indian Vet. J.*, 77: 172-174

Singla, L.D., Juyal, P.D. and Kalra, I.S. (1996a). Effects of levamisole on the clinical response of *Trypanosoma evansi* infection in cow-calves. *Indian Vet. J.* 73: 11-15

Singla, L.D., Juyal, P.D. and Kapoor, J. (1996b). Dot-Enzyme Linked Immuno Sorbent Assay for detection of *Trypanosoma evansi* in rabbits. *J. Vet. Parasitol.*, 10: 87-89

Singla, L.D., Juyal, P.D. and Sharma, N.S. (2010). Immune responses to haemorrhagic septicaemia (HS) vaccination in *Trypanosoma evansi* infected buffalo-calves. *Trop. Anim. Hlth. Prod.*, 42: 589–595

Singla, N., Parshad, V.R. and Singla, L.D. (2003). Potential of *Trypanosoma evansi* as a biocide of rodent pests. In Rat, Mice and People: Rodent biology and management. (Eds. Singleton, GR, Hinds LA, Krebs CJ, and spat DM). ACIAR Monograph No. 96. Canberra, Australia, 43-46

Songa, E.B. and Hamers, R. (1998). A card agglutination test (CATT) for veterinary use based on early VAT RO Ta T 1.2 *Trypanosoma evansi*. *Ann. Soc. Belg. Med. Trop.*, 68: 233-244

Sood, N.K., Singla, L.D., Singh, R.S. and Uppal, S.K. (2011). Association of *Trypanosoma theileri* with peritonitis in a pregnant cross-bred cow: a case report. *Veterinarani Medicina*, 56: 82-84

Soulsby, E.J.L. (1982). Helminths, Arthropods and Protozoa of domesticated Animals. 7th ed., ELBS and Bailliere Tindall. London, pp 809

Watson, E.A. (1920). *Dourine in Canada- History, research, suppression*. Dominion of Canada, Department of Agriculture, Canada.

Woo, P.T.K. (1977). Salivarian trypanosomes producing disease in livestock outside of Sub-saharan Africa. In: "*Parasitic Protozoa*". Vol. 1 Krier, J.P. (Ed.), Academic Press Inc., New York, pp. 269-296.

□□□

Chapter 12

Parasites and Parasitic Diseases in Fish Culture System

K.P. Jithendran
Central Institute of Brackishwater Aquaculture
75, Santhome High Road, Chennai - 600 028, India

Introduction

The fish production system in India has two main sources viz. culture fisheries- the fish grown in captivity and capture fisheries- the fish caught from the wild stock. There are also some intermediate forms of production such as culture-based fisheries, enhanced capture fisheries and capture based aquaculture. In culture based fisheries, fishes are stocked in reservoirs and lakes and caught back after they grow by utilizing natural food. Enhanced capture fishery means augmenting the fish stock in capture fisheries by stocking support. Under capture-based aquaculture fish seed collected from wild are grown in captivity. The major sources of fish production in India are: freshwater aquaculture, mariculture and coastal aquaculture with intermediate culture system based on culture based fisheries and enhanced capture fisheries of reservoirs/wet lands, marine capture fisheries of open sea, and inland capture fisheries of rivers estuaries and lakes. Of these, the first three hold huge potential to achieve a significant increase in fish productivity and production to meet the growing demand of fish as a protein source at affordable price besides providing livelihood for over 400 million people. At present, the three Indian major carps viz. catla (*Catla catla*), rohu (*Labeo rohita*) and mrigal (*Cirrhinus mrigala*) constitute the main contributor (90%) for freshwater aquaculture production with about half of the total fish production in the country followed by silver carp, grass carp and common carp.

Culture system with different combination of carps have been standardized to meet local requirements. Apart from culture of Indian major carps, opportunities exist for developing culture of magur (*Clarius batrachus*), many coldwater fishes like trouts and mahseers in hill states like Jammu and Kashmir, Himachal Pradesh, Uttrakhand, Sikkim and Arunachal Pradesh. Mariculture is also a fast growing enterprise with seabass (*Lates calcarifer*), grouper (*Epinephelus tauvina, E. malabaricus*), mullet (*Mugil cephalus*), red snapper (*Lutjanus argentimaculatus*) and many other marine fish species. Cobia (*Rachycentron canadum*) is also gaining importance as a promising marine fish species for sea farming in offshore grow-out cages. Coastal aquaculture, though dominated by shrimp species is also having potential for fish production with brackishwater species like seabass (*Lates calcarifer*), mullet (*Mugil cephalus*) and milk fish (*Chanos chanos*) either in pond, cage or pen culture (Figs 1-5). Fish production system which was practiced earlier as a traditional activity has grown into a commercial enterprise in late 1980's due to the thrust given to aquaculture. The growth of this sector has been phenomenal, contributing significantly to food security export earnings and employment generation. At present the country produces 4.6 million tons of fish and is the second largest producer of inland fish in the world and third in terms of total fish production contributing more than 1% to the country's GDP and 4.7% to the agricultural GDP. Apart from food sector, ornamental fish farming and trade is also developing rapidly in India. Recently brackishwater and marine aquarium is also drawing the attention of fish hobbyists in India.

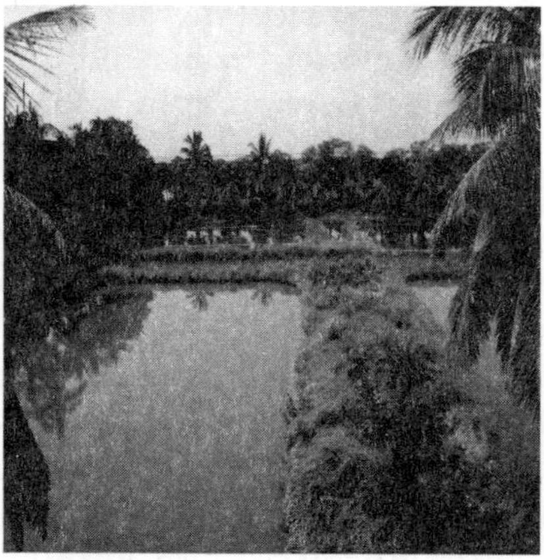

Fig.1: A fish culture pond in West Bengal

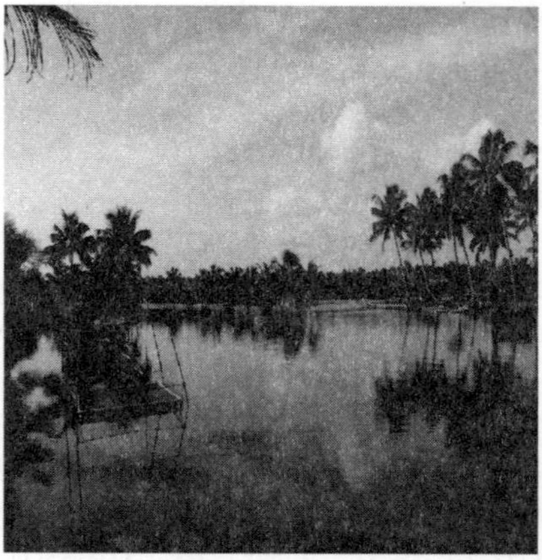

Fig .2: Cage farming of Asian seabass in Kerala

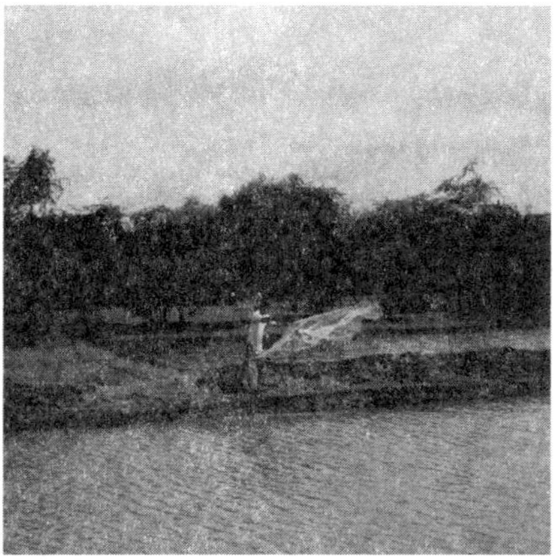

Fig. 3: A polyculture farm in West Bengal

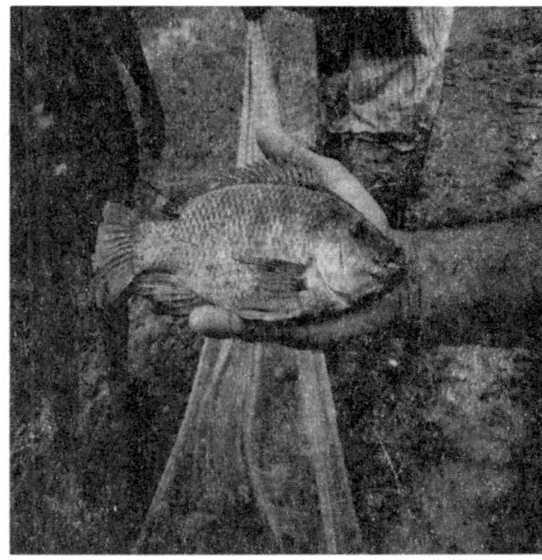

Fig .4: Cultured Tilapia fish in West Bengal

Aquaculture in the country holds tremendous potential to contribute towards the food security and for augmenting export earnings. The intensification of culture practices though helped to increase production levels, also led to the outbreaks of viral, bacterial and parasitic diseases. Many diseases result from intensification of culture practices without basic perception of the intricate balance between host, pathogen and environment challenging the sustainable development of aquaculture. Aquaculture environment that are suitable for growth and reproduction of cultured animals are also hospitable to potential pathogens. Like any other culture species, fish culture also has to deal with various pathogens like virus, bacteria, fungi and parasites. In wild, parasitism is a ubiquitous phenomenon in the marine environment. The effect of parasites on the condition and dynamics of wild populations are still poorly understood. A large volume of information on parasitic infections in wild fish is available in India, but the significance of these as a disease entity is vague. Readers are referred to recent compilation and checklist published by Abidi (2002). Parasitic diseases in fishes range from extremely pathogenic ones to those that are practically harmless and are broadly categorized into two major groups, protozoan and metazoan parasites. The present chapter deals with fish parasites and parasitic infections in wild and culture system that are of economic concern for production system and the emerging parasitic diseases in India and neighboring countries.

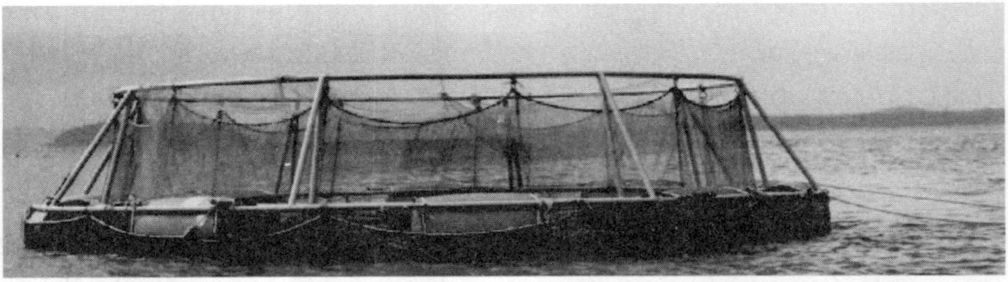

Fig .5: A cage design used for sea farming in India (CMFRI, 2010)

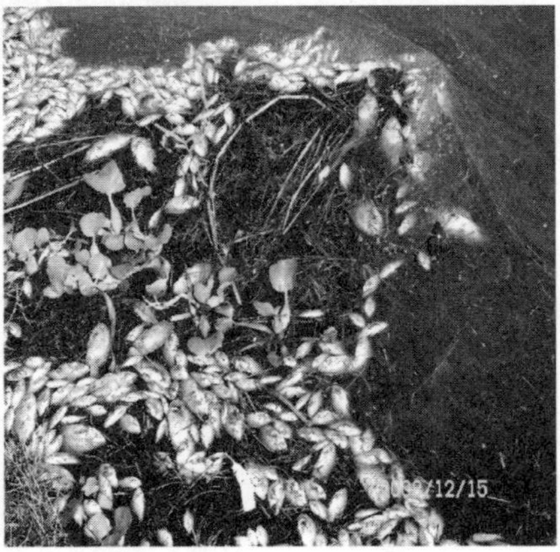

Fig.6: Mortality of cultured fish due to diseases, Andhra Pradesh

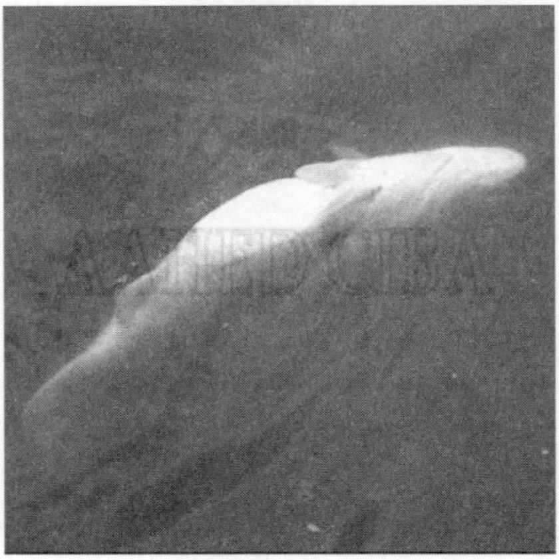

Fig.7: Seabass broodstock floating upside down with disease symptoms, Tamil Nadu

Diseases in aquaculture system

Disease is now a primary constraint to aquaculture production globally impeding both economic and social development in many countries. This is attributed to many factors such as intensification and diversification of aquaculture practices through translocation of broodstock, post larvae, fry and fingerlings, etc.; globalization of live fish trade including ornamentals and their products; the enhancement of marine and coastal areas through stocking aquatic animals raised in hatcheries; unanticipated negative interactions between cultured and wild fish populations; poor or lack of effective biosecurity measures; slow awareness on emerging diseases and above all global change in climate and human mediated movements of aquaculture commodities. Control of disease is complex and relies heavily on a combination of the following pathogen detection, disease diagnosis, treatment, prevention and general health management.

Parasitic diseases in fin fishes

Parasitic diseases are one of the most serious problems in fishes, though not of much concern among the wild fish stock because in most instances, no significant harm appears to be caused to them. However, parasites often cause serious disease outbreaks of among farmed fish. With the exception of cases of mass mortalities caused by outbreaks of parasites, assessment of the effects of parasite infection in natural fish populations is particularly difficult because of the presence of predators or scavengers which rapidly remove moribund or dead fish. Majority of the fish parasites belong to three major groups, protozoan, helminths and arthropods bring dominated by crustaceans.

Protozoan parasites

Protozoan parasites are either external or internal parasites, present in large numbers on the surface of the skin, gills or in the internal organs of fishes. They have direct life cycle and hence build up to very high numbers in a short time especially when fish are overcrowded. The most common protozoan parasite observed in fish culture system are ciliates although some obligate amoebic, flagellate and microsporidians (sporozoa) are also noticed.

Ciliate infections : Ciliates are external parasites with a direct life cycle and many are common inhabitants of pond reared fish (Figs 8-11). Most species get noticed once they become a problem due to excessive numbers on the host. Infection occurs in fishes when there is high level of organic matter in the water or poor water exchange and the stocking density is high.

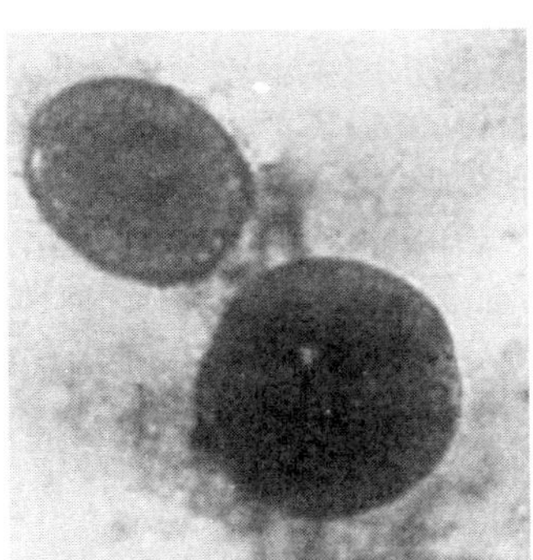

Fig.8: *Amyloodinium* spp.

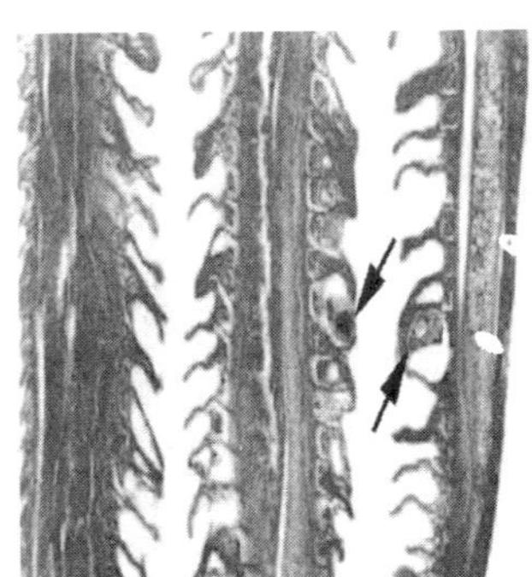

Fig.9: *Cryptocaryon* spp. on gills

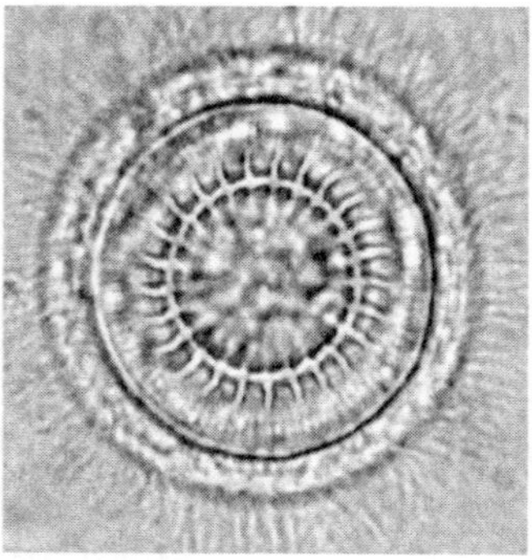

Fig.10: *Trichodina* spp. (fresh)

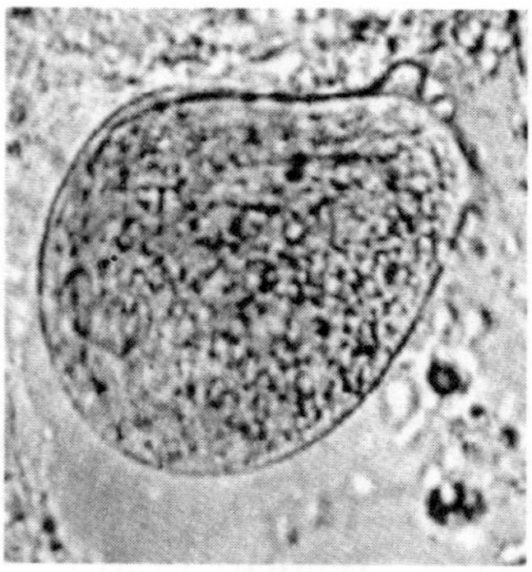

Fig.11: *Cryptocaryon* spp.

Ichthyophthirius spp. in freshwater and *Cryptocaryon* spp. in marine and brackishwater are the most common ciliates. Others are *Chilodonella, Tetrahymena, Trichodina, Ambiphyra, Apiosoma, Epistylis,* etc. *Chilodenella* is a large, heart shaped ciliate 60-80m with bands of cilia along the long axis of the organism. *Ambiphyra* and *Apiosoma* are sedentary ciliates commonly found on the skin, fins or gills of pond reared fish. *Epistylis* is a stalked ciliate that attaches to the skin or fins of the host in colonies.

Icthyophthirius multifilis : It causes icthyophthiriasis, also known as 'Itch' or 'white spot' and is probably the most significant protozoan disease which affects the early stages of all freshwater food fishes. They are up to 1 mm in size characterised by its large horse-shoe shaped nucleus. Incidences of large scale mortality are common in nursery and rearing ponds with numerous pin-head shaped white spots on skin, fins, and gills. In advanced cases the entire body surface of the fish becomes covered with such nodules resulting in severe mortality. The parasite feeds on the epithelial tissues and fluids of the fish causing simple hyperplasia of the epidermal cells around the site of infection. Stages of *I. multifilis* within the dermal tissues of the host fish are almost impossible to remove using chemotherapy. Hence control is targeted against the life cycle stages outside the dermal tissue of the host.

Cryptocaryon irritans : It is a pear shaped (0.3-0.5 mm in size) ciliate found often on the surface of the fish. Infection sets in when there is high stocking density and decreased water temperature.

Species affected : The pathogen, *I. multifilis* accounts for significant economic losses to the aquaculture of catfish, carp, tilapia, seabass, grouper, snapper, etc. and ornamental fishes, and epizootics in wild fish population can result in mass kill.

Gross signs: Symptoms typical of ciliate infection include skin, and gill irritation displayed by flashing, rubbing and rapid breathing. Infected fish show tiny white spots on the fins and skin when infection has reached the mature stage, increased mucus production; fish often rub against submerged objects.

Effects on host: The disease causes massive mortality within a short time. The parasite may destroy the skin and gills causing respiratory problems, secondary bacterial infection and mass mortality. Occurrence of this parasite is often linked with a drop in ambient temperature.

Diagnosis: Encysted organism appears as visible white spots on the surface of the fish. Microscopic examination of the mucous from skin and gills may reveal round or oval parasites with cilia and horse shoe shaped macronucleus typical of ciliates.

Prevention and control: *For 'itch'*

- An elevation of water temperature to 30°C for 6 hr. daily for 3-5 days.
- 0.05% salinity shock.
- 100 ppm formalin for 1 hr for 2-3 days.
- 25 ppm formalin and 0.1 ppm malachite green.
- Transfer of infected stock in previously dry parasite free tanks for 2-3 times at 3 day interval.

***For* Cryptocaryon**

- Copper sulphate bath (0.5 ppm) for 5-7 days with good aeration and daily replenishment of water. Long bath treatment with 25-ppm formalin, for 5-7 days with good aeration and replacement of treated water daily.
- Preferred treatment for *Epistylis* is salt (0.2%) as an indefinite bath or a 3% salt dip.

Trichodina spp. : One of the most common ciliates found on the skin and gills of pond reared fish. Serious pathogens affecting the fry at low saline water with body shaped like hockey puck with its characteristic movement, which makes them fly through the water like a flying saucer. They mainly live on gills, skin with rings of chitinous teeth and spiral cilia around cytostome. *Trichodina* has a circular body 100 μ diameter with cilia around the perimeter. The infection sets in when there is high level of organic matter in the water or poor water exchange.

Species affected : Catfish, carp, tilapia, mullet, milk fish, seabass, grouper, snapper, etc.

Gross signs : It infects mainly gills, body surface and fins and causes excessive mucus production on gills and body surface with frayed fins.

Effects on host : Low numbers are not harmful, but overcrowding or deterioration of water quality facilitates rapid multiplication and serious damage besides susceptibility to opportunistic bacterial infections. Clinically fish has pale gills with irritation of body and hence they rub body against objects. Fish becomes weak during heavy infection and there can be high mortality among young fish.

Diagnosis : Microscopic examination of wet mounts of gill filaments and mucous from skin reveals saucer shaped parasite with cilia. Characteristic darting movements and presence of a toothed, circular disc within the body makes the identification easy.

Prevention and control : Easy to treat but the correction of the environmental problem is of prime importance.

- Salinity shock using 2-3% salt solution for 2-5 min. for 3-4 days
- Freshwater bath for 1 hour for 3 days
- Short bath with 200-ppm formalin for 30-60 min. for 3 days.

Amoebic infections : Amoebae are considered as serious pathogens of cyprinid fish. Most of the amoebic parasites are opportunistic pathogens, which lead a free life normally.

Causative agents : Some species of the genera *Entamoeba* cause kidney inflammation in trouts, while those of *Acanthamoeba* infect tilapia fish.

Life cycle : Direct and multiply very fast in numbers on debilitated fish.

Species affected : Cyprinids

Gross signs: Infected fish show respiratory distress, dropsy and anaemia.

Effects on host : Cause nodules in visceral organs, and enlargement of kidneys and spleen. Lamellar hyperplasia and hypertrophy, cellular infiltration and necrosis have been reported.

Diagnosis : Amoebae are readily detectable in wet mounts of infected tissues; however species identification is a matter of specialized job.

Prevention and Control : Good hygiene and husbandry besides treatment with saltwater or formalin baths are suggested.

Flagellate infections : Flagellate protozoans infect fish externally and internally. They infect both freshwater and marine fish and are characterized by one or more flagella to aid in a whip like or jerky motion. Majority of the flagellates are considered harmless; however some of them are well known parasites in fishes.

Causative agents : Dinoflagellates are external microscopic parasites with flagella for movement (eg. *Amyloodinium*). It is usually attached to the gill filaments or body surface of affected fish. Infection occurs in low saline water with high level of organic matter and high stocking density of fish. *Amyloodinium ocellatum*, a dinoflagellate causes 'velvet disease' in marine fishes. Primarily a parasite of the gills, later on spreads throughout the body imparting a velvety appearance to the fish and may even invade tissues. Lack of specificity and direct life cycle makes the infection to reach the level of fatal epizootics. *Piscinoodinium* sp. and *Crepidoodinium* spp. are similar to *Amyloodinium* spp. in all aspects and are found to infect freshwater fishes. *Hexamita* is small intestinal parasite commonly found in the intestinal tract of freshwater fish. Trypanosomes are flagellate parasites found infecting the blood of both freshwater and marine fishes with leeches as intermediate hosts. Most of the species are considered less pathogenic but sometimes heavy infection can lead to mortality with clinical signs of sluggishness, pale gills and anaemia. *Trypanoplasma* are biflagellate blood parasites similar to trypanosomes, infecting freshwater fishes. *Cryptobia* spp. causing cryptobiasis is also a biflagellate affecting fresh and marine fishes. Ichthyobodosis caused by *Ichthyobodo* spp. is also a dangerous infection, attacking the entire body surface and gills causing high mortality in freshwater fishes. Non-specific nature and direct life cycle coupled with high stocking densities usually result in fatal epizootics in culture conditions.

Life cycle : The life cycle is direct. The trophont detaches from the host fish, encysts and undergoes a series of divisions to produce free swimming infective stages to infect fresh hosts.

Species affected : Serious disease conditions affecting cat fish, carp, tilapia, seabass, grouper, snapper, etc. among food fishes and occasional mortality in marine ornamental fishes (*Abudefduf bengalensis*) kept under captive conditions.

Gross signs : Fish often come to the water surface or gather near the zone of aeration. Pale gills and darkening of the body surface are also noticed.

Effects on host : Destroy gills and skin, high or mass mortality, if not treated. Sick fishes are dark in colour and extremely thin.

Diagnosis : Diagnosis is by the squash preparation of mucous from gills, skin and fins in case of external parasites and intestinal contents in case of internal parasites.

Prevention and control : Most of the infections are easy to control. Copper sulphate bath (0.5 ppm) for 3-5 days with good aeration and a daily replenishment of water. Short bath treatment with 200 ppm formalin for 1 hr with good aeration is also recommended.

Sporozoan infections : Sporozoans, as a group are spore forming endoparasites, accommodates the largest number of fish parasites. Generally their life cycle consist of three stages, merogony, gamogony and sporogony and in many forms an intermediate host is also involved. Major groups infecting fishes are microsporidians and coccidians.

Microsporidians: Microsporidians which are also obligate intracellular parasites forming oval spores with an average size of 6 μm in a wide range of fishes. The infection manifests itself when there is poor water quality and poor nutrition.

Life cycle: The life cycle is direct and infections occur on ingestion of spores either as free spores or via a vector or predation. After ingestion, the infective sporoplasms are released and they enter the target host cell where the parasite undergoes vegetative development to produce characteristic cyst like structure of host origin (xenoma). Large numbers of spores are released from xenoma on host cell rupture.

Causative agents: Many species exist but most important fish microsporidians are *Pleistophora* spp. and *Glugea* spp. (Figs 12-15).

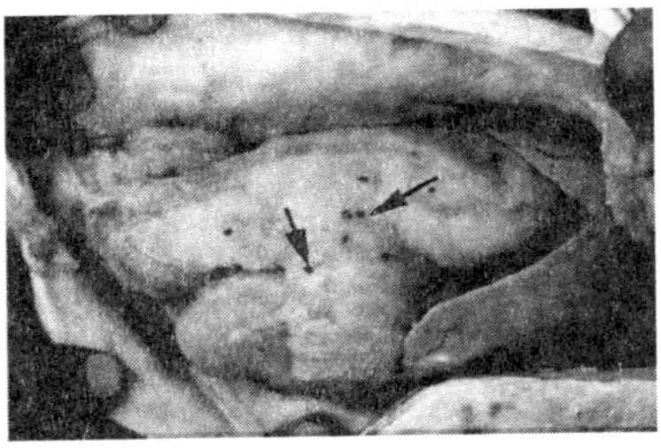

Fig.12: Microsporidian(*Glugea* spp.) nodules (xenoma) in the visceral organs of grouper (*Epinephelus tauvina*)

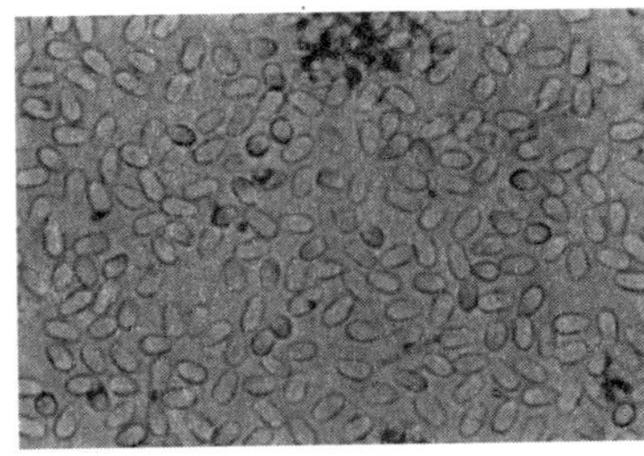

Fig.13: Fresh spores of microsporidian (*Glugea* spp.) from grouper, *E.tauvina* (1000x).

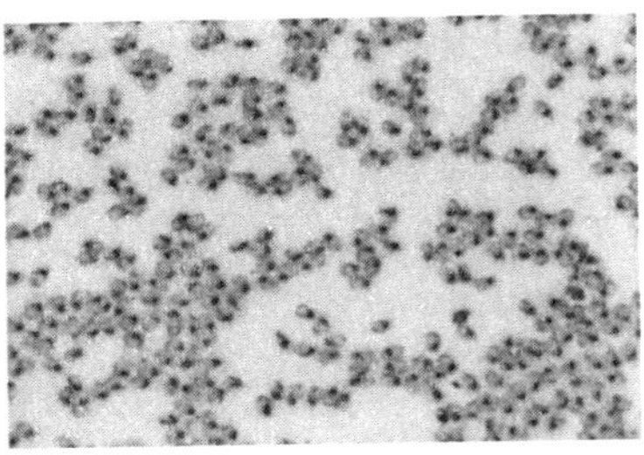

Fig.14: Giemsa stained microsporidian (*Glugea* spp.) spore from grouper, *E. tauvina* (1000x)

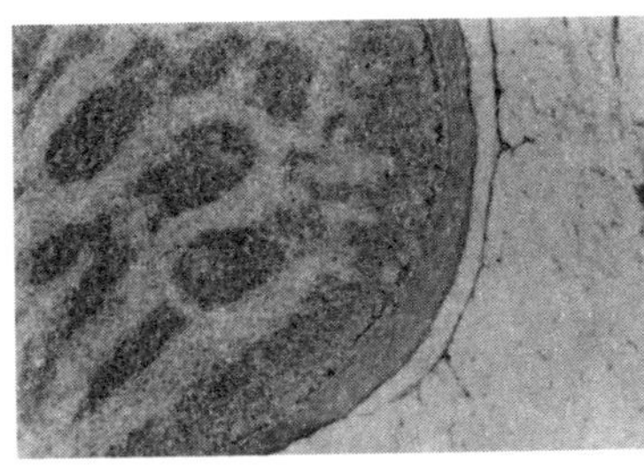

Fig.15: Histological section showing the *Glugea* spp. xenoma in the adipose tissues of grouper, *E. tauvina* (40x).

Species affected : Ranges of wild and cultured fish are susceptible.

Gross signs: No visible signs of infection except the finding of cysts like xenomas during necrosis of fish.

Effects on host : Infect various internal organs like intestinal wall, ovary, fat tissue, etc. The growth and proliferation of the microsporidian within the host cell results in complete destruction of the cells. The development stages and mature spores gradually replace the cell contents until the host cell becomes a mere envelope containing the parasites. Host tissue is damaged by pressure atrophy, which elicits proliferation of the connective tissue around the parasite mass forming a brown or blackish cyst-like structure of various size and shape, called as xenoma.

Diagnosis : The main diagnostic stage of the parasite, the minute unicellular spore measures 3-10 m with a single coiled polar filament.

Often they form small pea sized nodules of different sizes and colours on the affected tissues and are filled with pear shaped transparent spores.

Prevention and control : Good water exchange and management interventions. No treatment is available.

Coccidians: Most of the coccidian species have low pathogenicity and do not cause significant disease, but there is increasing evidence that they are potential pathogens. The most common infection in fish are intestinal. Other infection sites include reproductive organs, liver, spleen and swim bladder.

Causative agents : Main species belong to the genera are *Eimeria* and *Goussia.*

Life cycle : The typical life cycle may be direct by the ingestion infective oocysts which release sporozoites and invade host cells in the gastrointestinal tract. After several stages of development within host cells typical to each species, oocysts with sporocysts are released through host faeces to continue the life cycle.

Species affected : Catfish, tilapia, seabass, grouper, mullet, snapper, ornamental fish, etc.

Gross signs : Lethargy, poor feeding, emaciation and mucous strands protruding through anus

Effects on host : Typical coccidian pathology affecting the intestinal epithelial lining.

Diagnosis : Suspected fish shows mucous strands in the faeces and intestinal haemorrhages. Confirmation requires microscopic examination of intestinal contents for the presence of characteristic coccidian oocysts.

Prevention and control : No recommended treatment is available except the removal of affected fish from husbandry system and good and hygienic management practices.

Metazoan parasites

Compared to protozoan, metazoan parasitic diseases are less pathogenic. They have a multicellular organization but largely do not have the ability to multiply within host's body. Hence intensity of infection depends on the number of initial infective stages. Diseases caused by myxozoans, parasitic helminths, crustaceans and leeches are grouped under this category.

Myxozoans : Myxozoan comprises more than 2180 spp., most of which are fish parasites, and infect any tissue and group organ and cause disease in a wide variety of fishes (Figs 16-28). Myxozoans earlier classified under protozoans are internal microscopic parasites composed of unique morphology and several shell valves. The average size of the spore is 10 um. They are obligate parasites of tissues of various organs (histozoic) or live freely in cavities like gall bladder, abdominal cavity (coelozoic), having an indirect life cycle involving a vertebrate (fish) and an invertebrate (annelid) intermediate host. Severe infections can result in death of the fish. The myxozoan infections in fishes occur when there is poor water quality, high stocking density, feeding with infected trash fish and lack of quarantine measures. Many species of myxozoans were also recorded from marine ornamental fishes, such as Sergeant major, *Abudefduf bengalensis* and Blue damsels, *Pomacentrus caeruleus* (CMFRI, 2009).

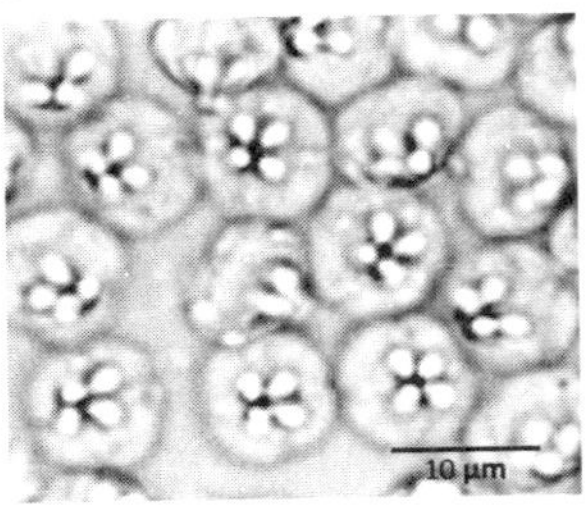

Fig.16:

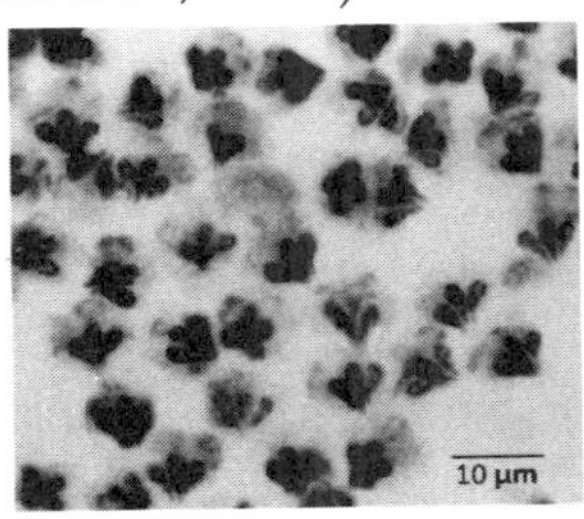

Fig.17:

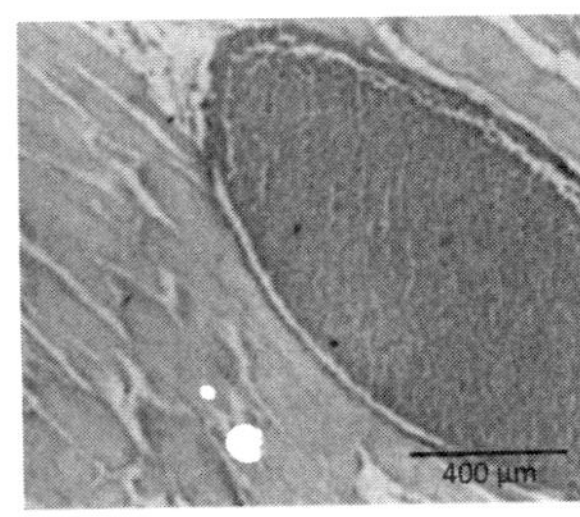

Fig.18:

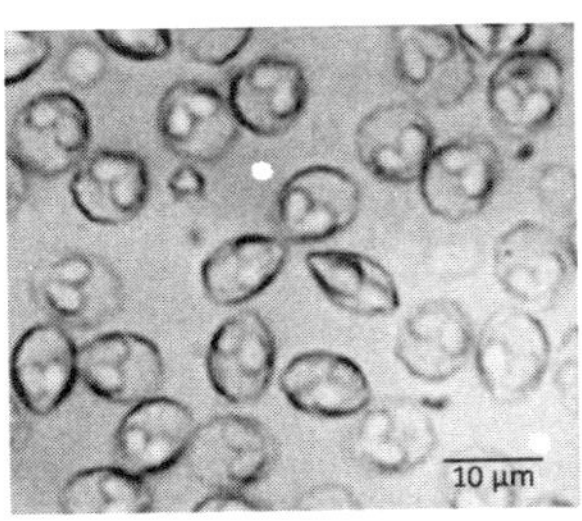

Fig.19:

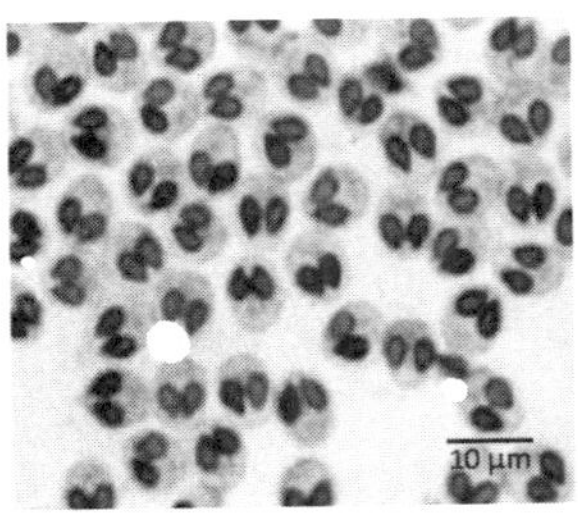

Fig.20:

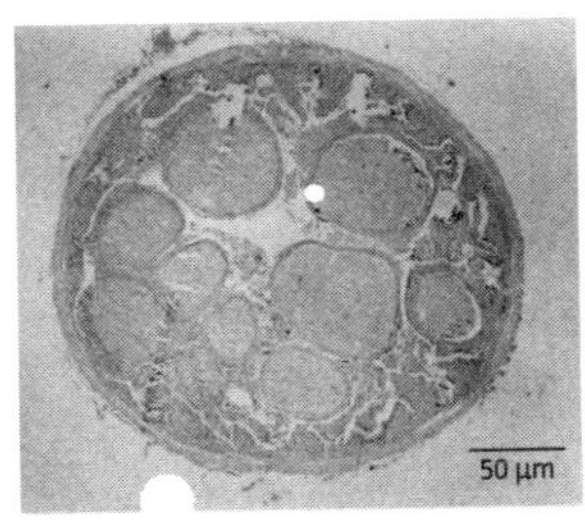

Fig.21:

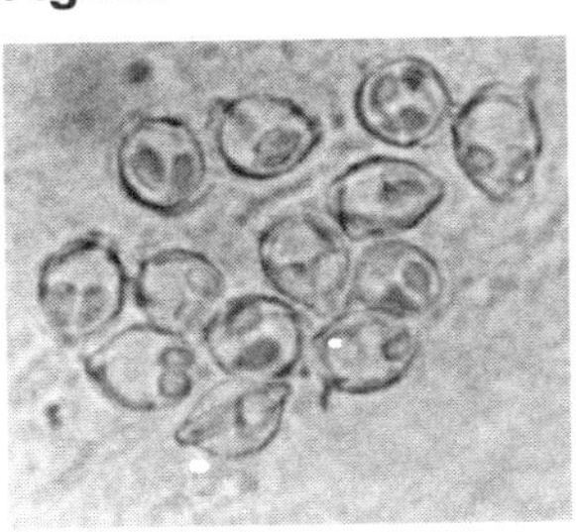

Fig.22:

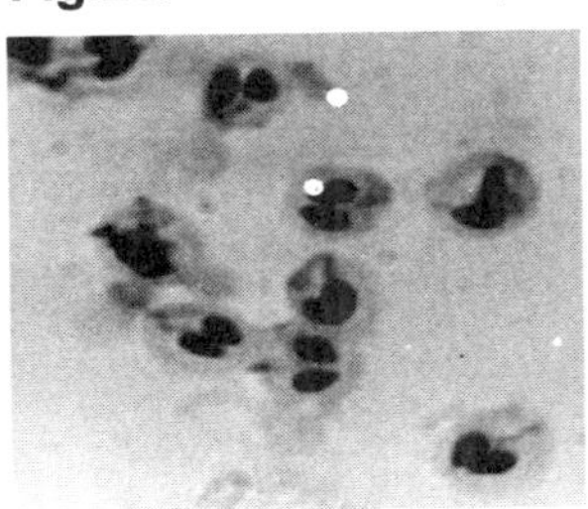

Fig.23:

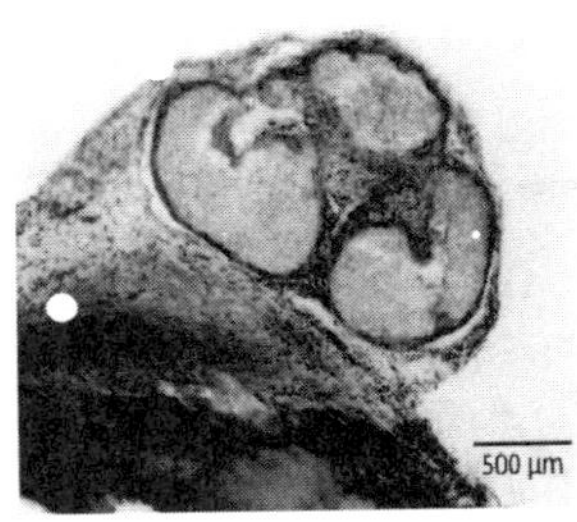

Fig.24:

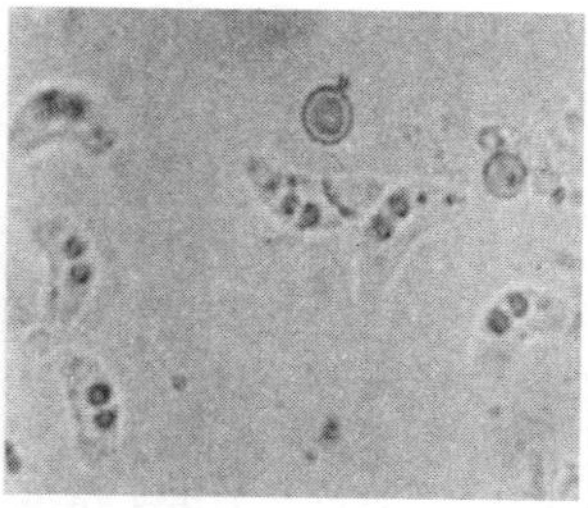

Fig.25:

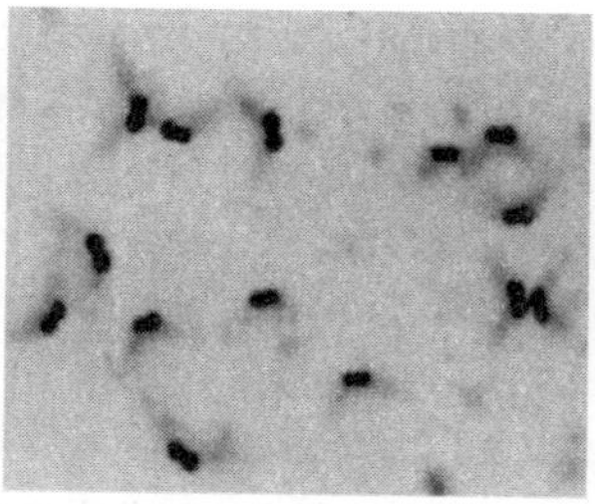

Fig.26:

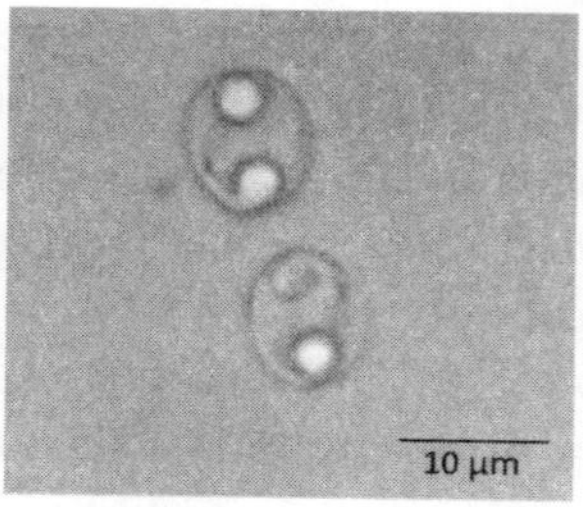

Fig.27:

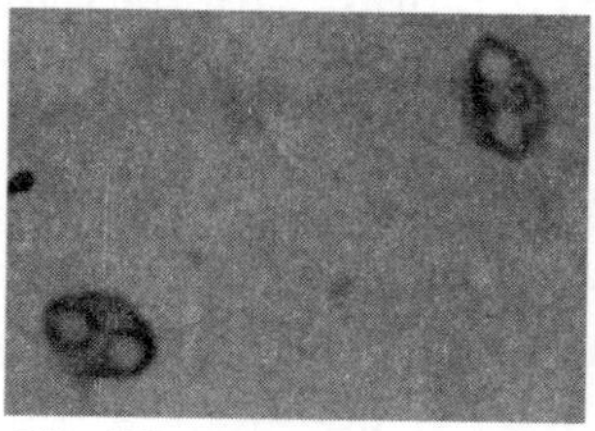

Fig.28:

Fig.16: Squash preparation of cysts recovered from skeletal muscle of *M. cephalus* showing freshspores of *Kudoa* spp. (x1000).

Fig.17: *Kudoa* spores stained with Giemsa (x1000, note the deeply stained polar capsules and less dense sporoplasm).

Fig 18: Histological section of infected muscle showing *Kudoa* cyst (x100)

Fig 19: Squash preparation of cysts recovered from intestine of *M. cephalus* showing fresh spores of *Myxobolus* spp. (x1000)

Fig 20: Spores of *Myxobolus* spp. stained with Giemsa (x1000)

Fig 21: Histological section of intestine showing *Myxobolus* spp. cysts filling the intestinal lumen (x100)

Fig 22: Fresh spores *Myxobolus etropli* infecting bulbus arteriosus of *Etroplus suratensis* (x1000)

Fig 23: Spores of *M. etropli* stained with Giemsa (x1000)

Fig 24: Histological section of the bulbus arteriosus showing cysts of *M. etropli* (x100)

Fig 25: Fresh spores of *Ceratomyxa etroplusi* infecting gall bladder of *Etroplus suratensis* (x1000)

Fig 26: Spores of *Ceratomyxa etroplusi* stained with Giemsa (x1000)

Fig 27: Fresh smears of gall bladder fluid showing *Myxidium* spp. in *Epinephelus tauvina* (x1000)

Fig 28: Spores of *Myxidium* spp. from *Epinephelus tauvina* stained with Giemsa (x1000)

Causative agents : Some of the common genera of myxozoans are *Hennegua, Myxobolus, Myxidium, Ceratomyxa, Kudoa, Sphaerospora, Zschokkella,* etc.

Life cycle : Involve a complex life cycle with an invertebrate intermediate host (oligochaetes, polychaetes, etc.).

Species affected : Almost all fish species; wild, cultured, and ornamental fishes with some degree of host and site specificity.

Gross signs : No apparent visible clinical symptoms. But visible white or blackish cysts can be seen on body surface, gills, fins and internal organs in affected fish.

Effects on host : The parasites invade all major organs and form cysts or freely floating mass called pansporoblast. They destroy gills and all major target organs according to the species. Severe infestations by these parasites can result in disease and/or death of the host fish. Each parasite is somewhat species specific as well as organ specific.

Diagnosis : By observing the characteristic spores with or without stains (Giemsa, Methylene Blue) within the cysts in various organs or as developmental stages. Histology also allows visualisation of the distinctive spores.

Prevention and control : No effective treatment, but prevention is possible by efficient water exchange, avoid feeding of trash fish and quarantine measures.

Trematodes or flat worms

These are relatively large external or internal parasites with adhesive structures for attachment to the host. Monogeneans are external parasites with specialized posterior attachment organs characteristic to each species and require a single host, while the digeneans are internal parasites occurring mostly in the intestinal tract and need more than one host species for completion of their life cycle.

Monogeneans comprise 'skin' and 'gill' flukes infecting skin, gill and fins of fishes (Figs 29-35). Monogeneans are capable of multiplying in large numbers in short time due to their simple life cycle involving a single host. They are often found threatening to young fish with massive mortality. Gill flukes are again ectoparasites, 0.5-1 mm long and the infection is a sign of high stocking density and poor sanitation. Skin flukes are 2-6 mm long. The most common skin flukes encountered are *Benedenia* spp., *Dactylogyrus* spp., etc. These infections are common when there is high stocking density, poor water exchange and overlapping generations of cultured fish.

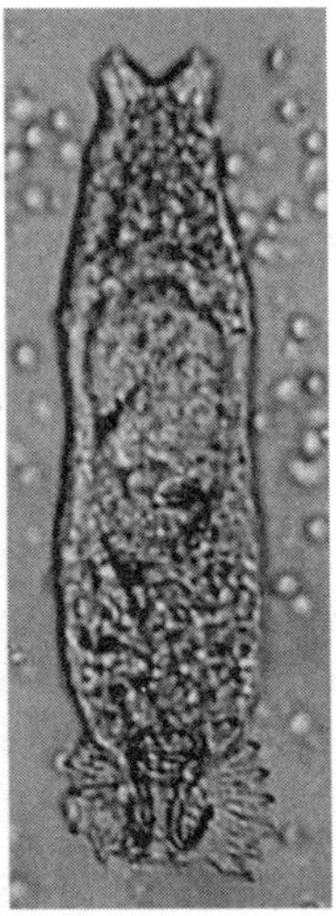

Fig.29: Various species of monogeneans in fish *Gyrodactylus* spp from mullet;

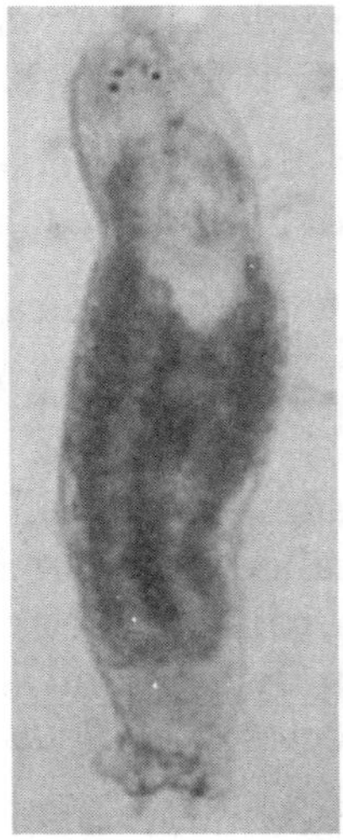

Fig.30: *Dactylogyrus* spp.from mullet;

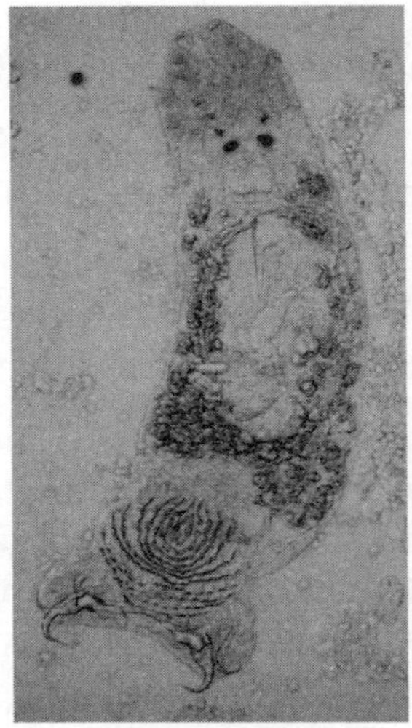

Fig.31: *Diplectanum* spp. from seabass;

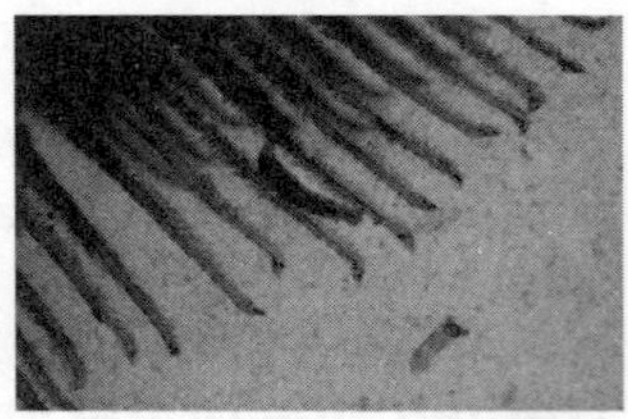

Fig 34: A monogenean parasite on seabass gills

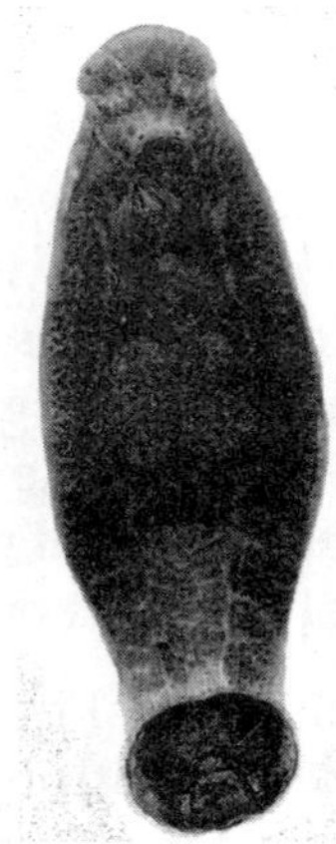

Fig.32: *Benedinea* spp. from grouper;

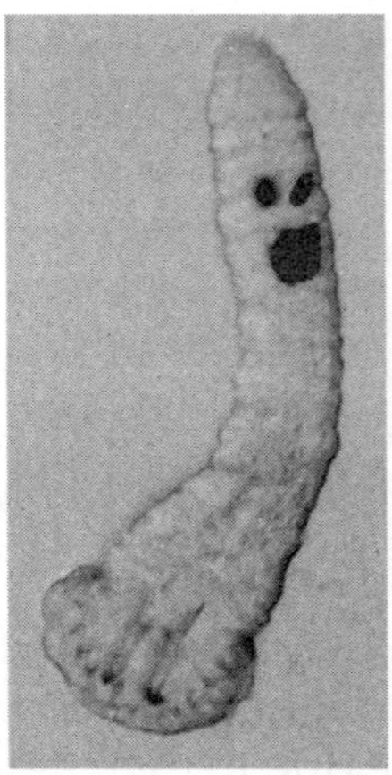

Fig.33: *Dactylogyrus* spp. from mullet)

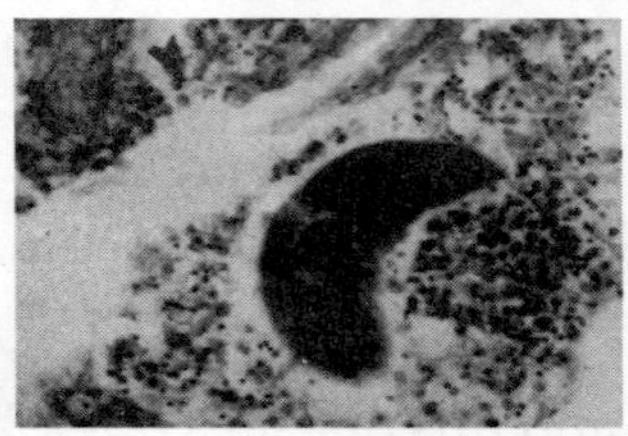

Fig 35: An unidentified fluke in gill section(Courtesy: Dr. P.K. Sahoo)

Causative agents : The most common monogenean parasites in fishes are *Dactylogyrus, Gyrodactylus, Diplectanum, Benedenia,* etc. among predominantly among marine and brackishwater fishes and *Diplozoon, Bifurcohaptor* among many freshwater edible fishes.

Life cycle : Monogeneans are either oviparous or viviparous with a single host and hence transmission is direct. Life cycle is simple involving hermaphroditic adults, eggs and larva. The eggs of many viviparous monogeneans possess long filaments to aid in attachment to substrates and other fish which hatch to free swimming stage to seek fresh hosts. Species of *Gyrodactylus* are viviparous in which the larva is retained in the uterus until it develops in to a functional preadult, inside which a second larva is already formed with a third larva inside that and a fourth inside the third like Chinese boxes, a condition called 'polyembryony'. When fish are living closely together, as in a cage or pond environment, it is easy for the adult worms and larval stages to move from one fish to another thus spreading the infection at an exponential rate.

Species affected : Catfish, carp, tilapia, seabass, grouper, mullet, pearl spot, etc.

Gross signs : Mainly affect body surface, gills, fins and rarely eyes as well. Fish shows lethargy, excessive mucus production on gills and body surface accompanied with opaque eyes, skin lesions, etc. The fish rub its body against submerged objects during heavy infection. High or mass mortality due to the rapid multiplication of the parasite in culture system have been recorded.

Effects on host : Gill flukes mainly affect gills and hence show pale gills and poor appetite, erratic swimming behaviour due to irritation and heavy mucus production on gills. In *Dactylogyrus* infection, the colour of gills becomes pale and produces excessive secretion of mucus. Damage is usually done by the attachment organs as well as by feeding activities. Small and weak fishes are easily infected although massive infections of adult fishes are also reported. The parasite damage the host's tissues leading to secondary bacterial infections. Often high or mass mortality due to the rapid multiplication of the parasite is reported in captive condition. Eye infection leads to blindness.

Diagnosis : Gross and microscopic examination of mucous from skin and gills for the worms with posterior adhesive organs armed with hooks and spines. The presence of eggs with long coiled filament is also diagnostic feature in the genus *Diplozoon, Diplectanum,* etc.

Prevention and control: Short bath treatment with freshwater for 10-30 min. or short bath treatment with 200 ppm hydrogen peroxide for 60 min. or 100-200 ppm formalin, with strong aeration.

Digeneans are mainly intestinal parasites and vary in size according to the spp. A large number of digenea have been recorded parasitizing various fish species (Figs 36-39). However, only a few have been found to cause concern in fish culture systems. Adult trematode may infect the intestine or gall bladder of fishes and are generally harmless as the pathology is restricted to irritation and inflammation at the site of attachments. However, larval trematode, the metacercaria, which invades and encysts in various organs, causes lot of damage. *Diplostomulum* or eye fluke is a larval digenean that develops in the eye of may warm water fish species. The visible signs are opaque, white lens. In India, metacercarial stages of *Diplostomum* spp. have been reported to cause black spot disease in carp nursery and rearing ponds.

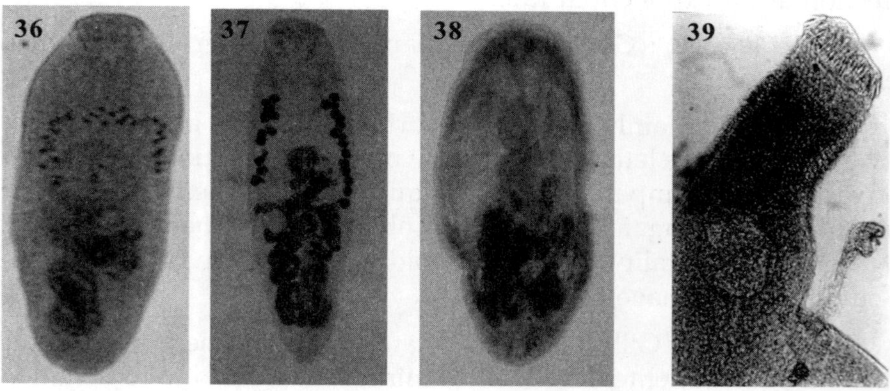

Fig.36-39: Digenean Parasites of Intestine (Unidentified)

Causative agents: Many species which are of non-significant nature are observed among wild fish. *Lecithochirium* spp., *Pseudometadena* spp. and *Bucephalus* spp. were found in many species of fishes. *Diplostomum* is known to be pathogenic in fishes.

Life cycle : As the digeneans complete its life cycle involving at least a molluscan host and one or more fish host where it is found as adults. The life cycle involves fishes either as the primary host or an intermediate host (by harbouring the larval forms, metacercaria) of several digenean spp. of other animals and man.

Species affected : Catfish, carp, tilapia, seabass, grouper, snapper, etc.

Gross signs : *Diplostomum* spp. in case of heavy infection may cause blindness. Yellow grub disease, black spot diseases, etc. are also caused by metacercaria in fishes which encyst in tissues.

Effects on host : Affected fishes have black ovoid patches on the body surface. These pigmented patches are cysts of metacercaria and is the diagnostic feature of the disease.

Diagnosis : Metacercariae are visible in various tissues and adults in intestine.

Prevention and control : No treatment method is effective although anthelminthic drugs are of use. As the digeneans complete its life cycle involving at least a molluscan host, controlling of molluscan host in the culture facility would reduce the transmission cycle (larval stages) of the parasites.

Cestodes or tapeworms

Though cestodes are found inhabiting the digestive tract of wild fishes they do not pose serious problems in cultured fish. Fish also act as intermediate hosts for other tapeworms of higher vertebrates.

Causative agents : *Ligula intestinalis* is a large visceral tapeworm found in pond cultured and some wild populations of many fishes. *Caryophyllaeus* and *Khawia* spp. are encountered in carps. Tapeworm larva (plerocercoid) burrows through the stomach wall into the body cavity and grows. Plerocercoid of *Diphyllobothrium latum* is capable of human infection and is of zoonotic importance.

Life cycle : Aquatic cestodes require at least two hosts. Fish may act as either a second intermediate/parataenic or as final host depending upon the species. The first intermediate host is usually a copepod, where in larval stages released from ingested tapeworm eggs develops as infective form of the tapeworm.

Species affected : Catfish, carp, tilapia, seabass, grouper, snapper, etc.

Gross signs : Clinical signs include emaciation, anemia, discolouration of the skin and susceptibility to secondary infections. Fishes are found to harbour pleurocercoides (larval form of tape worms) in brain, heart, spleen, kidney and gonads, which are harmful to the hosts.

Effects on host : The adult parasites live in the intestinal tract of vertebrates and are usually not considered as serious pathogen. In heavy infection, visible sign is greatly swollen belly due to the blocking of intestine. Intermediate stages live in a variety of body locations in both vertebrate and invertebrate hosts causing tissue reactions.

Diagnosis: Diagnosis of cestodiasis is dependent upon demonstration of the parasite within the intestinal tract/body cavity of the fish.

Prevention and control : There are no known treatments for larval cestodes. Praziquantel is being used in aquarium industries.

Nematodes or round worms

Nematodes are mainly the inhabitants of intestine and body cavities of fish and are large enough to be seen by the naked eye ranging from a few millimeter to several centimeters (Figs 40-45). Fish act as definitive as well as intermediate hosts. Adults seldom cause pathogenicity, but larval stages cause serious tissue damage and even death. Anisakiasis caused by the larvae is a serious problem in marine fishes. Larvae of *Philometra* spp. by its feeding and migration causes inflammation and haemorrhage of swim bladder. Very large nematodes like *Philometroides marinus* recorded from *Rachycentron canadum* reach up to 80 cm may affect the health status and thereby the reproductive performance in broodstock fish.

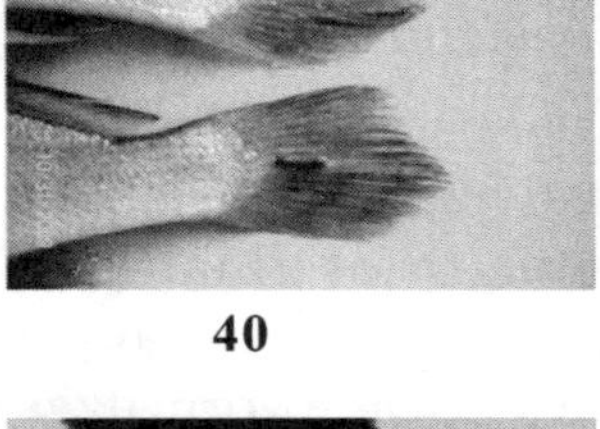

40

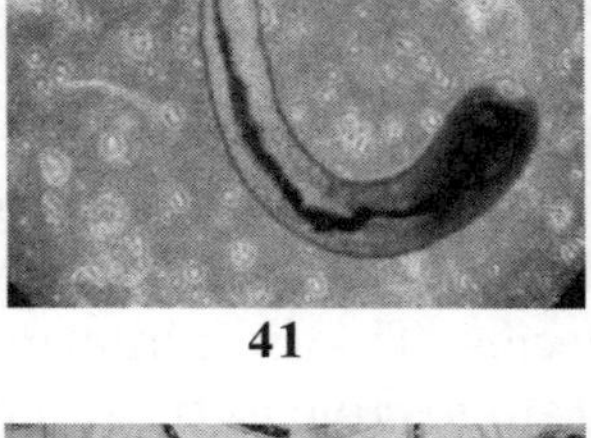

41

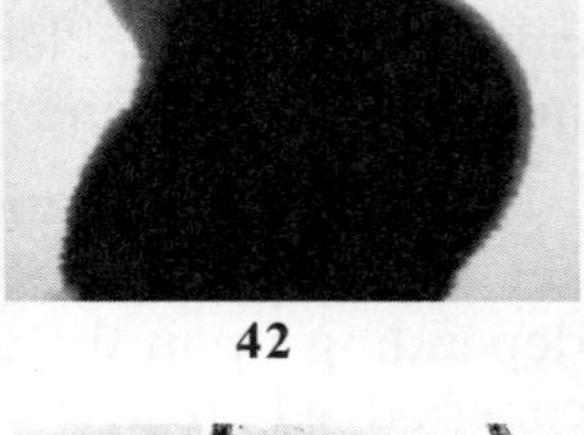

42

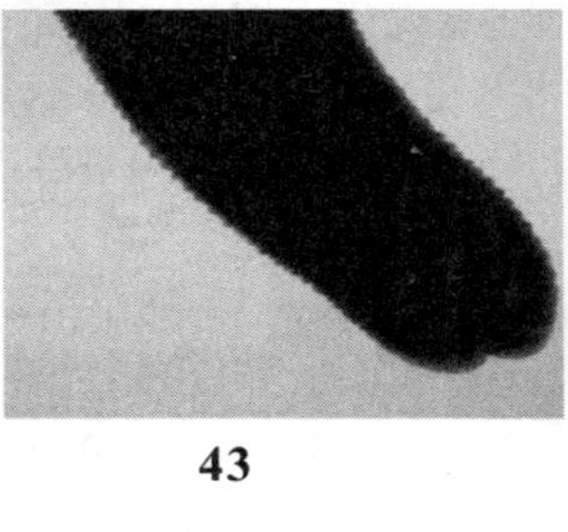

43

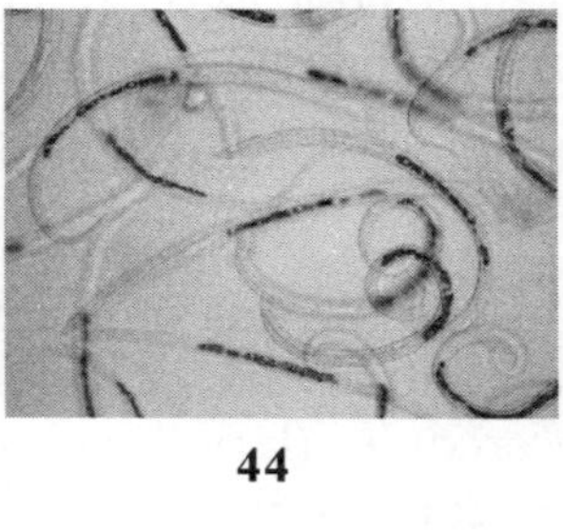

44

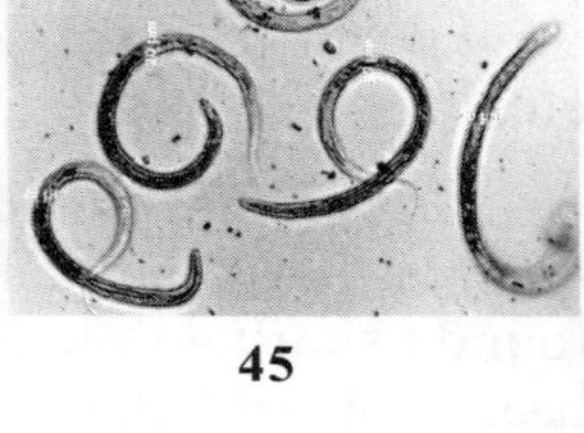

45

Fig.40: *Philometra* spp. in sub-cutaneous nodules on caudal fins.

Fig.41: Adults of *Philometra* spp. infected sub-cutaneous portion of caudual fins of *Otolithes ruber.*

Fig.42 & 43: Anterior and posterior end of adult nematode, *Philometra* spp. collected from *Otolithes ruber.*

Fig.44 & 45: Larvae of *Philometra* spp. specimen from *Otolithes rubber* (*Courtesy:* Dr. S.N. Sethi).

Causative agents: *Cucullanus, Camellanus, Spirocamellanus, Anisakis, Philometra, Philometroides*

Life cycle: Dioecious; most nematodes in fishes have complex lifecycle involving at least two hosts,

Species affected: Siganids, Sciaenids, catfish, seabass, grouper, snapper, etc.

Gross signs: In case of parasites in the stomach and intestine, the affected fish is emaciated and have discoloured body which is some time swollen depending on the degree and species of infection.

Effects on host: May impair feeding, resulting in emaciation and mild mortality,

Diagnosis: Gross examination and dissection of the viscera or intestine with liquefied contents and worms.

Prevention and control: Elimination of intermediate hosts, drying and disinfection of culture facilities. Prevention is possible by maintaining hygiene in the fish tank.

Acanthocephalans

Comprises worms with an anterior proboscis covered with many hooks and hence referred as are 'thorny' or 'spiny headed' worms with aquatic life cycles; fish as final or parataenic hosts and crustaceans as intermediate hosts. Adults feed on the intestinal walls of vertebrates, especially freshwater and marine fishes. They are often encountered in culture system as majority of the broodstock fishes are sourced from wild. Some of the species like *Serrasentis nadakali* reported from captive cobia (*Rachycentron canadum*) are large measuring more than 10 cm and resemble a tapeworm due to pseudo segmentation of the body. Very heavy infection of acanthocephalan parasite *Tenuisproboscis* spp. in red snapper, *Lutjanus argentimaculatus* are detrimental to the broodstock health (Sanil *et al.*, 2011) and may affect the reproductive performance of captive cobia broodstock (CMFRI, 2010).

Causative agents : Medium to large sized parasite, most common species are *Acanthocephalus, Neoacanthorhynchus, Tenuiproboscis.*

Life cycle : Worms are dioecious endoparasites; males usually smaller than females. Eggs are released by female worms directly in water via the host faeces, the ciliated larvae called acanther infects first intermediate host (usually a crustacean and develops into a cystacanth which in turn finds it way on ingestion by a fish to act as a primary host or even as parataenic host before reaching its final predator host fish.

Species affected : Catfish, carp, tilapia, mullet, seabass, grouper, milk fish, snapper, etc.

Gross signs : The parasite is attached to the intestinal mucosa, emaciated body but no visible external symptoms.

Effects on host : The parasite causes necrotic hemorrhagic ulcers in the intestine of the host. Pathogenicity is mainly due to the mechanical injury caused by the attachment of spiny proboscis on the intestinal wall leading to inflammation and tissue necrosis.

Diagnosis : Identifiable only during necropsy examination with characteristic sac like worms with retractile and thorny proboscis.

Prevention and control : Control of intermediate hosts and quarantine of new stocks for prevention.

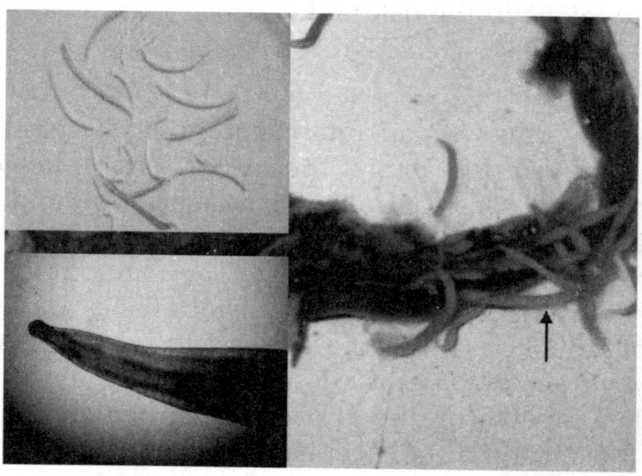

Fig.46: Neoechinorhynchus agilis in mullet gut

Crustaceans

Parasitic crustaceans (Phylum: Arthropoda) resemble in their general morphology with other crustaceans in having segmented body, covered with exoskeleton and jointed appendages. There are three parasitic groups comprising mainly external parasites in cultivable finfish in the class Crustacea; the Branchiura, Copepoda and Isopoda (Table 1). Members of the Branchiura and Isopoda are relatively large and both sexes are parasitic, while Copepods (the most common crustacean parasites) are generally small even microscopic with both free living and parasitic stages in their life cycle. Infestation by these parasites in the wild do not manifest in serious disease outbreaks. Males of parasitic copepods die after copulation in the pre-adult stages, that is usually seen attached to the fish is the mature female with distinctive paired egg sacs at the posterior end.

Parasitic copepods have a complex life cycle with different larval stages; between each of which is a moult. Eggs hatch to release free-swimming nauplius larvae. After a succession of naupliar stages they moult to form copepodid stages. In primitive groups of parasitic copepods such as ergasilids, the copepodids are free swimming. Copulation occurs during the free-swimming stages, after which the males die. The female is left to seek, attach and mature on a marine or freshwater fish host with the help of the prominent claw like second antennae. In more evolved copepods such as the caligids some or all of the copepodid stages may be parasitic including adult male. Caligid copepods generally have direct life cycle, consisting of a free-living planktonic nauplius stage, free swimming infective copepodid stages, attached chalimus, pre-adult and adult stages. In case of *Lernaea* spp., the eggs released by the female hatch in 1-3 days with subsequent nauplii larvae. The nauplius metamorphoses into first or second copepodid stage in 4-16 days. No further development occurs unless it attaches to a host. Larvae pass through five successive copepodid stages before attachment. Copulation occurs during the fourth copepodid stage and the male dies similar to the *Ergasilus* spp. Although *Argulus* spp. cannot survive without a host for long period, they may swim freely looking for new host. Unlike other crustaceans, there is no sexual dimorphism; eggs are not carried by the females in egg sacs, but leaves its host to deposit its eggs to submerged objects. Larvae do not hatch as nauplii but as copepodid stage with thoracic appendages to follow a series of subsequent larval stages by progressive development of the dorsal shield and abdomen, the maxillary suckers

Table 1: Common crustacean parasitic infection in brackishwater finfish in coastal and estuarine zones.

Subclass/ family	Genus	Characteristics
Branchiura		
Argulidae	*Argulus* sp.	Body broad and flat covered anteriorly with dorsal shield with a pair of compound eyes,hooks and barbs,which it uses to attach to the fins, gills and skin of its host, second maxillae usually form prehensile suckers.
Copepoda		
Caligidae	*Caligus* sp. *Lepeophtheirus* sp. *Anuretes* sp	Transparent, cephalothorax covered dorsally by a sub circular shield, with a pair of suckers on the frontal edge of the body and four pair of legs, vestigial abdomen in some species, found in large numbers on gills and body surface with different stages of life cycle in the same host
Ergasilidae	*Ergasilus* sp.	Cephalothorax constituting half or more of body length, the second antennae are modified for clinging to the host, moderate to large numbers on gills with rigorous feeding action and movements
Lernanthropidae	*Lernanthropus* sp.	Few in number but large in size, feed on gill tissues and blood, seriously damage the tissues
Lernaeidae	*Lernaea* sp.	Body unsegmented, with its anterior part deeply embedded in host tissue with the help of a hold fast organ,infect nostril, skin, fin, gills, buccal cavity
Isopoda		
Cymothoidae	*Cymothoa* sp.	Entire dorsal surface of body divided into many narrow segments, eyes are sessile, parasite immovably attached to surface, buc cal or branchial cavity of fish.

and reproductive organs. Thus, transmission of parasites within the system is by physical contact with infected animals or by the free living infective stages after reproduction. Many species simply glide from one fish to other. Many parasites are transferred to culture system by way of water, live feed, wild fish, contaminated farm implements, etc. Hence control methods may vary greatly depending upon the farm conditions, the type of parasites and its life cycle stages.

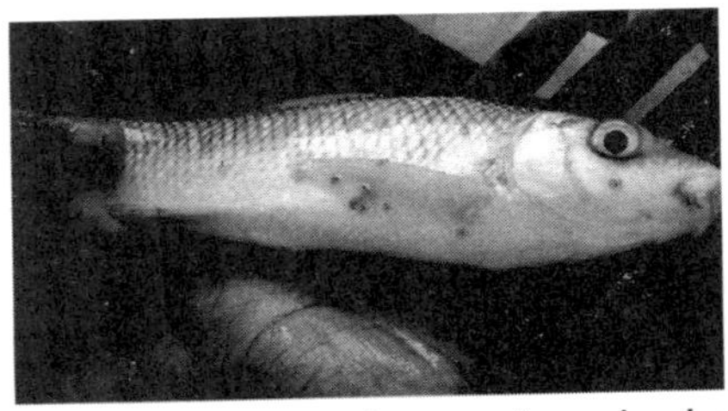

Fig.47: *Argulus siamensis* on body surface of Carp fish, *Labeo rohita* (*Courtesy:* Dr. P.K. Sahoo

Branchiurans : Members of the family Argulidae represented by genus *Argulus* commonly called as 'fish lice' is an important parasites of fish (Fig 47). It has a broad, flat oval body with hooks and barbs, which it uses to attach to the fins, gills and skin of its host. They are one of the most widespread and dangerous ectoparasites in fresh water fish ponds causing large scale fish mortality. Argulosis is a major problem in many areas of Orissa and Andhra Pradesh where freshwater aquaculture is concentrated and the infection has emerged as a significant problem in composite fish culture ponds in India (Mishra, 1991) and considered as lethal pathogen in semi-intensive and intensive aquaculture (Saurabh *et al.*, 2010).

Causative agents : Argulus siamensis, A. indicus, A. foliaceus

Life cycle : Branchiuran parasites on fishes are usually found in the walls of the branchial cavity and not permanently attached to their hosts, but can crawl on their surfaces and can slowly swim leaving one fish to another. Sexual dimorphism is not marked. Both sexes are parasites and lead a direct lifecycle. After mating the female deposits the eggs on a suitable substrate, such as aquatic plants. The eggs hatch, develop and infect fresh hosts and metamorphose to adults.

Species affected : Catfish, carp, etc.

Gross signs : Fish suffering from argulosis exhibit behavioural abnormalities including lethargy, irritation and loss of appetite. Infected fish may show increased flashing, agitation and excess mucous production.

Effects on host : They damage the fish directly by extracting blood and vital tissue fluids from the host with their modified mouthparts.

The mode of feeding of *Argulus* involves secretion and injection of relatively large quantities of digestive fluids, which are toxic to the fish. The sting of one fish lice can kill a small fish. Feeding sites become hemorrhagic and ulcerated and provide access to secondary infections by other pathogens. Mucous is secreted when skin, fin and gills become infected.

Diagnosis : *Argulus* spp. can be diagnosed by naked eye with characteristic two spots on the body.

Prevention and control : The only way to prevent *Argulus* infection is to deny parasite's access to the cultivable fish. Since both adults and larval stages are active swimmers, it is difficult to prevent them from entering the pond. Appropriate filter designs might prove more efficacious to check the degree of infestation. Treatment with organophosphates, formalin or potassium permanganate will eradicate adults. Juveniles can be treated with 2% salt bath. Draining and drying is good option for larger system.

Copepods

The most important copepods affecting fish are *Caligus* (sea lice), *Ergasilus* (gill maggots) and *Lernaea* (anchor worm). They are ectoparasites infecting skin, fins and gills (Figs 48-51). The intensity of copepod infestation generally increases in rainfall and late spring and decline in winter and summer due to the lack of recruitment and parasite death. This is a major problem in cage cultured brackishwater fishes but the economic impact of this disease is not known.

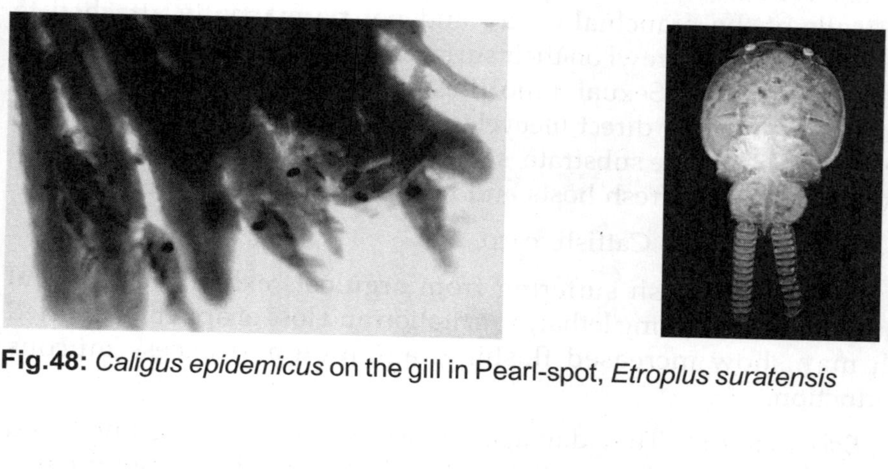

Fig.48: *Caligus epidemicus* on the gill in Pearl-spot, *Etroplus suratensis*

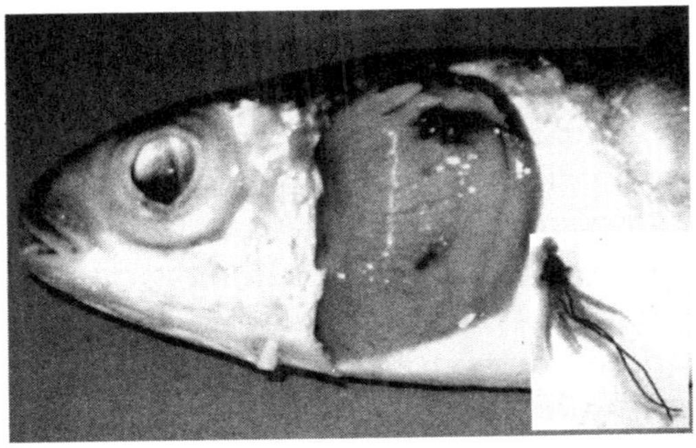

Fig.49: *Lernanthropus shishidoi* on the gills in Mullet, *Mugil cephalus*

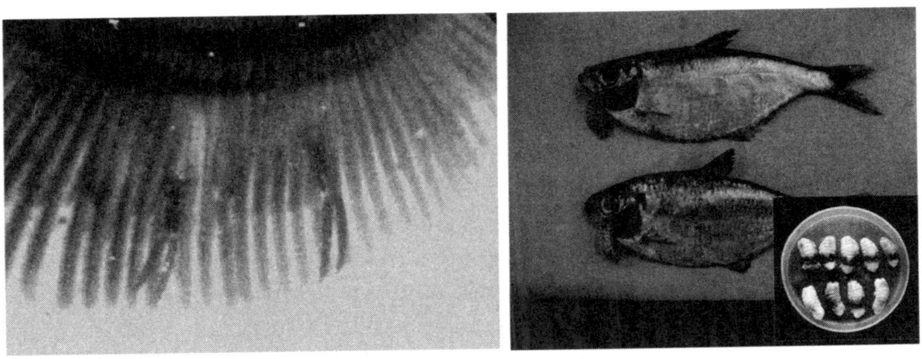

Fig.51: Cymothoid parasite attached to the gill chamber in wild marine fish (Courtesy: Dr. S.N. Sethi)

Caligus spp. or 'sea lice' is a common copepod parasite under Caligidae infesting a wide range of fish species in the coastal and estuarine zones although other lesser known species viz. *Lepeophtheirus* and *Anuretes* spp. are reported from marine fishes in Indian subcontinent. Three species of *Caligus, C. epidemicus, C. orientalis* and *C. punctatus* are the potential major pathogens in the development of cage culture. *C. orientalis* seriously affects wild population as well. When they first infect a farmed fish population they cause extensive irritation and nervous activity.

Ergasilus spp. also known as 'gill maggot' are found on the body surface, gills and branchial and nasal cavities of many fish species including seabass, grouper, mullet, pearl spot, tilapia, etc. where it feeds on blood and epithelium. Heavy infestations can result in mechanical damage, patechial hemorrhage, impaired respiration, epithelial hyperplasia, and anemia with growth retardation. Severe gill damage is caused by the feeding activity of the copepod and this often leads to fish death. Proliferation of this parasite is observed in summer.

Lernanthropus spp. is relatively large, reddish in colour, firmly attached to the gills, inflicts serous damage to the gills by way of erosion, desquamation and necrosis of the secondary lamellae near the site of attachment. The grasping action of the mandibles and the maxillae results in the exposure of blood vessels and hemorrhages. This serious pathogen is frequently encountered in many species of wild fish and cultured sea bass, mullet, etc. and is relatively difficult to control.

Lernaea spp., better known as the 'anchor worm', this species affects a large number of warm water fishes. Adults are visible to the naked eye. Although *Lernaea* (eg. *L. cyprinacea* in carps and a number of freshwater fishes including ornamental fishes) is typically a freshwater copepod; it has been reported from brackishwater fish also. Different fish species were reported to have varying levels of susceptibility to *Lernaea* infection under natural environment and culture conditions. The parasite seems to have an affinity for the heart region of small fish and kills them by piercing the heart or other vital organs. The female lernaeidid copepod has long filamentous body with trailing attached egg sacs. Morphological modifications include the head, which is a rounded knob inserted into the musculature of its fish host; one or two pairs of anchors to hold it in position. Damage to the fish host includes haemorrhagic and ulcerated lesions with potential for secondary infections, anemia, retarded growth, loss of weight and loss of equilibrium.

The destructive activity of *Lernaea* spp. is due to its relatively large size and its mode of attachment and feeding. As the maximum damage to the fish is caused by the adult parasite which remain attached to the host tissue with an anterior holdfast organ and also by the developmental stages that remain attached to the host, any reliable and effective prophylactic measure should aim to kill the free living stages of the parasites at nauplii and copepodid stages before it gets attached to the fish host. *Lernaea* is extremely difficult to control because only the free-living larvae are susceptible to treatment. The adult female produces three sets of eggs; these eggs produce larvae over a four week period. Since the larvae remain free living for about one week, it is necessary to treat it once a week for four weeks to eliminate this parasite.

Life cycle : Copepods have direct life cycle, consisting of a free-living planktonic nauplius stage, free swimming infective copepodid stage, attached chalimus, pre-adult and adult stages. In most cases, it is the attached chalimus stage that causes significant pathological lesions leading to mortality when present in large numbers. The pre-adult and adult stages are not very invasive and cause minor tissue damages.

Species affected : Tilapia, seabass, mullet, grouper, pearl-spot, snapper, etc.

Gross signs : Excessive mucus production and signs of irritation including frequent flashing.

Effects on host : Feeding on the fish skin, mucous and blood, these lice can cause small hemorrhages and sores, erode the skin and expose the underlying tissue to secondary infection. In disease situations, death is caused by the development of secondary infections exacerbated by stress, osmoregulatory failure and in the case of the gills, respiratory impairment. It is well recognized that parasites act as mechanical vectors of the pathogens though they are not an obligatory host.

Diagnosis : Parasites can be seen on skin or gill scrapings. Anchor worms are clearly visible to the naked hanging from the body and *Ergasilus* spp. seen attached to the gills.

Prevention and control : Parasitic copepods with relatively narrow host ranges such as *Ergasilus* are easier to control, especially where there are few wild hosts present. The species with broad host ranges and/or abundant wild hosts (e.g. *Caligus* spp.) in the vicinity of aquaculture sites are generally difficult to control because of recurrent infestations from carrier hosts. In pond culture, overcrowding and poor water quality had been cited as factors responsible for the development of parasitic copepod diseases. The important management techniques to be followed are rearing different batches in separate tanks, pond drying, removal of all probable hosts from the stocking sites prior to stocking so that all infectious stages die due to lack of hosts, quarantine prior to stocking and introduction to the rearing system and frequent cleaning of holding tank/nets. The parasites can be controlled by fresh water bath for 10-15 min or by chemical treatment using 1000 ppm hydrogen peroxide or 100-200 ppm formalin for 30-60 min. Some of the treatments commonly applied in marine/brackishwater fishes are shown in Table 2. Strong aeration must be provided during treatment. Drying of unused tanks also helps to destroy the developing stages. Treated fish should be transferred to clean parasite free facility. In all cases, infected fish should be quarantined to avoid cross-infection. Complete draining and disinfection of the system may be the option to break the life cycle. Generally copepod infections are treated with organophosphates. Dichlorvos has been found to be effective against the *Caligus* and *Ergasilus* at a concentration of 1 ppm. *Lernaea* spp. is very difficult to control due to different stages of life cycle showing different susceptibility to chemicals. Further, the concentration of these chemicals required to kill the developmental stages are toxic to fish. Successful control in freshwater ornamental fishes using gradual shift to salinity of about 10 ppt has been reported. Temperature dependant development of larval stages and the lethal effects of even low salinity on larval stages etc. can be utilized for the control of fresh infections in the system. Eradication of copepods using freshwater bath is also suggested.

Table 2: Common treatment against copepods in marine/ brackishwater finfish

Drugs / chemicals	Dose	Type of treatment, duration
Formalin	100-200 ppm	Short bath; 30-60 min
H_2O_2	1000 ppm	Short bath; 30-60 min
Dichlorvos	0.75 - 1 ppm	Short bath; 60 min
Caprylic acid	I mM	Short bath; 5-10 min

Isopods : Isopods are large parasites (6-50 mm in size) with its body divided into many narrow segments, with a pair of large eyes. They are protandric hermaphrodites, living on the skin in the gill chambers or in the mouth of the host fish. *Cymothoa* spp. has been reported as a serious problem in fishes kept in captivity or cages besides wild tropical marine fishes.

Causative agents : *Cymothoa indica* is a common parasite under this class found commonly in the gill chamber, buccal cavity or body surface of many fishes. *Nerocila* spp., *Aegas* spp., *Gnathia* spp. and *Cirolana* spp. have been found to cause mortality in cage cultured seabass. Others commonly observed in wild fishes are *Joryma* spp., *Glossobius* spp. and *Agarna* spp.

Life cycle : Parasites are generally found in male female pairs. Female were found to have thousands of young larval forms, which could spread to other fishes under high stocking density. They have a short free-living planktonic phase; juveniles and adults are exclusively parasitic living on the skin, buccal cavity and gill chamber of the fish.

Isopods absorb their nourishment directly from the host's body and depend upon their hosts for feeding.

Species affected : Tilapia, seabass, grouper, mullet, pearl spot, snapper and many species of marine fishes.

Gross signs : The affected fish rub its body against objects and inflict injury. If buccal cavity of small fish is occupied by large number of parasites, there is difficulty in feeding and thereby emaciation is often found.

Effects on host : No much mortality has been reported, the damages caused by them resemble that of other copepods but the most serious effect of isopod infection is destruction of host tissue resulting from the pressure of the parasite's body. Fishes with *C. indica* infection in the branchial chamber showed loss of weight, loss of fat content, changes in the water content of various tissues and significant reduction of respiratory surface area of the host fish.

Diagnosis : Diagnosis is usually done by gross and microscopic examination of scrapings from skin, gills, fins, etc. from affected fishes and by observing general clinical symptoms. Pre-disposing factor for transmission of crustacean parasites is poor water exchange and thus sufficient water exchange can prevent their proliferation.

Prevention and control: No specific control or therapeutic measures against isopods have been in practice except the manual removal of the parasite; by implementing optimum management practices during culture as infection in the planktonic phase is the common feature. Formalin bath 200 ppm for 30-60 min. can reduce the gravity of infection. Manual removal and destruction of the parasites were also found to be effective in larger fishes.

Leeches

Leeches are large annelid parasites with pseudo-segmented body, 8-15 mm long and with anterior and posterior suckers used for feeding and movement (Fig 52). Found on body surface, fins, mouth, gill chamber, eyes, etc. Leech infestation is associated with poor maintenance facilities and poor water quality in pond.

Causative agents : Many species in freshwater and marine fish including *Pontobdella* spp., *Zeylanicobdlla* spp.

Species affected : Catfish, carp, tilapia, mullet, seabass, grouper, snapper, etc.

Life cycle : They have a direct life cycle with immature and mature stages being parasitic on hosts.

Gross signs : Mainly affect body surface, fins, eyes and rarely gills. Brownish-black parasites attached in patches in the affected area. The fish rubs its body against objects during heavy infection.

Effects on host : Pathogenic effect is related to the number and size of leeches leading to chronic anemia. The feeding and attachment sites of the parasite damage the host's tissues leading to hemorrhagic lesions and possibly secondary bacterial infections.

Diagnosis : Visible to naked eye as being attached to fins, gills, and skin.

Prevention and control: Manual removal of the parasite from the affected fish after segregation or short bath treatment with 50-100 ppm formalin for 1 h with strong aeration and subsequent transfer of treated fish to a clean, parasite free tank. Ponds with heavy leech infestation require drainage, treatment with chlorinated lime followed by drying to destroy the adults and eggs.

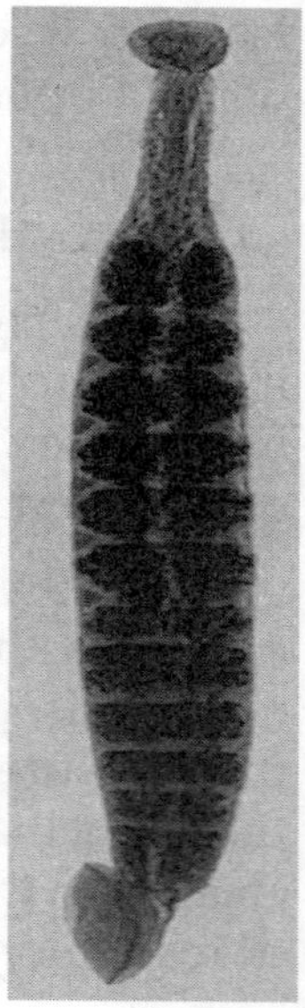

Fig.52: An unidentified leech from Grouper fish

Parasitic zoonoses of fish origin

Fish borne zoonotic parasites or ichthyozoonoses transmitted by fish and shell fish products pose major public health problems in many countries. Though the transmission of these parasites through fish caught in the wild has been well documented, the association between cultured fish and human infection has gained the attention only recently. There is a complete lack of priority for parasites of zoonotic significance and this remains an unexplored area even though some parts of the country face these problems. Major fish borne parasitic zoonoses in India are listed in Table 2. Food safety issue is a growing concern especially in the export sector as majority of the fish products are being exported as frozen items. The zoonotic parasites of fish origin also vary from freshwater, brackishwater and marine ecosystem. Many zoonotic parasites enter human by way of consumption of raw aquatic vegetation/tubers, etc. In India, food borne zoonosis in general and the fish borne in particular are comparatively very less prevalent than in South East and Far East countries mainly because of the traditional culture of cooking and serving. However, eating raw or undercooked fish, crustacean, snail, etc. is a delicacy in certain ethnic communities, and people. A single factor responsible for fish born zoonoses could be lack of hygiene (poverty, lack of personal hygiene, scarcity of potable water, consumption of raw or undercooked food) and/or favorable climatic conditions for parasite growth and transmission. So the incidence of helminthozoonosis can be minimized substantially, if people are provided with clean drinking water and hygienic living conditions. Besides, people need to be made aware and educated of risks of infection by way of consumption undercooked fish/crab. The future impact of these fish-borne zoonotic parasites may be linked closely to the expected growth of aquaculture in Asia. However, there is disagreement on the relative importance of pond cultured fish versus wild caught fish in the epidemiology of human infection.

Fish borne parasites come from three main groups: digenetic trematodes (species under families Opisthorchiidae, Heterophyidae), cestodes (species under family Diphyllobothriidae) and nematodes (species under family Anisakidae, Gnathostomatidae). Generally, human infection takes place through the consumption of raw, undercooked or otherwise under-processed fish containing the infective stages of the parasites. Dermal exposure by introduction of infectious agents into open wounds or abrasions through handling of infected fish or infected water is also possible.

A large number of freshwater fish species can transmit the infective trematode metacercariae, the fish belonging to cyprinidae (carps) being the most common. *Chlonorchis, Opisthorchis, Paragonimus, Heterophyes, Haplorchis, Metagonimus*, etc. are examples. Aquaculture being the world's most important food sector dominated by Asian countries, fish-borne trematodiasis is also most prevalent in Asian region.

Cestode, *Diphyllobothrium latum* causes a mild disease in about 20 million individuals per year with recent increase in cultivated fish as well, due to consumption of raw fish in ethnic dishes such as sushi, sashimi, ceviche, and other similar products (Figs 53-55). The parasite has a complex life cycle with piscivorous animals and man, as primary host and copepods as the first intermediate host, and a predatory freshwater or salt water fish as the second intermediate host.

Table 3: Fish-borne parasitic zoonoses

Sl. No.	Name of the parasite (Host)	Name of the parasitic stage infective to man	Source of infection to man	Mode of infection	Remarks
			Trematodes		
1.	*Heterophyes heterophyes* (dog, cat, man)	Metacercaria	Freshwater fish, *Mugil cephalus* and others	Ingestion of raw or undercooked fish	Human cases have not been diagnosed in India
2.	*Opisthorchis tennuicollis* (dog, cat, man)	Metacercaria	Cyprinid fish	Ingestion of raw or undercooked fish	Human cases have not been diagnosed in India
3.	*Clonorchis sinensis* (dog, cat, pig, man)	Metacercaria	Cyprinid fish	Ingestion of raw or undercooked fish	Human cases have not been diagnosed in India
4.	*Paragonimus westermani* (dog, cat, pig, cattle, goat, tiger, man)	Metacercaria	Crabs (*Potamon* sp. In India) or Cray fish	Ingestion of raw or undercooked crustaceans, Contamination of food through utensils and hands	'Lung fluke' infection, a public health problem existed in Madras, West Bengal, Assam and Manipur; recent reports from NEH only.

5.	*Pseudamphistomum truncatum* (pig, man)	Metacercaria	Freshwater fish, *Leuciscus rutilus*	Ingestion of raw or undercooked fish	No reports of human infection in India
6.	*Echinochasmous perfoliotus* (dog, cat, fox, man)	Metacercaria	Fish	Ingestion of raw or undercooked fish	No reports of human infection in India
			Cestodes		
7.	*Diphyllobothrium latum* (dog, man)	Plerocercoid	Freshwater fish, particularly large predator fish and others (barbel, parch, trout etc.)	Ingestion of raw or undercooked fish harboring plerocercoids	'Broad fish tape worm' of man and other animals, No reports of human infection in India in recent years
8.	*Spirometra* spp. (dog, cat, man)	Procercoid & Plerocercoid stages	Cyclops, containing procercoids and fish, tadpoles, frogs containing plerocercoids	Accidental ingestion of intermediate host (s)	'Sparganum' a disease caused by the larval stage of the species *Spirometra* have been reported recently from Rajasthan

			Nematodes		
9.	*Gnathostoma spinigerum* (dog, cat, man)	L_3 encysted in viscera and muscles of freshwater fish (*Ophiocephalus* spp. *Clarius* spp., eels), frog etc.	Inadequately processed fish, frog, or other second intermediate hosts and paratenic hosts	Ingestion of infected fish, frog; rarely direct penetration of the skin by the infective larvae	Reported from animals; Infective larvae of the nematode may be found in freshwater fish (*Ophiocephalus punctatus*) in viscera and muscles, Reports of human case dates back too 1945.
10.	*Anisakis* spp. (Marine animals, man)	Infective larvae in a variety of marine fish and also in anadromous and freshwater fish.	Raw or semi cooked fish	Ingestion of infected fish containing infective larvae	Cause 'herring worm disease' in human, mainly a common problem in many European, American and Asian countries; but there is no incidence of this disease in India.
11.	*Angiostrongylus contonensis* (rat, man)	Infective larvae	Intermediate hosts (slugs, snail) and many paratenic hosts like prawn, crab, frog etc.	Ingestion of food containing raw or undercooked infected intermediate and paratenic hosts.	'Lung worm' of rats; Only accidental human parasites through aquatic animals. Human cases with eosinophic meningitis reported in India.

12.	*Dioctophyma ranale* (dog, man)	Infective larvae	Paratenic hosts like frog, fish harbouring encysted infective larvae	Ingestion of frog or fish carrying infective larvae	No reported cases in India.
			Protozoa		
13.	*Entamoeba histolytica* (man and animals as reservoir hosts)	Mature cysts	Food (fish) and water contaminated with faeces of infected man, animals	Ingestion of food (fish) and water contaminated with mature cysts.	Mechanical contamination only
14.	*Giardia lamblia* (man and animals as reservoir hosts)	Mature cysts	Food (fish) and water contaminated with faeces of infected man, animals	Ingestion of food (fish) and water contaminated with mature cysts.	Mechanical contamination only
15.	*Balantidium coli* (pig, man)	Mature cysts	Food (fish) and water contaminated with faeces of infected man, animals	Ingestion of food (fish) and water contaminated with mature cysts.	Mechanical contamination only
16.	*Cryptosporidium* spp. (Domestic, wild animals, aquatic animals (?), man)	Sporulated oocysts	Food (fish?) and drinks contaminated with sporulated oocysts	Ingestion of food (fish) and water contaminated with oocysts.	Mechanical contamination only

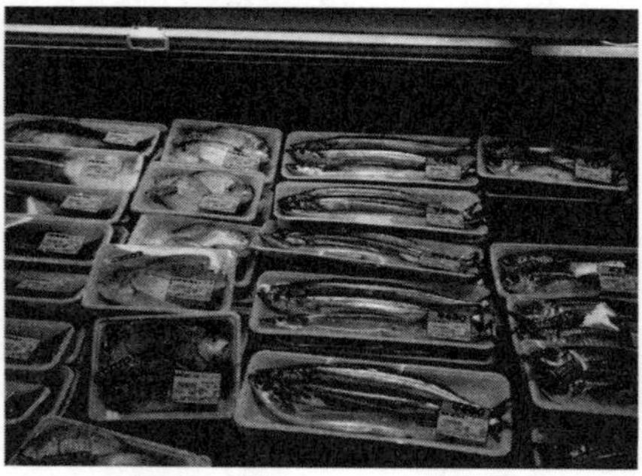

Fig. 53:

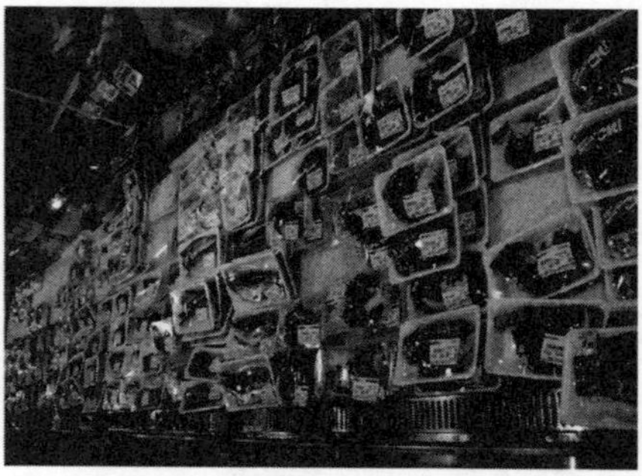

Fig. 54: Ready to cook fish and other aquatic animal products in Asian market

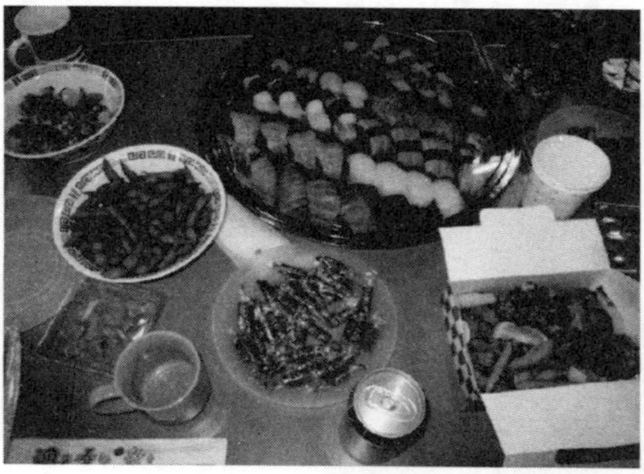

Fig. 55: Largely raw or semi-cooked/ processed delicacies like 'sushi' on dining table.

Nematodiasis dominated by Anisakiasis refers to infection with larval stages of fish nematodes of the genera *Anisakis, Contracaecum,* etc. Anisakiasis is a serious zoonotic disease caused by the consumption of raw or undercooked fish dishes containing the larvae of parasite with clinical entity of acute or chronic infection. Gnathostomiasis caused by *Gnathostoma* spp. in man is considered as an accidental hosts where the condition 'larva migrans' is one of the known symptoms. The life cycle is complex involving intermediate, parataenic and finals hosts.

Prevention and Control : About 18 million people are affected by fish borne trematodes alone and are geographically confined to population living in low and middle income countries called as 'hot spots' of fish borne zoonoses including parts of India. No much information on fish borne zoonotic metacercariae from brackishwater and marine fish though these parasites are common in country's freshwater fish.

Fish borne parasites are derived from the consumption of raw fish, or fish dishes or products that have not been cooked or have not been processed sufficiently to kill the parasites in farm. Apparently, the control is easy with consumer education campaigns, mass education, besides the consumption of well cooked/processed fish products. Application of HACCP principles in the production system where each stage is evaluated for the existence of hazards and risks for public health is a tool that has the potential to assumes safety of cultivated fish at risk of infection with zoonotic fish borne parasites.

Emerging parasitic infections in cultured fishes

There are parasitic infections which assume clinical significance and cause pathological condition in farmed fish. A couple of examples worth mentioning include apicomplexan parasitic diseases such as coccidiosis and cryptosporidiosis. Piscine apicomplexan parasites of significance belong to the genera *Cryptosporidium, Eimeria, Goussia,* etc. These parasites have been known to infect many fish species and cause chronic disease with gradual mortality. The pathogenesis of piscine coccidiosis has been reported in many fish species such as carps, gold fish and cat fishes. However, not much clinical significance was attached to these infections in culture conditions till recently. Among production animals, cryptosporidiosis causes significant economic losses and remains a potential zoonotic condition. In contrast, there is scanty literature regarding piscine cryptosporidiosis, despite infection being increasingly reported in dozens of species of marine and freshwater fish during the last decade (Baragahara *et al.*, 2011; Gabor *et al.*, 2011). However, recently, some reports of severe outbreaks of diseases in *Lates calcarifer* juveniles with high prevalence of *Cryptosporidium* and *Eimeria* were reported from Vietnam (Gabor *et al.*, 2011; Gibson-Kueh *et al.*, 2011). The origin of these infections remains unknown though using trash fish as feed is suspected to be the cause. Same is true with the taxonomy and zoonotic potential of *Cryptosporidium* of fish origin. In India, the sector is largely unaware of these infections due to inadequate capacity building in diagnosing these infections in culture facilities.

Another area requiring attention is the parasites in aquarium fishes as most of the trade is by breeding the exotic fishes in India. Live fish trade by import and export may increase the possibility of transboundary movement of parasites across geographical regions. Though this sector is dominated by freshwater ornamentals, originated from backyard/cottage units from rural India, some species of hatchery produced marine (*Amphiprion, Premans*) and brackishwater (*Scatophagus*) ornamental fish seeds are now available. There is need for health management studies during culture operations in non-native environment and the potential transfer from wild to cultured animals and *vice versa*.

Issues in fish parasitology research in India

Fish diseases are major constraints in the sustainability of aquaculture industry in coastal states of India. Diseases of aquatic animals and biosecurity measures for managing risks of aquatic animal disease outbreaks have received less attention than livestock diseases. Intensification of aquaculture production systems continues to create new paradigms for disease expression, and new knowledge of disease pathogenesis is fueling and refining our surveillance needs. Further increasing globalization and trade volume of the aquaculture sector has created new mechanisms by which pathogens and diseases may be introduced or spread to new areas. Trans-boundary movement of aquatic animals contributes to faster spread of various diseases. Considering the importance of Parasitology research in India in cultured fish species it is a fact that there is lack of detailed studies on epidemiology, host-pathogen relations and paucity of such studies with regard to parasites. The researchable issues related to the discipline and also short-term and long-term priorities are listed below. There is a need for the networking of Fish Parasitologists, need to identify research priorities in the area of fish parasitology with a blend of biotechnology application for the diagnosis and control of important fish parasites. Further, fish parasitologists should strengthen their affiliation to the discipline, considering the limited manpower in this specialized area, either independently through an identified research project at the institute level or on a collaborative mode with other fisheries research institutes or with other institutions engaged in fish parasitology research.

Voluminous research work on fish parasitology has been undertaken by many general universities; however most of this information has never been compiled. Food safety issue is a growing concern; especially in export sector as majority of the fish products are being exported as frozen items. Further, there is also a need for the establishment of a national network of fish parasitologists and a national surveillance system for parasite diseases in the country. Host-parasite interactions, taxonomy, diagnosis, prophylaxis, epidemiology and economic losses associated with these parasites should be considered as priority areas for future research. Establishment of national surveillance system for parasitic diseases in fishes could also be considered for augmenting the research programme. The following is the list of the thematic areas in the field of fish parasitology for prioritization.

Area I: Taxonomy

- Parasite profile of commercially important finfish-a least investigated area
- Exploration of fish parasites diversity and digital documentation

Area II: Epidemiology

- Establishment of national surveillance system for aquatic parasitic diseases.

Area III: Host-parasite interactions

- Application of molecular tools in the control of important parasites affecting fish
- Host-parasite relations using molecular tools

Area IV: Diagnostics

- Development of molecular detection tools for OIE listed fish parasites.

Area V: Therapeutics and Prophylaxis

- Development of novel therapeutics and prophylactics against parasitic diseases.

Acknowledgements

The author is thankful to Dr. P.K. Sahoo, National Fellow (ICAR), Central Institute of Freshwater Aquaculture (Bhubaneswar, Orissa) and Dr. S.N. Sethi, Scientist, Madras Regional Centre of CMFRI (Chennai, Tamil Nadu) for providing some of the photographs.

References

Abidi, R. (2002). Fish pathogens and diseases in India: A bibliography (1898-2001). Published by NBFGR, Lucknow (UP), India, pp. 500

Badul Huq, M.A., Srinivasan, M. and Murugan, M. (2006). Observations on parasites of *Epinephelus malabaricus* (Bloch and Schneider). *Indian J. Fish.*, 53: 459-461

Baragahare, R., Becker, J.A., Landos, M., Slapeta, J. Dennis, M.M. (2011). Gastric cryptosporidiosis in farmed Australian Murray cod, *Maccullochella peelii peelii*. *Aquaculture*, 314: 1-6

CMFRI (2009). Annual report, CMFRI, Cochin, pp.122

CMFRI (2010). Cadalmin, CMFRI newsletter, 125, pp. 28

Cruz-Lacierda, E.R., Toledo, J.D. Tan-Fermin, J.D and Burreson, E. (2000). Marine leech (*Zeylanicobdella arugamensis*) infestation in cultured orange-spotted grouper, *Epinephelus coioides, Aquaculture*, 185: 191-196

FAO (2010). The state of world fisheries and aquaculture. Rome, FAO, pp. 197

Gabor, L.J., Srivastava, M., Titmarsh, J. Dennis, M., Gabor, M. and Landos, M. (2011). Cryptosporidiosis in intensively reared barramundi (*Lates calcarifer*). *J. Vet. Diag. Investig.*, 23: 383-386

George, P.V. and Nadakal, A.M. (1981). Observations on the intestinal pathology of the marine fish, *Rachycentron canadum* (Gunther) infected with the acanthocephalid worm *Serrasentis nadakali*. *Hydrobiologia*, 78: 59-62

Gibson-Kueh, S., Yang, R., Thuy, N.T.N., Jones, J.B., Nicholls, P.K., Ryan, U. (2010). The molecular characterization of an *Eimeria* and *Cryptosporidium* detected in Asian seabass (*Lates calcarifer*) cultured in Vietnam. *Vet. Parasitol.*, doi:10.1016/j.vetpar.2011.05.004

Gibson-Kueh, S., Thuy, N.T.N., Elliot, A., Jones, J.B., Nicholls, P.K. and Thomson, R.C.A. (2011). An intestinal *Eimeria* infection in juvenile Asian seabass (*Lates calcarifer*) cultured in Vietnam- A first report. *Vet. Parasitol.*, doi:10.1016/j.vetpar.2011.05.004

Hemaprasanth, Raghavendra, A., Singh, R., Sridhar, N. and Raghunath, M.R. (2008). Efficacy of doramectin against natural and experimental infections of *Lernaea cyprinacea* in carps. *Vet. Parasitol.*, 156: 261-269

Hemaprasanth, Singh, R., Raghavendra, A., Sridhar, N., Raghunath, M.R., and Eknath, A.E. (2011). Comparative susceptibility of carp fingerlings to *Lernaea cyprinacea* infection. *Vet. Parasitol.*, 178: 156-162

Jithendran, K.P., Natarajan, M. and Azad, I.S. (2005). Management of monogenean parasites in brackishwater finfish. *Aquaculture Asia,* 10: 38-41

Jithendran, K.P., Vijayan, K.K., Alavandi, S.V. and Kailasam, M. (2005). *Benedenia epinepheli* (Yamaguti, 1937), a monogenean parasite in captive broodstock of grouper, *Epinephelus tauvina* (Forskal). *Asian Fish. Sci.,* 18: 121-126

Jithendran, K.P. and Kannappan, S. (2010). A short note on heavy infection of acanthocephalan worm (*Neoechinorhynchus agilis*) in grey mullet, *Mugil cephalus. J. Parasitic Dis.,* 34: 99-101

Kabata, Z. (1985). Parasites and diseases of fish cultured in the tropics. Taylor and Francis Ltd, London, pp. 316

Kumaraguru Vasagam, K.P., Rajkumar, M., Trilles, J.P. and Balasubramanian, T. (2006). A note on *Lernaea cyprinacea* (Crustacea, Copepoda, Lernaeidae) parasitizing the cultured Sailfin molly *Poecilia latipinna* and their control with salinity treatment. *J. Fish. Aquatic Sci.,* 1: 284-290

Lavilla-Pitogo, C.R. and Cruz-Lacierda, E.R. (2002). Diseases in aquaculture-IV. Proceedings of the fourth symposium on diseases in aquaculture, Nov. 22-26, 1999, Cebu City, Philippines

Leong, T.S. and Wong, S.Y. (1986). Parasite fauna of sea bass, *Lates calcarifer* Bloch, from Thailand and from floating cage culture in Penang, Malaysia. In: Maclean, J.L., Dizon, L.B. and Hosillos, L.V. (eds). The first Asian fisheries forum, Asian fisheries society, Manila, Philippines, pp. 251-254

Lima dos Santos Carlos, A.M. and Howgate, P. (2011). Fish-borne zoonotic parasites and aquaculture- a review. *Aquaculture* (in press)

Lom, J. and Dykova, I. (1992). Protozoan parasites of fishes. Elsevier Science Publishers, Amsterdam, Netherlands, pp. 125-157

Maharajan, A. (2009). Diseases of Asian sea bass, *Lates calcarifer* (Bloch) under farming. *Fishing Chimes,* 29 (7): 28-31

Mehlhorn, H. (1988). Parasitology in Focus: Facts and Trends. Springer-Verlag, Berlin Heidelberg, Germany, pp. 924

Mishra, B.K. (1991). Observations on the susceptibility of the hybrid, *Labeo rohita* x *Catla catla* to *Argulus siamensis* infection in composite culture ponds. In: Proceedings of national symposium on new horizons in freshwater aquaculture, CIFA, Bhubaneswar, India, pp. 184-185

Nagasawa, K. (2004). Sealice, *Lepeophtheirus salmonis* and *Caligus orientalis* (Copepoda: Caligidae) of wild and farmed fish in sea and brackishwaters of Japan and adjacent regions: a review. *Zoological Studies,* 43: 173-178

Nagasawa, K. and Cruz-Lacierda, E.R. (2004). Diseases of cultured groupers. Southeast Asian fisheries development center, Aquaculture department, Iloilo, Philippines, p. 81

Narasimhamurti, C., Kalavati, C. and Saratchandra, B. (1980). A new myxosporidian *Myxosoma microspora* n. spp., from *Mugil cephalus*. *J. Fish Biol.*. 16: 345-348

Paperna, I. and Baudouy-Laurencin. (1979). Parasitic infections of the sea bass *Dicentrarchus labrax* and the gilthead sea bream, *Sparus aurata* in mariculture facilities in France. *Aquaculture*, 16: 173-175

Paperna, I. Diamant, A. and Overstreet, M. (1984). Monogenean infestations and mortality in wild and cultured Red Sea fishes. *Helgolander Meresunters*, 37: 445-462

Pillai, N.K. (1985). Fauna of India- parasitic copepods of marine fishes. Technical and General Press, Calcutta, pp. 900

Prabha, C. and Pillai, N.K. (1986). Additions to the copepods parasitic on the marine fishes of India. On twenty six species of caligids. *Rec. Zool. Surv. India, Occas. Pap.*, 79 : 1-139

Rajkumar, M. Perumal, P. and Trilles, J.P. (2005). *Cymothoa indica* (Crustacea, Isopoda, Cymothoidae) parasitizes the cultured larvae of the Asian seabass *Lates calcarifer* under laboratory conditions, *Dis. Aquatic Org.*, 66: 87-90

Rajendran, K.V. and Janardanan, K.P. (1992). *Ceratomyxa etroplusi* sp. n. (Protozoa: Myxozoa) from the gall bladder of the brackishwater fish, *Etroplus maculatus* (Bloch). *Acta Protozoologica*, 31: 177-180

Rajendran, K.V., Thirunavukkarasu, A.R. and Santiago, T.C. (2000). Mortality of captive broodstock, *Lates calcarifer* (Bloch) due to monogenetic parasite, *Diplectanum latesi* (Tripathi, 1957). *J. Aquaculture in Tropics*, 15: 199-206

Rajendran, K.V., Vijayan, K.K. and Alavandi, S.V. (1998). Cardiac myxosporiosis of Pearl spot, *Etroplus suratensis* (Bloch), due to *Myxobolus etropli* sp. nov. *J. Fish Dis.*, 21: 169-176

Rajendran, K.V., Thirunavukkarasu, A.R. and Abraham, M. and Kailasam, M. (1999). Diseases and pathogens of seabass, *Lates calcarifer* (Bloch). *Fishing Chimes*, 19 (8): 16-18

Rattan, P. and Parulekar, A.H. (1998). Diseases and parasites of laboratory reared and wild population of banded pearl spot *Etroplus surantensis* (Cichildae) in Goa. *Indian J. Marine Sci.*, 27: 407-410

Ravi, V. and Rajkumar, M. (2007). Effect of isopod parasite, *Cymothoa indica* on gobiid fish, *Oxyurichthys microlepis* from Parangipettai coastal waters (South-east coast of India), *J. Environ. Biol.*, 28: 251-256

Roberts, R.J. (2001). Fish Pathology, 3rd edn., W.B. Saunders, London, pp. 472

Sanil, N.K., Asokan, P.K., John, L. and Vijayan, K.K. (2011). Pathological manifestations of the acanthocephalan parasite, *Tenuiproboscis* sp. in the mangrove red snapper (*Lutjanus argentimaculatus*) (Forsskål, 1775), a candidate species for aquaculture from southern India. *Aquaculture*, 310: 259-266

Sanil, N.K., Vikas, P.A., Ratheesh, T.B. George, K.C. and Vijayan, K.K. (2009). Mortalities caused by the crustacean isopod, *Cirolana fluviatilis*, in tropical, cage-cultured Asian seabass, *Lates calcarifer*: a case study from the southwest coast of India. *Aquaculture Res.*, 40: 1623-1633

Santos Carlos, A.M. Lima dos and Howgate, P. (2011). Fish borne zoonotic parasite and aquaculture: A review. *Aquaculture*, (in press)

SEAFDEC (2001). Health management in Aquaculture (eds. Gilda Lio Po, Celia, R. Lavilla and Erlinda, R. Cruz-Lacierda), SEAFDEC, Philippines. pp. 55-73

Seenappa, D. and Manohar, L. (1980). *Myxobolus vanivilassae* n. sp. parasitic in *Cirrhina mrigala* (Hamilton). *Proc. Indian Acad. Sci.* (*Anim. Sci.*), 89: 485-491

Seng, L.T. and Colorni, A. (2002). Infectious diseases of warm water fish in marine and brackishwaters. In: Diseases and Disorders of Finfish in Cage Culture (eds. Woo, P.T.K., Bruno, D.W. and Lim, L.H.S.), CABI Publishing, CAB International, Wallingford, UK, pp. 193-230

Shailesh, S. and Sahoo, P.K. (2010). Non-specific immune response of the Indian major carp *Labeo rohita* Hamilton to infestation by the freshwater fish louse *Argulus siamensis* (Wilson). *Indian J. Fisheries*, 57: 45-53

Sobhana, K.S. (2009). Diseases of seabass in cage culture and control measures. In: Course manual: National training on cage culture of seabass. Imelda, (eds. Joseph and Joseph, Edwin, V. and Susmitha, V.), CMFRI & NFDB, Kochi, pp. 87-93

Sourabh, S., Sahoo, P.K., Mohanty, B., Mohanty, J., Jena, J.K., Mukherjee, S.C. and Sarangi, N. (2010). Modulation of the innate immune response of rohu *Labeo rohita* (Hamilton) by experimental freshwater lice *Argulus siamensis* (Wilson) infection. *Aquaculture Res.* (in press)

Southwell, T. and Prashad, B. (1918). On some Indian myxosporida. *Rec. Ind. Mus.*, 15: 344-348

Steunhagan, D., Oesterreich, B., Korting, W. (1997). Carp coccidiosis: clinical and hematological observations on carp infected with *Goussia carpelli*. *Dis. Aquatic Org.*, 30: 137-143

Sudhakar, S., Anbalagan, T., Veerappan, P. Soundrapandian, P. and Arumuam, R. (2009). Nematodes parasites from sciaenids fishes of Parangipettai, southeast coast of India. *Curr. Res. J. Biol. Sci.*, 1: 6-10

Thapa, S., Jyrwa, D.B. and Tandon, V. (2011). A new report on the occurrence of monogenean parasites (Monogenoidea) on gill filaments of freshwater fishes in Meghalaya. *J. Parasitic Dis.*, 35: 80-84

Thirunavukkarasu, A.R., Mathew, A. and Kailasam, M. (2004). Hand book of seed production and culture of Asian seabass, *Lates calcarifer (Bloch)*. Bulletin No. 18, pp.58

Tripathi, Y.R. (1952). Studies on parasites of Indian fishes: I. Protozoa Myxosporidia together with a checklist of parasitic protozoa described from Indian fishes. *Rec. Ind. Mus.*, 50: 63-89

Tripathi, Y.R. (1957). Monogenetic trematodes from fishes of India. *Indian J. Helminthol.*, 9: 1-149

Tripathi, Y.R. (1959). Studies on parasites of Indian fishes. 5. Acanthocephala. *Rec. Ind. Mus.*, 54: 61-99

Vinoth, R., Ajithkumar, T.T., Ravichandran, S., Gopi, M. and Kumar, R. (2010). Infestation of copepod parasites in the food fishes of Vellar estuary, southeast coast of India. *Acta Parasitologica Globalis*, 1: 1-5

Yamaguti, S. (1935). Studies on the helminth fauna of Japan. Part 8. Acanthocephala, I. *Jap. J. Zool.*, 6: 247-278

Yamaguti, S. (1963). Systema helminthum. Vol. V., Acanthocephala. Interscience publishers, New York, pp. 1-423

Yang, R., Reid, A., Lymbery, A. and Ryan, U. (2010). Identification of zoonotic *Giardia* genotypes in fish. *Int. J. Parasitol.* (in press)

Zanguee, N., Lymbery, J.A., Lau, J., Susuki, A., Yang, R., Ng, J. and Ryan, U. (2010). Identification of novel *Cryptosporidium* spp. in aquarium fish. *Vet. Parasitol.* (in press).

□□□